# Dancing

One Family's Story
of Faith, Strength,
Courage and Love

**Karen and Michael Turnbull**

# *Dancing in the Rain*

Karen and Michael Turnbull

Copyright © 2020
by
Karen Elizabeth Turnbull
and
Michael William Turnbull

ISBN: 978-1-951943-59-2
eBook ISBN: 978-1-951943-60-8
LCCN: 2021904869
All Rights Reserved

Photo Credits:
Front Cover - Yong Dawson, May 5, 2013
Back Cover - Amanda Ventling, March 7, 2020

Layout & Design by Jim Sommer
Edited by Michael Turnbull
Final Design by Melissa Howard & Norm Miller

For Jim Sommer

For our boys, Evan and William

To all the well-wishers, we are forever grateful.
The comments included are a small portion of the love and
support we received. During our journey our website had over
4,000 comments and over 28,000 visits!

An instant. What does that even mean? A second, a breath, a heartbeat, a snap? In an instant life can turn upside down, inside out and backwards. It goes from walking in the door after work, excited to see your family, to sitting on the couch looking at your partner, your soul mate, your husband and hearing him say, "I have cancer." An instant. Everything changes.

So then what? You hear the words, your brain processes it, your heart skips, your stomach flips and then, if you're me, you plan. You start to take action. Because we have two choices: A) Do nothing. B) Take action. I'm a take action kind of girl. I've never been one to sit by and wait for things to happen. You can't work as a professional dancer in New York City without taking action. I guess life set me up well for this next dance.

The book you're holding is our story. It is our truth. Nothing sugarcoated, nothing exaggerated. Just us. The story of Karen, Mike, Evan and William Turnbull. We've come to be known as Team Turnbull. Others see us as the family that fought through it when all the odds were against us, but to us we're just getting through, moving forward one step at a time.

This book is many years in the making. It was never intended to become a book at all. It was actually just my blog, simply my way of communicating with everyone without becoming overwhelmed and exhausted. But it became much more than that. It became my outlet, my journal, my way to get my thoughts out. It was my dad, Jim, who said, "Karen, this story needs to be shared. It has to be preserved." So he took what started out as a blog and began to turn it into this book. To get it to this stage has not been easy. To read back over journal entries and comments and to look at the pictures has been emotional and difficult. But here it is. Here we are.

If this book has found its way into your hands, then my hope is … that if you are needing some sort of healing this helps, if you are needing some small tokens of faith you find some here, if you are feeling lost and alone then maybe this will help you feel a little less so. This is not a self-help book. It's not a magical healing account or anything earth-shattering. It truly is just our story. Thank you for joining us on the dance.

Karen

# Contents

1. The Journey Begins — 3
2. Dark Skies Ahead — 64
3. The Storm Intensifies — 116
4. A Break in the Clouds — 211
5. Scattered Showers — 250
6. Dancing in the Rain — 265
7. Signs, Symbols and Voices — 288
8. Index: Comments — 296

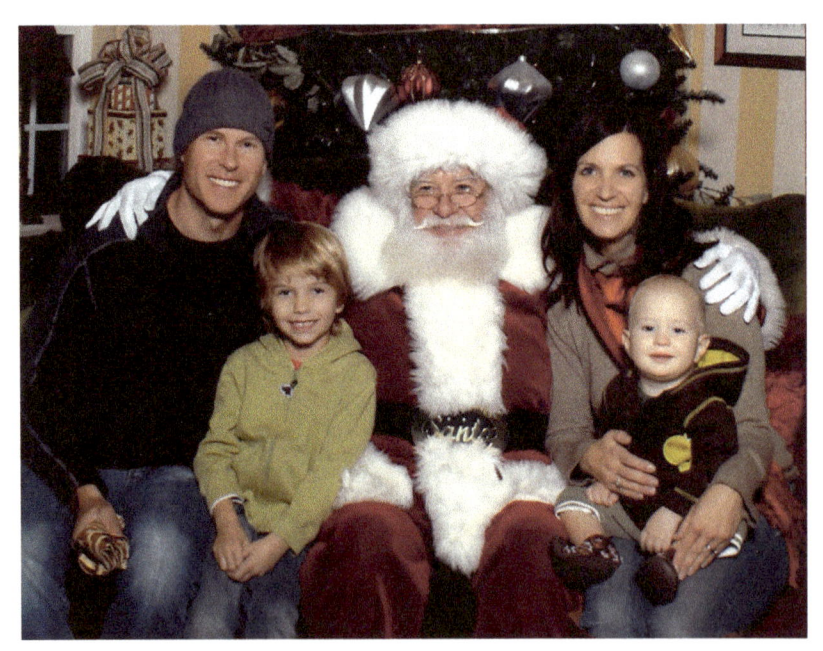

*Two months before diagnosis*

# CHAPTER ONE

## The Journey Begins

### 2013

### PET Scan

*By Karen Turnbull — Mar 23, 2013*

*This first entry was written after diagnosis as our team was being assembled...*

On Monday, March 18th we met with Dr. Robert Wang to discuss Mike's case. After two hours with this man we both felt confident that he could do what needed to be done. He is in it for the cure! He is a calm, wise man who is honest but kind. He has quickly assembled a team of doctors for us. We met with a radiation oncologist, Dr. Toy, on Thursday and he also spent over two hours with us. Mike and I were amazed by the amount of information Dr. Toy gave us and his respect for Dr. Wang has reassured us that we made the right choice. Friday we saw an oncologist, Dr. Obara, who will also be a part of our team. Basically we will not know how extensive follow-up treatments will be until after the pathology reports come back from the surgery.

The worst part of Friday was that no one told us ahead of time that after Mike's PET scan he needed to stay away from children for twenty-four hours. We were livid. (Kind of an important piece of information when there are two small children at home!) We managed to work it out and get through the day, thanks to friends keeping me and the boys busy. Mike was going to stay in a hotel, but due to March Madness Vegas hotel rooms were literally sold out! So Mike stayed quarantined in the downstairs bedroom and the boys and I stayed out and about.

Surgery is scheduled for next Saturday, March 30th. It will be a long and involved process, taking about seven hours. Dr. Wang says he is in no hurry and will take as much time as he needs to get it all out and preserve the structure of Mike's neck. He will also try to preserve his ability to play trombone, which of course comes second to curing him. So I think that brings us up to date. We feel very blessed to be surrounded by so much love and support and the best thing anyone can do for us is to keep Mike and his surgeons in your thoughts and prayers.

We will beat this!

# My Story

*By Michael Turnbull — Mar 29, 2013*

Hello All. We are incredibly grateful and we feel very blessed and fortunate to have the love and support of our many friends and family members as we navigate this illness. It is difficult to respond to all the calls, texts, emails, cards and general well-wishes, so we have decided to set up this page as an efficient means of keeping everyone informed. Our friend Brian encouraged us to do so, as it was helpful to him while he dealt with his own, even more complicated issues. Thanks for checking in and we will continue to keep you posted.

We are still in the process of learning about my disease, and the doctors on our "team" are gradually narrowing their diagnoses, so there are still some uncertainties and I may not have all the facts straight. I'll give it a shot, though!

In December, while performing with Donny & Marie at the Pantages Theater in Los Angeles, I (along with a good portion of the cast and crew) came down with a bout of bronchitis. A visit to an urgent care facility resulted in a prescription for a course of antibiotics, although the doctor I consulted with recommended I hold off on taking them as she was uncertain whether it was a viral or bacterial infection. The symptoms persisted, however, and as I was coughing consistently and forcefully during this period I coughed up a small amount of blood. I figured this was just a result of irritation, so I took the antibiotics and things seemed to clear up. I had some time off in January and did not notice any significant symptoms, but when I returned to work in February the hemoptysis (coughing up blood) also returned. This time it was frequent and substantial. My loving and alarmed wife encouraged me to see our general practitioner, and it wasn't until I did so that I realized I hadn't had a physical in five years, since a few months after our oldest son Evan was born. The doctor found nothing wrong with me and all the blood work he ordered came back clean a few days later, but when

I mentioned the hemoptysis he suggested I either go straight to the ER or have a chest x-ray at a nearby radiology center.

In addition to the aforementioned issues, I have had a lump or protrusion on my throat for several years. (We are uncertain as to when this developed). My cricoid cartilage is more pronounced than normal and is similar in appearance to the laryngeal prominence (Adam's Apple), only smaller. The lump has never bothered me, so I naively assumed it was a result of repetitive strain injury or overuse syndrome. Occasionally after a four-hour salsa gig my throat will be a bit sore, but considering the pressure involved in playing trombone at high volumes and having done so for thirty-five years I thought my occupation was the culprit. When I pointed out the protuberance to my physician, he also ordered an ultrasound of my neck. The chest x-ray yielded nothing unusual but the ultrasound revealed a large mass on my thyroid, which I now know is pushing the cartilage outward.

At this point I was referred to an otolaryngologist (ENT), who prescribed a stronger course of antibiotics as a precaution. He assumed the two issues were unrelated, as it is extremely rare for a thyroid tumor to cause pulmonary problems. When the hemoptysis worsened again he also suggested I go either straight to the ER or to a pulmonologist. I also needed to see a cytologist for a thyroid/lymph biopsy, but as he is regarded as the best in the state he was backlogged for several weeks and the bleeding seemed to be the more pressing concern. The pulmonologist decided to perform a bronchoscopy, so I underwent the procedure on February 28th. He found no issues in the bronchi but did discover a tumor on my trachea, which was determined to be the source of the bleeding. The tumor was biopsied and sent to a local pathology lab. They forwarded the samples to the Cleveland Clinic for further evaluation, so it was a while before we had any results.

Meanwhile, I took a week off, the bleeding ceased, and I was able to get in with the cytologist. He performed a Fine Needle Aspiration biopsy of my thyroid as well as two adjacent lymph nodes, and the pathology report came back positive for a Hürthle Cell Neoplasm. These can be benign, but as it has metastasized to the lymph nodes and I have an adjacent tumor on my trachea, the assumption is I have Hürthle Cell Carcinoma, which has invaded the tracheal cartilage. The ENT referred me to two surgeons: the chief of head and neck surgery at UCLA, who was unavailable, and Dr. Robert Wang, the chief of head and neck surgery at University of Nevada.

From what I understand, there are four main types of thyroid cancer. Hürthle Cell Carcinoma is usually classified with the follicular group, but it is a distinct type that makes up only three percent of all thyroid cancers. In only around ten percent of those cases does it invade the lymph nodes, and in only a handful of those does it affect the trachea. As Brian said on his history page, "I guess I'm special." Many otolaryngologists perform thyroidectomies, and some have done over one thousand. Once the lymph nodes are involved a neck dissection is necessary, which reduces the pool of qualified surgeons. A tumor on the trachea also requires a tracheal resection or reconstruction. Apparently, only a handful of surgeons in the country are experienced, qualified and willing to take on such a procedure. Lucky for us one of them happens to be in Las Vegas.

Dr. Wang was the first person in this process to go into detail with us about the disease, the treatment and the recovery. He answered all of our questions and was informative, patient and kind. According to his peers in the medical community, he is a pioneer in his field and the only surgeon in town able to perform this surgery. He practices as an ENT but is also a surgical oncologist. The other doctors we spoke to said he is too modest to mention that credential and some of them follow his surgical reports. One oncologist went so far as to say that without traveling east to Johns Hopkins, UPMC Pittsburgh, Mayo Clinic or a few other head and neck surgery hospitals, Wang is the best we will find. He has also assembled a team of other highly qualified doctors: a radiation oncologist, Dr. Beau James Toy, and a hemotological oncologist, Dr. Gregory Obara. All three of these men spent over two hours with us during our initial visits, so we are confident we are in good hands.

I have none of the common risk factors for thyroid cancer (female, Asian, smoker, low iodine diet, advanced age, family history, exposure to radiation as a child, victim of nuclear fallout as in Chernobyl). Doctors are asking me about radiation exposure and I cannot recall any significant events. The staging guidelines for thyroid cancer follow a cut-off age of forty-five. Had I been diagnosed last year, I would be considered Stage I despite the metastasis. Since I turned forty-five in November, however, I am considered Stage IV. Also, the pathology reports from the thyroid and tracheal tumors vary slightly, so until the surgery and resulting pathology reports are completed we will not know for sure what our treatment protocol involves. So far in this approximately six-week adventure, I've had two chest x-rays, two CT scans (chest and neck), two ultrasounds of the neck, two nasal endoscopies, a bronchoscopy, an FNA biopsy, a PET scan, multiple blood tests, four days of fasting and an EKG.

The irony here is that I feel great, as healthy as ever. I guess that is the insidious nature of cancer in general, in that most patients are unaware of what's going on until it is sometimes too late. Although hemoptysis is a side effect of a well advanced case, it was also the signal to get myself examined. I was informed that the bronchoscopy would further irritate the trachea and therefore cause increased bleeding, but in fact the bleeding ceased immediately afterwards! I've been told by all parties involved that if I do not have the affected tissue removed it will kill me, so I am scheduled for a seven-hour surgery this Saturday at Mountain View Hospital. (Yes, that is tomorrow. I had every intention of publishing this entry earlier. Turnbull is Scottish for procrastination). Dr. Wang scheduled me on his day off so he would have no other procedures the same day, and got me in as soon as possible. His office staff has been amazing in regard to scheduling, referrals, insurance, obtaining test results, etc. His wife, Dr. Annabel Barber, is his surgical assistant and she has been wonderful to us as well. The majority of the surgery time will be spent carefully identifying, marking and moving structures in order to preserve as much integrity as possible. There are between two to three hundred lymph nodes in the neck (depending on who you talk to) and I will have as many as one hundred removed. I will undergo a bilateral radical neck dissection, total thyroidectomy, nodal dissection, and tracheal resection.

If you've made it this far, I apologize for being long-winded, but this was the only way to answer all the questions I've been asked lately. As I stated what must seem like several pages ago, we are unable to express the love and gratitude we feel toward all of you for keeping us in your thoughts and prayers. Karen will keep this site updated with posts detailing my progress, and I will write when I am able.

Thanks again for everything!

> *Jason H*
> *Mike, I'm just completely floored by all this without a real clue how to respond. True friends like you and Karen only come along a couple times in life, and I just hate that this whole thing is happening - hate it. But, if there was or is to be any people in the world who I think could overcome some awfulness like this, it is definitely you and Karen. Stay strong for now, and I'm looking forward to all of us "Getting Strong" over a nice pint or two of Guinness in the near future. From my family to yours, much love.*

*Jeff W*
Hi, guys. This news obviously saddens me, but I've always believed people with positive attitudes (like the two of you!) face these challenges much better, and with better results, than average people. I can only imagine your loving family members are there to help and support in whatever ways they can. All I can do is wish you the best of luck, and try to encourage you with my family's personal experience. Hoping for the best for both of you!

*Christina P*
Hi, you two. Thank you for taking the time, energy and love to fill us all in. Please know that you have an army of supporters that will move the heavens for you, make a meal or simply say a prayer every day of healing. We are sending you all the love and hugs that your family can endure! We are here and we will be there in a heartbeat- just say the word. Love to all of you.

*Suzanne P*
Yes, Mike, you are special! And that is why eight years from now you will be able to sit and read your journey about the most life-changing event you will ever go through. I have faith in the healing powers, and I have faith in you, too. With much love and respect from one survivor to another. All hearts, prayers and healing energies are on you.

*Brian M*
Mike & Family, you have been in my thoughts all week since learning the news. You have such a gentle and joyful spirit, and legions of friends and colleagues whose lives you have touched pulling for you. I'll be sending good vibes tomorrow during the surgery and look forward to watching your good progress towards full recovery. As has been my MO since my own adventures in cancer land, "it's just a bump in the road." Much love.

*Bill C*
Hey, Mike. Sending you lots of positive healing energy, my friend. Take care and we'll be following your progress and recovery. Peace.

*Sharon H*
Dearest Mike, we are praying continuously for you ... all of us ... Jade, Ariane, Danny. I know you will be victorious in your fight. Sending you light, love and prayers. We love you so much.

*Hope M*
*Kick Cancer's Ass, Mike!!!!!!!!!! I'm thinking of you and I will be on the prayer circuit with everyone else this Saturday and EVERY day after that until you are fully recovered. We love you guys. We're here for you. :)*

*Birgit P*
*Mike, Rick and I are thinking of you as you are going through this very difficult time. I believe that you are in very good hands and with Karen by your side, things will be ok. We are sending you our best wishes, positive thoughts and strength, because that is all we can do.*

*Deborah P*
*Dear Mike & Karen, I want you to know that I have been thinking of you since Tiffany told me. Mike, you are a "special" kind of guy; honest, sincere, caring and unwavering in your positive attitude. Our thoughts and prayers are with you. Always here for you.*

*Mary P*
*Dear Mike, Karen and Kath, we are here or can be there for you and your family. Thank you for letting us be a part of your journey. Many hugs.*

*Kathy A*
*I have been praying, sending love and healing energy. You are all family to me. So sorry I can't be there in person but I will be in spirit. You are in great hands. Looking forward to your fast recovery. I love you both with all my heart. XOXOXOX*

*Jenny F*
*Mike, I'm sending all my most positive vibes to one of the smartest, classiest, funniest guys I've had the pleasure of knowing. You are a gem. I know Karen will be simply the best for you and you deserve no less. I'll be thinking of you every moment tomorrow. Hugs.*

*Jen K*
*Mike, Karen & boys- You are in my prayers EVERY DAY!!! You both are amazing people and will get through this!!! We love you both and are here for anything you need!!! Lots of hugs for tomorrow!!!*

*Cathy M*
*We are holding you in our hearts and sending bundles of Colorado healing energy your way as you navigate this journey. Our prayers and thoughts are with you for strength and an uneventful recovery. Your team is highly skilled and we're confident that they will give you the very best of care. Even though they've just met you, surely they must realize how important and well-loved you are to all who call you friend. We are with you, Mike!*

## The Obvious?!
### By Michael Turnbull — Mar 29, 2013

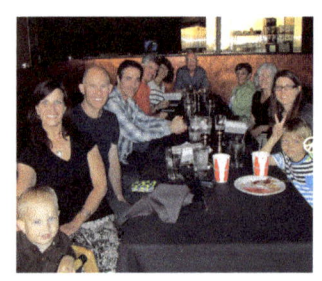

I've tried to educate myself enough to be prepared, but not so much that I freak myself out. Various people have advised for/against scouring the Internet for both reasons. Here's my favorite piece of information, gleaned from a well respected medical site. It was on a list of what to expect post-op.

*Family dinner the night before surgery*

"Your neck may be sore."

## Surgery
### By Karen Turnbull — Mar 30, 2013

Well, we are on our way. We have been blessed with wonderful hospital staff this morning. Everyone has been so kind and done all they can to calm Mike (and me). Dr. Wang came and met with us before surgery. His calm manner and knowledge of the task at hand eased our fears. Mike is definitely in good hands and the anesthesiologist assured us that he would feel no pain and would be taken good care of. (Dr. Wang informed us later that the anesthesiologist is highly trained and specializes in intricate procedures. My feeling is that Dr. Wang chooses those he wants in the room with him and will take only the best. I am grateful for that!)

I am surrounded with love and support and I thank you all so much for the love, prayers, thoughts, etc! Keep them coming! For now, we patiently wait. I am here with my amazing mother-in-law Kathy, sister-in-law Wendy, and brother-in-law Mark so I am in great company! Also, a special thank you to Pastor Marta for waking early, driving to the hospital and praying with us. Your kindness has truly touched me and my family!

### Eric T
*I love you, Mike. Sending healing thoughts and strength to you.*

### Nate K
*Mike, I had no idea any of this was happening, so thank you for sharing it with all of us. I'd wish you luck but you don't need it. If there's one thing trombonists are inherently great at, it's persevering against all odds. Knock this one out of the park, brother, and I'll look forward to our next chance to jam together! Much love.*

### Stacia F
*Well, you know friends from your past are going to start appearing. And that's ME! I keep up with you guys through mutual friends and I am certainly with you on this. I send light and healing strength to you. And anything else you need. LOVE from New York.*

### Gil K
*Thoughts and Prayers are with you! You got this, my brother!*

### Darelle H
*Well, if you were ever wondering why, in the big scheme of things, you and Karen ended up in Las Vegas, I guess the fact that one of the only qualified and willing surgeons to do a tracheal resection or reconstruction is there could be it. Dear brother, you are in my thoughts and my heart. I will meditate, pray, whatever you want to call it, to send you positive vibes. Stay strong. You are such an important part of our lives and hearts, so stop being so special, get well and go back to being boring, healthy and happy!!! I love you and your beautiful wife and your pretty babies!!!*

### Rob M
*Hey Mike, when you are done screwing around at the hospital, get your butt back on stage because we miss you and your antics. Karen, thank you both for setting up this web site. We need to be updated but we don't want to pester you. And Dr. Wang and Dr. Toy? You sure you went with these guys because they are the best at what they do? Because it sounds like you just like their names. Both of you take care and hug those babies for Etsuko and I.*

*Michael M*
Mike, I just got a CaringBridge email from Karen. Wow. I'm wishing you the most complete of recoveries. You are a lovely guy and a great musician. I thought about you out of the blue yesterday, and the night we all hung out with your dad. You are certainly in my heart and my thoughts.

*Ed R*
You both are in my prayers and I have asked Shirley to give it her best with everyone in heaven.

*Mark M*
Jessi and I are thinking about you guys. Hang in there!!

*Frank S*
Mike, just in case I don't get to see you again before I leave, I'm so glad I got to see you and the entire family yesterday! You're going to get through this, with even more great stories to tell (we relived a few yesterday :)). I love you dearly, my brother!

*Kim B*
Mike and Karen, you both have been in my thoughts and my prayers since I heard the news. Just seeing your photo here makes me smile and miss you. You will get through this! The power of prayer is amazing and you have a lot of people praying for you and your team of doctors.

*Sara O*
Praying that God's hand is guiding the surgeon's hands. Praying for divine healing. Sending love and hugs to you and your family.

*Shari B*
Mike & Karen, when I think of the two of you it always brings a lightness to the room. Your positive attitude, nurturing ways, deep down goodness mixed with an incredible sense of humor makes anyone around you feel good. You and your precious little boys are such a wonderful part of our family. I just wish we lived closer to each other so that we could help in any way possible. Please know that I'm a phone call/email/text away if you need anything! Thank you so much for setting this up so that we can be kept in the loop! It also reflects the huge amount of people who love and care about you! You will beat this, Mike!!! All our love.

*Beth S*
Karen, I am so sorry to hear of your family's struggle right now. I am thinking of you and praying for your husband and the best possible news you could hear. I am so happy that you are keeping us updated and I will check in every day.

*Frank L*
Mike and Karen, sending you loving thoughts and prayers. You are in our hearts, always.

*Karen Mc*
Our prayers are with you all.

*Brie D*
Wish I could ACTUALLY be there, but I'm there in spirit. Love you guys.

*Melissa M*
Can't stop thinking about you guys. Prayers are most definitely with you! Love you guys so much!!!

## Update

*By Karen Turnbull — Mar 30, 2013*

The nurse just came out to tell us that Mike is doing very well but they are not yet done. They have completed the neck dissection and now it is on to the thyroid and we are guessing the trachea. Not sure how much longer but we are taking this to mean that our skilled surgeon is being extra careful and thorough. He had told us this morning that he would send samples to pathology as he goes as he wants to be sure to get it all out. We have been blessed with beautiful visits from friends as we patiently wait. The love is overwhelming!

## Thank God!

*By Karen Turnbull — Mar 30, 2013*

It is 6:43 PM. Mike is out of surgery and in recovery! He is breathing on his own and will spend the night in ICU for close monitoring. Dr. Wang said he got clear margins, which means he got it all! He removed many lymph nodes, the entire thyroid, part of the parathyroid and a large portion of the trachea and reconstructed it. He was able to move the healthy part of the parathyroid to his arm where it will function and regulate his calcium levels. Dr. Wang said Mike is doing well and trying to talk (although they don't want him to yet). He also commented that during surgery he was thinking about preserving Mike's ability to play trombone. I have tears of joy that we got through the day. Thank you all for your prayers and love and PLEASE keep them coming as I know they are working!

We love you all so much!

### Dan F
*What wonderful news! God surely directed this surgeon. I'm beyond happy to hear all of this, Karen! I'll see you both soon. Love to you and your family!*

### Matt J
*Hallelujah!!! Amazing. Not intubated and on a vent??? Incredible. Go Mike, Go!!!*

### Tammy C
*So glad Mike had such an amazing surgeon that was guided by God!! What a blessing! We are continuing to pray for complete healing and restoration. Love to you all!!*

### Marianne M
*Thank you God for the miracle today! Mike and Karen, words cannot express how much you and the boys mean to us! We are so very thankful that we can be here to support you through this trying time.*

### Laura T
*We're so relieved to hear the surgery went well! We've been thinking about you all day and we're so thankful to you, Karen, for keeping us all posted. Have a peaceful and restful night and know that we're sending even more love your way.*

### Shelley Dr
*We're so happy things went well today. Thanks for keeping us updated. We've been checking throughout the day and continue to send love and prayers your way!!!!!*

*Mark S*
*I had no idea Mike was ill. I believe it has been a slap upside the head to each of us who know and work with him. He has always been the most gentle of men and seems interested in people and their lives. I am returning that at this time. I am now most interested in his recovery and updates as they are available. Please let him know my thoughts are with him and his family during this difficult time.*

# My Hero
*By Karen Turnbull — Mar 31, 2013*

Got to visit briefly with Mike tonight and he was talking and even joking! He is pretty woozy from all the anesthesia but looks good. He will stay in ICU through the night. He is truly amazing! For all you musician friends you will appreciate this: when told that the doctor was working to make sure he could play trombone again he said, "I don't know if I want to. Maybe I should try drums!" All I can say is I love him with all my heart!

Goodnight. More to come tomorrow.

*Shari B*
*Oh, Karen. Thank you for sharing that last entry for the night. It made me smile to know his sense of humor is definitely in tact! Love you!*

*Kate P*
*I wish I had the words to convey how strongly I'm pulling for you, Mike! Sending lots of positive vibes your way!*

*Frederick W*
*Mike rocks!*

*Frank L*
*Best Easter gift ever!!! Sending you so much love!! Xoxo*

*Tom P*
*Positive thoughts your way on this beautiful Easter morning! Much Love.*

*Megan S*
Sending you the very best. I understand what you are going through. You are in our thoughts and prayers and we wish you a speedy recovery.

# Ouch

### By Michael Turnbull — Mar 31, 2013

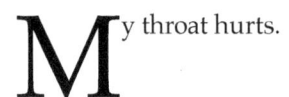

My throat hurts.

*Brian M*
Mike: Master of the obvious, huh? I should think your throat f-ing hurts! Don't be afraid to push the little button, it is your very special friend during these first days after surgery. As for drums, I have seen you play them and you are a natural talent (no surprise). But I suspect you'll have that cursed sackbut back to your face before long. I was thinking this morning about your proclivity to scale tall objects or go on other little adventures, from which you always managed to extricate yourself safely. Maybe you were just preparing for this? Love you and your amazing family and so happy that you are through the first big step.

*Shelley Dr*
Mike Turnbull: the master of the understatement. Did you ask the nurse for a cough drop? Hang in there, Mikebull!

*Gabriel F*
Awesome Resurrection Day, Mikey!! Happy Easter to you and your family. See you soon, bro!!

*Karen B*
Michael, I was Karen's teacher a long time ago. She is a very special person and I know she is caring for and about you beautifully. Just stopping by to add my good wishes for a full recovery of all faculties and capacities.

*Dan S*
Sore throat in hospital = Unlimited Popsicles and Ice Cream!!

*Pam Ra*
To Mike, Karen, and the two cutest boys I have ever seen, it was

so nice to see and hug you all last week. "Clear margins." That is music to all of our ears! I remember Mike once saying he was going to try out for the Blue Man Group and I thought he would be perfect for that. If the drums don't work out, he could reconsider this option. I love you all and I am so happy (understatement) that the surgery was a success. Un abrazote muy fuerte.

*Kelsey P*
I am so happy to hear all the great news. Thinking about you and love you lots. Hugs and kisses to my big and little cousins.

## Out of ICU

*By Karen Turnbull — Apr 1, 2013*

Mike is out of ICU and in a regular room. He is doing well, although it is very painful to swallow and he feels pretty beat up. All is good though and the doctor checked to make sure there was no nerve damage. I am headed over there now to check and see how he is today. Easter was lovely and we definitely celebrated the miracle we received this weekend. The road to recovery will be long but one step at a time. Mike and I are overwhelmed with the support we have been given.

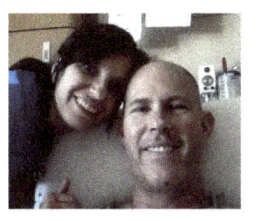

Thanks again for all the love.

*Soeren J*
Mike, I'm so glad to hear you're doing ok so far!! I can still barely believe any of this is happening, but it's great to see that your sense of humor wasn't controlled by your thyroid. ;-) (I hear that humor is very important in the recovery process) Best of luck going forward!! Coni and I are both thinking of you.

*Brenda M*
Hi Mike, I read every word of your My Story and Journal. You were very thorough and informative! Wow, my friend, you have been through a lot already and when I saw you on Friday, you had the biggest smile and positive attitude I've ever seen! I'll keep the prayers coming for quick recovery and healing! God bless you and your family! Now get back to work soon! :-) Looking Up.

### Les K
*Awesome news! Mike, you rock! Sending a huge hug to you, Karen and boys. God bless you and may you continue to have a smooth, tranquil recovery. Brother, you are an amazing soul and friend! I love you man ... Peace & Light.*

### Rocco B
*This is incredible news. We are all so happy to hear that you pulled through this unimaginable procedure. The power of prayer continues to be with you and your family. Thank you, Dr. Wang and staff for helping our friend. Blessings to you all. We love you, Michael, and we are all hoping that you're blessed with an easy recovery. See you very soon!*

### Rosita P
*Dear Mike, we are so happy you are progressing. God might be a little overwhelmed listening to our prayers for you and your family over and over again. We love you and look forward to see you ... please take care of yourself. God bless you dear!!!*

### Jodie M
*All of us at New Song Academy will be happy to see you back on your bike with the boys in tow. Many prayers for strength and a full recovery!*

### Devonee M
*Hi, Mike!! So wonderful to see your family at school today! Evan and William have so much love surrounding them right now while you are in the hospital. They are being adored and hugged often:) We are praying for you so much! We are so thankful that the surgery went so well and are now praying for a quick recovery for you! You are so strong and we know you will fight this battle with amazing strength! Lots of hugs sent your way.*

### Anne-Corinne B
*Dear Karen and Mike, our thoughts and prayers are with you and we're hoping and praying for a speedy recovery! We heard from our family (who all adore you!!!). It is good that you have been in such great health prior to this, and this strength helps to recover from your surgery. Everything you report is very sound from a surgical perspective; you are in good hands. Our hearts go out to you.*

# Young Frankenstein

*By Michael Turnbull — Apr 1, 2013*

Insert favorite quote here: ("It's Alive!" or "Puttin' On The Ritz!")

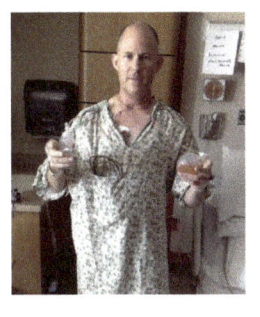

# Amazing News!

*By Karen Turnbull — Apr 2, 2013*

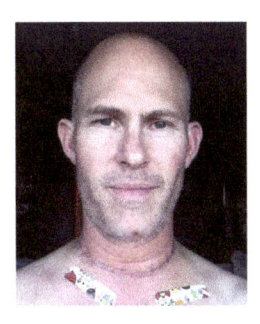

Less than forty-eight hours from the end of surgery, Mike was discharged and sent home! He is truly amazing! It is midnight, Monday, April 2nd and he is sleeping in his own bed! He was able to take a shower, eat some ice cream for his sore throat and crawl into his own bed with about twenty pillows around him to support his body and head upright. His only restrictions are no neck extensions so as not to pop any trachea stitches, no lifting anything over fifteen pounds and no trombone for a while. His pain medicine is Tylenol! Unbelievable!!!

Sleep well all ... I will! :)

*Brian M*
Mind-blowing news. Overjoyed to hear Mike is already at home!

*Angela C*
Hi, Karen and Mike! So excited and amazed that he's home already!! Please let us know if you need anything! Congratulations! What a trooper!!

*Frederick W*
Seriously, Mike rocks!

*Frank L*
The best news ever!!! Beyond thrilled. Sending you all buckets of love. So much to be thankful for. All our love.

*Teri C*
What amazing news! God does some incredible things through the power of prayer. May you continue to amaze us, Mike. Karen, thank you for the detailed updates. They are so appreciated.

*Ellen So*
So glad to hear this news! Did they really let you leave? Or did you just decide to take a walk and explore the neighborhood? Welcome home!!

*Karine Z*
You continue to amaze us, Mike. Truly incredible! We are so very happy to hear this!!! We're sending our love!

*Cathy M*
Well done, Mike!! This is great news! So glad you are home with your family. Continue to amaze us with your progress in recovery and we will keep up with our prayers and well-wishes. You are truly a WARRIOR and we are in awe of your strength. Our love to you, Karen, Evan, William, your Mom, Wendy, etc.

*Matt J*
Hi, Mike. Tylenol as in acetaminophen???? Incredible!! Back home, I got a smile right now that bisects my face.

*Melin F*
We are so happy and relieved. The outpouring of love will continue. Even though we don't see you any more you are always in our

*thoughts. You both have been so kind to Darelle that you will always have a place in our hearts. Take care of one another and love those two beautiful boys. Our prayers will be right there with you as your life returns to normal. Best wishes.*

*Lisa L*
*Mike is such a wonderful man. I know that if anyone can beat this, he can. He is truly blessed to have such a supportive family. He (and the family) will continue to be in my prayers.*

*Tim C*
*Mike, it's been a LONG time, but I'm thinking of you and so happy to see everything went so well in surgery. I can't believe you are home already after that, but it bodes well for you. Rest well.*

## Finally Some Sleep
*By Karen Turnbull — Apr 3, 2013*

We got the clear today that Mike can be supine as long as his head stays lifted with pillows (we just can't let his head fall back into extension as the pressure on the trachea would be too intense), so finally he is getting some good sleep. Unfortunately, I will have to wake him at 11:30 PM to take his calcium pills, but hopefully he will be able to go back to sleep. Today it was great to have him home, although it was a bit challenging for me to figure out when to give him his pills, when and what to feed him and trying to help find a comfortable position to rest in. This will all work itself out, though, and I know we will find a groove. Luckily I had been juicing for him for the past month so I have that pretty well down. (Unfortunately our juicer decided to break tonight but it looks like I just need to order a part - in the meantime I have a loaner coming tomorrow ... thank you Danny and January!) The boys are thrilled to have their daddy home and they have been extra gentle with their healing hugs!

Goodnight!

*Karine Z*
*Karen, these updates complete my days. Thank you for taking the time, despite how full things are right now. We are so happy to hear about Mike's continued progress. It's so amazing! Get yourself some rest. Even rock stars need to sleep! Love you tons!*

*Les K*
*The weight of this experience must be unimaginable but you guys hang in there. We're all spiritually here for you, hoping to help lighten the load. Godspeed.*

*Gary A*
*So glad to hear you are on a path to recovery. As a cancer survivor, I know the difficulty of not knowing or understanding all that is happening around you. Sort of like sight-reading without key signatures or metric markings. Sounds like you have an amazing team to guide you through this temporary modulation. Recover at a decent pace ... 120 bpm ... and lay out on the unisons.*

*Kenny A*
*Hey Mikey, I know you'll pull through all this and have a full recovery! It's in your nature to overcome things! You're one of my best friends and you have my prayers and love and positive vibes! I'm always here should you or your family need anything. You're gonna come out of this just fine, and we're gonna have many more adventures, whether climbing on rooftops, drunken singing songs in taxis, or running across yachts in Monte Carlo!! Love you, my brother!!*

# A True Hero

*By Karen Turnbull — Apr 4, 2013*

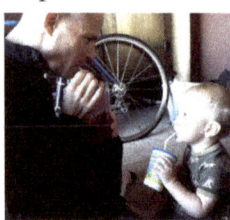

Well, Mike is continuing to shock and amaze us all! Today he was much more alert and active. He had a nice visit with our good friend Danny and even came downstairs and outside to enjoy the gorgeous day for a while. He and William had a "smoothie party" and sweet little William kept checking to make sure daddy drank it all. It is not nearly as painful to swallow and so he is eating more and I am very glad that I made the boys baby food because I am able to get a little creative with some food purées. Also, our dear friend Suzanne had suggested aloe vera juice as it had helped her when she received chemo and had mouth and throat sores. Thank you Suzanne, because it really does seem to be soothing! The grand finale for the night was that Mike joined us all downstairs to hear Evan read a Dr. Seuss book to us. Never did I think he would be doing so much just four days after surgery. He is truly amazing and I am so proud of his positivity and determination to recover quickly! Keep the energy and prayers coming. It inspires him every day to know that so many people are pulling for him.

Thank you all so much!

> **Hope M**
> *Sounds fantastic. Not to diminish your progress, Mike, but Evan read a Dr. Seuss book?????? Awesome. :)*
>
> **Nancy W**
> *You are one tough dude, Mike! I'm amazed at your rate of recovery and the gifts of certain surgeons. Stay a steady course and heal well.*

# Gratitude

*By Michael Turnbull — Apr 4, 2013*

### • Things I am grateful for •

**Small things:**
The ability to swallow without severe pain. Being given the go-ahead to lie supine, rather than propped at forty-five degrees. The absence of Jackson-Pratt drains, intravenous needles, catheters, EKG monitors, adhesive tape, pneumatic compression stockings, heart rate monitors, oxygen sensors, blood pressure cuffs, etc. Being free of anesthesia and prescription pain medicine (since discharge I've only been alternating acetaminophen and ibuprofen). The ability to walk outside. Being able to watch the mountain view sunrise from our home rather than from Mountain View Hospital.

**Not-so-small things:**
The lack of intubation upon awakening from surgery, since if I couldn't breathe on my own I would have remained intubated until I could do so. The ability to speak (although barely), control my facial muscles, and raise my arms above my head, all three of which could have been compromised due to nerve damage. That the projectile vomiting I just engaged in (a stomach virus has been running through my family all week; guess who's turn it was tonight?) as I was about to publish this entry did not rupture the sutures in my trachea.

**Huge things:**
My surgeon, Dr. Wang and his wife, Dr. Barber, and their entire team. They quite literally saved my life. All of you, my friends and family,

the most wonderful, generous, supportive, kind-hearted people on the planet. My children and the chance to watch them grow up and cherish each moment with them. My wife Karen, the best nurse in the world, a born nurturer, caregiver, teacher and mother, a shining beacon of light and love and a real Angel on Earth. God (or whichever higher power, spiritual being, life energy, guardian angel or positive vibes you believe in, and for summoning them and sending their healing my way.)

*Shari B*
*Mike, if I didn't think it was possible to think more of you or have a better appreciation for the incredibly good person you are, you proved me wrong. Your "gratitude" entry was so meaningful and I so appreciate that you shared such heartfelt thoughts. I love you so much, Mike, and I'm so thankful that you are doing so well, have such wonderful doctors, have a huge amount of friends and family that surround you with love and support, and furthermore, an amazing wife and children that bring you so much love and joy that fill your soul. We love you and miss you.*

*Les K*
*Hang in there, buddy. Sorry about the stomach bug (let's hope it's done). Thanks for your effort to keep us informed and for the awesome journal entry. Stay strong. I love you, brother. Karen is such a blessing!!!*

*Karine Z*
*We are SO grateful for YOU, Mike! And yes, your amazing wife as well! So grateful that you are healing this well (despite the stomach bug) We love you.*

*Katey J*
*So great to see all of the positive things happening during your healing (aside from the stomach bug!). You are an inspiration to those who are following your journey. We keep you all in prayer and hope today continues to see you feeling stronger and continuing to enjoy your family.*

*Laura T*
*Just a few of the things I'M grateful for: My amazingly talented, generous, funny, insightful, smart and unbelievably brave nephew, Mike; His extremely loving, beautiful, strong, caring and dedicated wife, Karen; And their two incredibly adorable, intelligent, clever,*

*squeezable boys. I'm so sorry that the flu found you! I was hoping that it would skip right over you. I hope you're feeling better today and that you can continue on your road to recovery unencumbered! We love you all and think of you constantly.*

## Bad Time for a Stomach Bug!

*By Karen Turnbull — Apr 5, 2013*

If there was a really, really, really bad time to get a vomiting stomach virus I would say it is probably right after a full neck dissection! Somehow we got through it and hopefully there is no more! Poor Mike, talk about bad timing! Once again Dr. Wang was a voice of calm. His answering service put me straight through to him and he talked us through it and assured us that Mike's sutures should be fine.

When it rains it pours.

> *Rosita P*
> *Ohhhh no, Mike, not now. Please hang in there. I know you will get through this. Let me tell you that you are an inspiration for a lot of people, including me. I'm so thankful to have you as my friend and a big shout-out to your beautiful wife.*
>
> *Tammy C*
> *So sorry you had to endure the flu on top of all that you have been through! I pray there are no more storms that come your way so that you can experience some calm in your journey to complete health. You are always in our thoughts and prayers!*

## Visitors

*By Michael Turnbull — Apr 6, 2013*

I was in quite a bit of a fog during my brief stay in the hospital, but I do remember a few special people coming to visit me.

**Pastor Marta**
Our son Evan attends a small kindergarten at a church in our neighborhood. We are able to walk there and the student/teacher ratio is very low. Evan loves his teachers and classmates. We are acquainted

with the pastors there, Pastor Dave and his wife Pastor Marta, but we are not parishioners. Pastor Marta drove across town very early on Saturday to pray with my family at my bedside just prior to surgery. She did this on Easter weekend (if not her busiest weekend, definitely her second busiest) and did so unprompted. We were not even aware she knew of my condition until a couple of days prior. Unsolicited acts of kindness such as this deserve to be recognized, and it helped put us all at ease.

**Brook**
A colleague of Karen's at Las Vegas Academy, Brook might be as much of an angel as my wife. They could be sisters. (Speaking of which, Karen's real sister Marianne is definitely an angel. She is still here helping take care of our kids.) I know her presence was calming to Karen and much appreciated.

**Gil**
My colleague with Donny & Marie, Gil and I have been standing next to each other most nights for the past two and a half years (he says he isn't cutting his hair until I return) and have become good friends in the process. He lives only ten minutes from the hospital so despite his busy schedule he said he would visit me every day. Fortunately for him that only ended up being twice! It meant a lot to me to have him there and I know he kept our musician friends informed of my progress. He brought cards signed by the entire company, as well as a sizable donation collected from my coworkers. I don't know how to thank everyone, except to say it is hugely appreciated and I'm lucky to work with such great people.

**Frank**

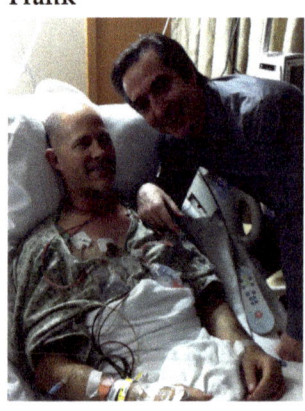

*Frank Strauss*

One of my dearest friends anywhere, Frank is like a brother to me. We spent nine years on the road together with Tom Jones. I called him a few days before surgery to tell him what was going on, and before I could say anything he said he'd been meaning to call me to let me know he'd be in town that weekend. I said we probably wouldn't be hanging out much! Frank worked for Melissa Manchester before Tom, and now she occasionally uses him as a sub. He was arriving the day before my surgery and leaving two days after, and he was playing at a casino hotel only ten minutes from my hospital. I picked him up Friday and he had dinner with my entire family. He and Brian played at our wedding so he knows them well. Sunday he came to visit and made me laugh as usual. Frank lives in Philadelphia and only plays with Melissa a couple of times a year, so it's hard to believe this was all just a coincidence. Thanks for always being there when we need you, brother.

I truly believe these special people helped with my speedy recovery. Also, as Karen mentioned in her post and even though I didn't get to see them, thanks to **Tom, Jeneane** and **January** for visiting the hospital as well. I know that meant tons to Karen and I'm sorry I missed you. (I think I was cut open at the time!) And thanks to another great friend **Danny** for visiting me at the house several times this week. (Thanks for the conversation and the Kruger Omni Healing, buddy!) You've gone out of your way to help a friend and it is so very much appreciated ...

Ok, I'm back to edit this post a day later, as the rest of the D&M horn section, **Rocco** and **Rob**, came by today. Fellow trombonist **Randy** did as well. Rocco, thanks for the olive oil (first pressed from your family in Italy? Wow!). Rob, great to see **Etsuko** and the kids as well. You and Rocco crack me up, and you're cool! Randy, great conversation but now my throat hurts from talking so I guess I need those popsicles you brought! ... Two days later, more editing. Thanks **Mike** and **Kerry**! Mike, your soup is killer. Best thing I've eaten since surgery!

While I'm at it, I have to thank our family members. My mom and my sister stayed in a hotel next door to the hospital so they could be with me the entire time, and Karen's mom and dad and her sister and her husband stayed at our house so they could take care of the boys while Karen was with me. So thanks to **Kathy, Wendy, Jim, Betty, Mark** and **Marianne** (all of whom had to fly in from Denver or Pittsburgh, by the way. My mom's eight-day visit turned into over a month!). Karen and I have always said how fortunate we are to have not one but two great families.

We love you! We love you!

> **Dene R**
> *Hello, Mike. Your mom has kept me up to date on your progress. YOU are such a remarkable young man and you have no idea of how I have bragged on you and your accomplishments for years! Please know that I (as well as my church family in a little country church*

in Wilson, Oklahoma) continue to pray for you and your family. May God continue to bless you in your quest for good health. With love.

**Dawn K**
*So happy to hear you're continuing to feel better. I had no idea you were such an eloquent writer ... your last couple of posts have made me cry. You're amazing! Also, I hope you and Karen realize that it's no surprise you have both been shown such love and support through this time. It's because you are two of the sweetest people on the planet and deserve all the best. Love you, my sweet buddy!*

# Guestbook

*By Michael Turnbull — Apr 6, 2013*

I have to be honest. I just got around to reading everyone's guestbook posts early this morning during another restless night. I caught a few gems that Karen showed me during the week, but for the most part I had no idea so many people had contributed. I am overwhelmed. To know there is so much love and support out there for my family and me is truly heartwarming. I can't imagine what it is like to go through something like this alone. Thanks to everyone for all of your encouraging words.

I was amazed to see some of the names here! It has been many years since some of us have spoken, so it is really great not only to receive encouragement but just to hear from you! Thanks Tim, Steve, John, Brian, Gary, Fritz, Roxanne, Belinda, Laura, Nancy, Tom, Stephen, Debra, Clare, KC, Lanie, Stacia and anyone else I may have missed. Grab my email address from whoever sent you the link if you'd like to reconnect!

# One Week

*By Karen Turnbull — Apr 7, 2013*

Well, it is one week since surgery and every day has been a new adventure. In one week Mike has spent a night in ICU, a night in an oncology hospital room, came home (yippee!), figured out how to get some rest without moving his neck too much, drank about twenty pounds of fresh-juiced vegetables and smoothies, got the stomach bug (so much for all those nutrients), received the news from our surgeon that "clear margins" were achieved, ate solid food and last night joined us on the couch for family movie night! I would say it has definitely been a full week! We meet with Dr. Obara tomorrow to find out when the next part of this journey begins and what all will be involved. Dr. Wang was more than pleased with how Mike is recovering from the surgery and said in his opinion he got it all. He feels it is still worth doing the follow-up treatments of radioactive iodine as there is always a chance that one microscopic cell could be hiding somewhere. So we continue to recover and pray! We will do everything we can and the surgery was ninety-five percent of it.

Thank you again Dr. Wang! You are amazing!

> *Megan M*
> *It sounds like Karen's doing a great job being your nurse but if say around May 16th she needs to take a leave of absence I would have no problem giving up a week or two to come out there ... just an idea! But so happy to hear you're recovering so well! If you get bored my drawing skills have improved so we can play Draw Something! Can't wait to have a huge celebration in Hilton Head this summer! Love you guys and still praying for you, champ!*
>
> *Dan S*
> *Karen & Mike, I just wanted to say thank you for keeping us all up to date through this site over the past week. With the three hour time difference on the east coast, it has been nice to wake up each morning to read continuing good news (except for the flu, of course, but even that seems like it worked itself out ok). Thanks for sharing the pics as well. We're all tuned in out here. Continue healing and recovering. Looking forward to seeing you guys soon!*
>
> *Jill G*
> *Mike and family ... so sorry to hear that you are going through this ordeal but you have ALWAYS had a positive attitude and that will get you through it all. Continue to recover and we will pray for you and your family.*
>
> *Mike G*
> *Mike, so sorry to hear you are going through this. I LOVE YOU ALL and sent lots of healing love!*

*Michelle M*
*Mike, tell my mom I said "I told you so!", because when she called me and told me everything that was going on, I told her, "Well, knowing Mike, he'll end up coming out better than he was going into it!!" Who gets the stomach flu after having a full neck dissection and is still able to have smoothie parties and family movie nights? Only you! I never doubted for a second that everything would work itself out and you'd pull through - you are so incredible and we are all so lucky to have you in our family! I love you! And Karen, Evan and William, too! Praying for you constantly and knowing things are only going to go up from here, but know that I am always on your side cheering you on!! Love and miss you!*

*Frank S*
*Mike, I can't imagine that you would have thought you'd be this far along just one week after surgery. I can't wait until this is so far behind you that you think of it as a small bump in life's road. By the way, the way you handled this was truly inspiring.*

*Dave Ro*
*Mike! I just received your email about forty-five minutes ago and I've been poring through your journal. I am shocked with all you have been going through but am filled with such joy about your progress and spirit. You and Karen are both amazing and this is a true testament of the love and strength you both share. Please know that I will be sending all my positive thoughts your way ... even though you cracked on being a drummer!!! Peace and love to you, Karen, Evan and William.*

*Antonette L*
*Dearest Mike and Sweet Karen, I absolutely can't believe all that you have gone through in the last few months and I am so sorry I didn't know sooner to be there for your family. All of my prayers and positive thoughts will be with you guys. Please know that I am here to help with ANYTHING ... you know I'm a great babysitter, I cook, I clean and I know where lots of grocery stores are :-) Please lean on your friends (me). We love you and want to be here for you. All my love.*

# Oncology Appointment

*By Karen Turnbull — Apr 8, 2013*

Today we met with Dr. Obara, Mike's oncologist. We like him a lot and feel he is looking at Mike as an individual. He will be working with another doctor who is a nuclear medicine doctor. Together they will decide the next step. Mike's particular type is called Hürthle Cell and it tends to be a more aggressive type. The next step would be radioactive iodine treatment. However, sometimes Hürthle cells do not respond to this treatment. Fortunately, they can test for it first. Hopefully his body will respond to it as that would be a way to attack any cells that may be hiding. So for now Mike is on a low iodine diet and they will start regulating his thyroid stimulating hormone to get it at the optimal level for the treatment. We go back in two weeks to check his blood and see if his body will respond to the iodine, so now the prayers are that Mike's body will take up the iodine treatment. As far as his healing, he is doing amazing! He is laughing with the kids and truly finding joy in the small miracles of everyday life.

### Carolyn S
*Hi, Mike. Sending positive thoughts your way and you are in my prayers. I'm sorry you are going through this. Keep fighting!!!*

### Kathryn L
*Hey there, Mike. Holy Cow! What a whirlwind this must be. We're wishing you the easiest and fastest recovery and return to "normal" life. The love of your friends and family is impressive. You are a great guy! Hang in there and know that we are thinking of you. Love you, Mike.*

### Greg N
*Mike ... keeping you and your family in my thoughts and prayers. Hang in there, buddy!*

### Gail R
*Dear Mike and Karen, your family is in my thoughts and prayers. So glad to hear that the surgery went well and you are on the mend. Take care and I will look forward to seeing you all this summer. Tell Evan and William hello for me!*

### Dave G
*So sorry to hear of this illness, Mike!! From reading your journal it's easy to see you have strong support and a great attitude!! Hang*

in there, man, and I'll be thinking of you often!!!

**Brian P**
Hey, Mike. Thoughts are with you, my friend. Fight like hell and LiveStrong!

**Suzanne P**
I know this sounds crazy, and I didn't get it when people would say to me "that is the gift that cancer gives you, that you learn it is the little things that bring pleasure." It is truly the loved ones that we have in our lives, the smiles that they bring to us and the smiles we give to them. It is our relationships and the present moment that gives us the most satisfaction. It changes our perspective, even if we had a good one to begin with. Love you guys, hang in there and take one step at a time. You are doing amazing!!!! Hugs.

**Darelle H**
We will keep the prayers coming! You are both amazing and doing so well. We are all touched by you and feel grateful you are part of our lives. Much love.

**Nandita S**
Hi Mike and Karen! I love getting your updates and am so glad that both of you are feeling up to posting. My thoughts are with you, and I'm looking forward to when I get regular emails that say, "we're coming to town and can't wait to see you!" But until then, thanks for keeping all of us who are far away informed of how you are. Your voices come through so much in the journal! Big hugs.

# Insurance Ironies

By Michael Turnbull — Apr 10, 2013

Three or four days after surgery, as I was well into the process of recovering at home, we received a phone call from the office of the first otolaryngologist we visited during this odyssey. His assistant informed us she had just received notice that my insurance company was not going to cover my procedure if I had it performed at UCLA, but would cover it if Dr. Wang performed the surgery.

Thank God we were proactive and vetted our options, rather than waiting for that phone call. We had decided to have a consultation with Dr. Wang while we waited for word from the insurance company, both to get a second opinion and to have a back-up plan if we needed to stay in town. When Karen called Wang's office they scheduled us for the very same day, and upon meeting him we both knew he was the surgeon for us, for several reasons. Since there was a distinct possibility of going out of town at that point, we had been advised to run around and collect all films, slides, pathology reports, etc. so we could have everything with us when we traveled. For this reason Dr. Wang had no prior knowledge of my case, yet one of the first things he asked us was whether hemoptysis had initially alerted me to the problem. He was the first person to put all of the pieces together right off the bat. When he examined my neck Karen said his eyes were closed, yet through palpation alone he discovered a couple of affected lymph nodes that no one else had pointed out. He then proceeded to show us the same nodes on our films, which he had not yet examined at that point. His deliberate, steady hand with the endoscopy was also impressive and reassuring. Dr. Wang did not hesitate to schedule our surgery only twelve days later, and may have done so even sooner were it not for the fact that I needed a PET scan first. His team took over and referred us to the other doctors involved in addition to dealing with insurance on our behalf. Dr. Wang also scheduled me for a Saturday, so he would have no other procedures or distractions on the same day. Had I waited to travel out of state I may not have been seen yet, much less been ten days into recovery. Since the disease metastasized further than initially expected, we obviously made the right choice by not hesitating.

We also received a letter in the mail last week, just a few days after surgery, stating that a certain procedure was "experimental and medically unnecessary" and would therefore also not be covered by insurance. The procedure, Electromyography (EMG), is a diagnostic method of assessing the health of muscles and the nerve cells that control them (motor neurons). EMG results can reveal nerve dysfunction, muscle dysfunction or problems with nerve-to-muscle signal transmission. Dr. Wang had informed us of the risks associated with my surgery at our initial consultation, which included nerve damage and the resulting possible loss of muscle function in my face and/or arms and shoulders. He utilized the EMG procedure to monitor my nerve function and thereby avoid damaging the involved nerves, as he was attempting to maintain my ability to continue my occupation. Since I need the muscles in my face and arms to function in order to do my job, and I need to do my job in order to make contributions to my health plan and therefore pay the people who are performing the procedures, the "unnecessary" bit seems a bit exaggerated.

Joseph Heller, anyone?

*Dave Ri*
In honor of Michael Turnbull. who is a wonderful guy and an outstanding musician. Can't wait to throw down the funk with you at the Palms again soon.

*Kacia B*
Mike, we just heard about your ordeal, and are so pleased to read in your journal that you are recovering well from the surgery! We're sorry we haven't met Karen - sounds like you two make quite a team. Keep it up. We are wishing you all the best.

*Melin F*
You see, from the latest post, all things are put in alignment for the people who have great faith and are doing the right things in their lives. If you meditate/pray to whatever your higher power may be, you open the doors to the help you need and deserve. I'm so proud of you both for being proactive and diligent in Mike's recovery. The next steps will be a breeze compared to the surgery, so you're on your way. We send continued prayers and Swedish hugs to all of you.

## The Boss
By Michael Turnbull — Apr 11, 2013

How many people have a boss who would take time out of their busy schedules to visit you while recovering from a health event? And how many people have a boss with a household name? I have both! Donny Osmond paid a visit to our home today to see how I was doing. Very, very cool. Thanks, boss!

*Donny Osmond*

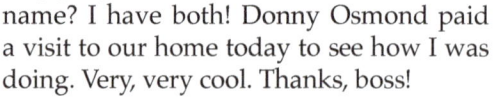

*Cathy M*
Well done, Mike! So happy to see Mr. Osmond realizes what a gem he has in you. Your progress and journey to health has been a true inspiration to us. Thank you for providing us with a great example to follow. Our prayers, thoughts and warm love are with you and your beautiful family.

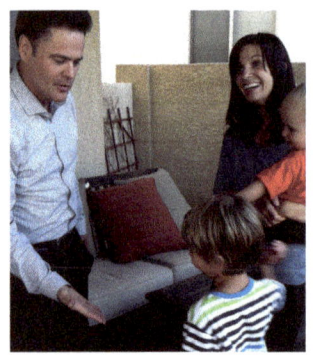

# Weekend!

*By Karen Turnbull — Apr 12, 2013*

I have to say I don't know if I have ever appreciated a weekend as much as I do right now! After returning to work, figuring out what a low iodine diet means, shuffling the kids to friends' houses, school, swimming and Taekwondo and fitting in homework, juicing, lunches, etc., I am so happy to just sit and be still! I am happy to say we have no plans this weekend and I am so excited to have a little relaxing family time. Mike's progress is remarkable! His scar is healing so well that in some spots it is already hard to see. His energy level is growing and he is really enjoying William's precious giggles and Evan's daily accomplishments, like riding his two-wheel bike like a pro! Mike got the clear today to stop the calcium pills, which means the parathyroid transplant into his shoulder is working. He is down to just his thyroid medicine and a vitamin D. Last Tylenol was a week ago!

We have been blessed with so much support it is remarkable. Thank you to our dear friends Devonee and Mike who have graciously watched William this week while I was at work even though it means dropping him off at 6:15 in the morning! And the amazing parents of Evan's kindergarten class who have provided home-cooked meals and organic fruits and veggies every day for us! And the wonderful friends who have taken time from their busy schedules to stop by for a short visit to check on Mike and see how he is doing. Knowing that so many people love us helps every moment of the day.

Thank you!!! Happy weekend!

> *Fran H*
> Hi, Mike and Karen. Just a message of encouragement from me and Chuck. We are so moved by the circumstances you find yourselves in and keep you in our daily prayers. This is a wonderful website and it has answered many of our questions. Having small grandchildren, we can appreciate the balancing act you must constantly endure while trying to stay afloat. God bless you with hope and strength!

# Details

*By Michael Turnbull — Apr 14, 2013*

Two weeks ago I underwent major surgery, and I am already feeling close to normal. Other than a few restrictions, such as no driving, no lifting anything over fifteeen pounds and no forceful exhaling (which considerably limits my employment opportunities), I am functioning regularly. Here are some more details about the experience, if you are interested. Thanks for reading!

The surgery ended up being ten hours long, as opposed to the projected six or seven. This was due to several factors such as thoroughness on the part of my surgeon (including preserving as much function as possible and performing real time pathology), and the fact that there was metastasis below the main thyroidal tumor in the central lymph nodes, which necessitated a central nodal dissection in addition to the previously mentioned procedures.

I have a sixteen-inch neck. The incision is ten inches long, more than sixty percent of the circumference. The medical grade superglue which was holding the incision together externally has mostly disappeared, while the subcutaneous sutures are probably just now beginning to dissolve. "You've got a bazillion stitches inside your neck."- Dr. Barber

I was offered both flu and pneumonia vaccinations before I was released from the hospital. I believe this is a standard, possibly state-mandated procedure. I was unsure whether to accept or not, until I sought the advice of my surgeon. His response: "If you contract pneumonia in the next two months while your trachea is trying to heal, that will be bad." I followed his advice. He also said, "Don't get them here. They'll charge you a fortune. Go to Walgreen's on your way home." The first day at home I was achier and more lethargic than I would have been were I only recovering and eliminating anesthesia from my system, but at least I got it all over with at once. Sometimes it is difficult to be a patient patient!

"The thyroid gland produces hormones which regulate the body's metabolic rate as well as heart and digestive function, muscle control, brain development and bone maintenance." Here's another: "They also stimulate mitochondria, which are the energy production centers of cells. The hormones control how much energy is used for body function or released as heat. In a general sense, they are responsible for virtually all metabolic activity in the body from appetite to nerve and cardiac function." Since my thyroid was removed, it took a few days before my body felt like it was functioning correctly. I imagine this will be a constant balancing act, monitoring TSH (thyroid-stimulating hormone) and adjusting the synthetic supplements accordingly.

At my follow-up appointment, one week post-op, Dr. Wang mostly reviewed the surgical pathology reports. He did not seem concerned with my progress whatsoever, as if my rapid recovery was expected. Of the approximately one hundred lymph nodes removed, seventy-one were large enough to biopsy. Ten came back positive for cancer. Of the four parathyroid glands, two were cancerous and removed, one was left as is and one was transplanted into my shoulder. When I inquired about the method utilized for performing biopsies during surgery, Dr. Wang informed me the tissue is frozen and stained. While not as accurate, it gives a good indication as to which tissue is affected. The remaining tissue is preserved in paraffin for final pathology.

As swelling decreases and nerves reconnect, feeling in the area is slowly returning. The area just under my jaw line or mandible is tingling, like a leg or arm does when circulation is cut off. The center portion of my neck is completely numb. It's an odd sensation trying to shave when you can't feel your neck.

My weight has been consistent my entire adult life, and has remained within a fifteen pound range until now. At the moment I weigh less than I did in high school.

Just under forty-eight hours after my surgery, Dr. Wang signed me out of the hospital. He had appointments all day as it was a Monday, so I knew I probably wouldn't see him until after 5:00 PM. Sure enough, at 5:30 PM he walked in and I happened to be standing. He asked if I had been walking around, which I had, and he performed a couple of nerve tests to make sure my arms and face were still functioning. Then he said, "Well, would you like to go home?" I responded, "Tonight?" and he replied, "There's no sense sitting around here." Karen and the rest of our family were across town at our house and I had to call to let them know I was ready to come home, which they were not expecting for at least another day. I mentioned to Dr. Wang that I was determined to heal quickly, but didn't necessarily expect to be released two days after a ten-hour surgery. He said it went "very well" and if it hadn't it would have been a completely different story.

An hour or so after that I saw Dr. Barber at the desk. She was dealing with other patients, but it was the first time I'd seen her since the surgery. She teared up and in her thick Texas accent said: "Hey! Ya look great! Yer a superstar!" I told her that her husband had just signed me out and she said, "Yeah, he just called and said to come on home. I guess he's in one of those get things done moods." I also joked around with her, acting like Frankenstein and saying it was too bad it wasn't October since I'd have a ready-made costume. She fired right back with: "We shouldn't a taken the bolts outta yer neck!"

*Karine Z*
*Mike, you're just incredible! Thank you for sharing such thorough details. We've been thinking of you everyday from Italy. Love to you guys!*

*Dwight S*
*Just read your latest entry. If you weren't such a good trombone player you could have been quite an excellent journalist! Not everyone can stand back and recount events and relay it with such expertise. Have you ever done this kind of thing before? I mean write, not have such a serious operation! Keep up the good work, Mike!*

*Heather B*
*Thank you for sharing your personal journey. When I blew out candles on my birthday yesterday, you and your family were a big part of my wishes. You are amazing and so is your family! Love from our family.*

## Follow-up Number Two

*By Michael Turnbull — Apr 19, 2013*

Today we met with Dr. Wang for my three week post-op follow-up. He continues to be pleased with my progress and actually lifted most of my restrictions! I am cleared to drive and lift William, our eighteen-month old. I need to wait at least another week before I can attempt playing, as any forceful exhaling could result in a hole in the trachea. Dr. Wang says my neck would fill with air and the skin would be like cellophane with bubbles underneath it. He said if that happened to "just stop" (!?). When I mentioned the numbness, he said there is no way to avoid cutting some nerves in a procedure such as this. When I mentioned the tingling, he said the nerves are reconnecting, which is good. He also asked if I could feel my earlobes and when I replied in the affirmative, said, "Oh good, we saved those nerves too." Another nasal endoscopy showed my vocal folds to be functioning well, and the surrounding tissue to have healed considerably, so the recurrent laryngeal nerve was not damaged. I don't have any high range when I try to sing, but my voice is loads better than it was a week or two ago.

While this is only the fifth time we've ever seen this man (consultation, surgery, release from hospital and two follow-ups), we feel we've been with him for years. He again spent well over an hour with us and had a clear answer for every question, which he backed up with statistics or study results. We were reminded why we chose him to perform the surgery and again feel blessed to find someone so skilled. Dr. Wang says I am recovering so rapidly because I am "young and healthy" (I wonder what the bill for that will be!), and I don't need to see him for another five weeks! He did, however, stress that I have a "bad" cancer and should do whatever I can to prevent it from recurring. Hürthle Cell* Carcinoma can be quite aggressive, as it is in my case. Wang mentioned that not only was it in my lymph nodes, but there was capsular invasion as well (meaning it penetrated the walls of the nodes and invaded the surrounding tissue.) I will probably be undergoing radioactive iodine treatment soon.

* "The Hürthle cell has consistently been the center of debate in the discussion of nonneoplastic and neoplastic lesions of the thyroid ever since it was first described in 1894 by Hürthle. In fact, the cells originally described by Hürthle are now considered to represent ultimobranchial body–derived parafollicular cells or C cells. The oncocytic cells that we now consider to be the follicular-derived Hürthle cells were actually described by Askanazy in 1898. Despite the fact that the cells originally described by Hürthle are likely not the Hürthle cells as considered today, the term has remained in the literature to describe follicular-derived epithelial cells with oncocytic cytology. Other terms for the Hürthle cells include oncocytic, eosinophilic and oxyphilic cells."

- Archives of Pathology & Laboratory Medicine

# Visitors, Round Two

*By Michael Turnbull — Apr 21, 2013*

Today I received an unexpected visit from some more friends from my days on the road. Kevin and Les rented a car, drove four hours from Los Angeles to Las Vegas, grabbed a bite to eat, visited with me for about an hour and drove the four-hour return trip home. Wow. It was great seeing you guys and your kind gesture is greatly appreciated. You never realize how connected you are to the people you share life with until something like this happens.

Also, four more guys from my current gig came by the house. Gabe (great conversation, bro); Dave (thanks for the nuts!), who is graciously covering me while I'm out and having to cover his own gig as well; Joey and family (thanks for the t-shirt!); and Jerry (I'm glad you're ok, too!).

I really enjoyed the visits and conversations with all of you guys, my fellow musicians and friends.

You're helping me heal!

# Absence

*By Michael Turnbull — Apr 27, 2013*

Hi everyone. We've been getting calls and messages asking if everything is ok, since we haven't posted anything here for a couple of weeks. Basically, no news is good news! We've been trying to get back to "normal" life (if that exists with two young, crazy boys) and have just been busy. I will try to backdate a few entries to get everyone up to speed on my progress, but otherwise no worries!

> **Mary Alice J**
> *We prayed that your family has peace. St. Anthony has come through so many times in our lives. It is nice to see he is doing the same thing for you. Keep up the good work. Enjoy the kids. And above everything, be nice to your nurse! We love ya.*

# One Month!

*By Karen Turnbull — Apr 28, 2013*

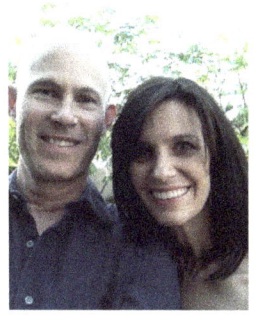

Well, we have made it to the one-month marker! Mike is doing very well and is healing great. We had an appointment with Dr. Wang on Friday, April 19th. He was very pleased with Mike's progress. We go back to see him in a month. Mike was cleared of restrictions with the exception of sudden or prolonged neck extension. He was even told he could "gently" try playing his trombone a little. He was warned, however, not to play too hard or the sutures could loosen and his neck would fill and puff up with air. We were told it would feel like crinkling Saran wrap all around his throat. When I asked what he should do if this happened we were simply told: "stop playing." This made us laugh! So for now Mike has decided a little more rest and recovery is probably best!

This week began a new adventure. Mike has appointments every day at Comprehensive Cancer Center for injections, pills and scans. Basically he is being tested and prepared for the radioactive iodine treatment. No date has been set for that yet. This week should tell the doctors if there are any remaining cells and how they respond to the iodine. We meet Friday with Dr. Obara to see how everything went. Praying for good results!

Mike's mom flew in yesterday to help with the kids and we are very grateful. The boys love their "Nana" and this makes it much easier for Mike to get some rest during the day. He is doing amazing, although each day brings some new challenges. As everything is healing he is experience tightness and new feelings of soreness. He has also been on a low-iodine diet for about three weeks now. This has caused some more eating challenges but we are trying our best. I have managed to make him some really delicious no-iodine granola that he can have with coconut milk which seems to be a favorite. I have also fed him so many veggies that he has actually talked about eating steak just to get some variety! It has probably been more than twenty years since he has had any!

We also got to go out on our first date since before surgery. We had a great time and enjoyed free tickets to Elton John! Mike's done so many cool things that he actually forgot he played for Elton John at his house! It was wonderful to spend some time together and feel somewhat normal. So, this pretty much updates everyone on the big news and we will post again soon. I am sure Mike will supply everyone with more details but this at least fills you all in. Again, we thank you all so much for checking in on him and sending the prayers and love. Keep it coming!

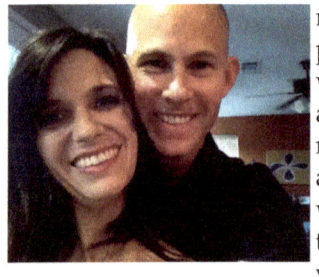

Also, thank you to our friends Mike and Devonee for taking our kids at 7:00 AM for the past two weeks so Mike could get some rest while I was at work. You truly saved us! I don't know how we would have managed without you!

And thank you to my beautiful angel of a sister, Marianne, who stayed with us for the first two weeks after surgery to take care of the kids. I thank God every day that He made us sisters! I love you!

> *Megan H*
> *Hi, Mike and Karen. My name is Megan and Jim is my husband. I wanted to reach out to tell you how relieved and happy we are that you are doing so well. Your odyssey is amazing and the grace in which you've handled both your diagnosis and recovery is inspiring. Jim and I are going through a similar ordeal, though Jim's treatment had (originally) been thoughtfully planned out and should have been fairly standard (if anything like "cancer treatment" can ever be considered such a thing). The universe decided that WE are not in charge and things have gone much differently than planned. Oy! Ironically (or NOT) ... April 8th was the day Jim's situation turned from controlled to critical. We saw you and your beautiful wife, Karen, at Comprehensive Cancer Center, there for your consultation with Dr. Obara. Jim was sitting in the lobby, in a wheel chair, looking like he'd been in a car crash when we saw you walk in. He tried to muster the strength to say "hey" but thought better of it. He was KIND of a mess and didn't want to rain on your parade, 'cause YOU, my friend, looked FANTASTIC! Jim was saying to himself, "That guy is amazing! That guy will be me!" Congratulations on your swift and fine recuperation from such an invasive surgery. Our positive thoughts and prayers have never wavered toward your complete, 100% recovery from cancer, your surgery and your treatment. You will blow that horn with a passion and gusto others*

*will never understand! Soon after that we will organize a jam session so you and Jim can play together. He will love that, from a musical perspective. I will love it for the simple, poetic justice of it all. I can think of a few more super-talented musicians who have told cancer to take a hike and they, too, can join the jamboree! It'll be the Kiss-Off-Cancer Quartet ... Plus! You are loved, you are inspired and you are warriors. Sent with love and admiration.*

**Les K**
*Mike!!! It was sooo good to see you and to be able to give you and Karen a hug;-). I think you guys healed me! Continued blessings, my friend. One Love.*

**Lou G**
*You are great, inspiring and should publish this memoir as a blueprint of hope, faith and healing for the ones facing adversity. But I know you won't consider this a big deal or heroic accomplishment. Thanks Mike, and glad you are healing, mending and in the middle of so much love.*

## Iodine, Here We Come

*By Karen Turnbull — May 4, 2013*

Well, it looks like more prayers were answered. Mike spent the past week getting thyroid hormone injections, an iodine pill and two scans. The scan results showed a "hot spot" on the right side of the neck. What exactly this is we don't know. It is possible it is just residual thyroid tissue and not necessarily cancerous. Our oncologist said it is basically impossible to not have some residual tissue left behind. The great thing is that it loved the iodine (which as I posted before is not always the case with Hürthle Cell), so whatever it is the next radioactive iodine treatment should attack it. The reasons to attack it are 1) if it is by chance a cancerous cell we want to get it now and 2) if it is not we don't want to give it the opportunity to develop into cancer. So, it looks like in about a week or two Mike will go to Sunrise Hospital to receive the radioactive iodine treatment. This will require a two-night stay in the hospital because he will be too radioactive to be around people. We will then have to figure out a means of quarantine for him so as not to risk interfering with mine or the kids' healthy thyroids. How exactly we do that we have yet to figure out. We will be meeting with our nuclear medicine doctor soon to figure out all the details.

We also met with the radiologist, Dr. Toy, who will administer the external beam radiation. This will probably happen in about three months. The scan was clear for the rest of his body which is more great news! So, this means Dr. Toy can specifically target the region of the neck that was affected and insure that there are no residual cancer cells left behind. Normally, external radiation is not necessary with thyroid cancer, but because Mike is special and his invaded the trachea we need to be a little more aggressive.

We have also learned how "bad" his cancer was and how "bad" things could have gone if not for such a skilled surgeon. Details no one spoke to us about before, probably out of fear of worrying us more than necessary. So, we are celebrating facts such as this: all detectable cancer is gone, Mike can speak, raise his arms, smile, turn his head, laugh and feeling to his neck is returning. All these things among others could have been compromised. We are forever grateful to the skilled hands and patience of Dr. Wang. This incredible man took ten hours to insure that Mike could return to his normal life. He will forever be considered an angel on earth to us.

We thank God daily for the miracles we have received!

> *Katey J*
> *We are so pleased to hear the latest update. You are right ... God is good and in times like these, it brings us closer to Him and makes us aware of all the miracles, big and small. We continue to pray for all of you!!!*
>
> *Yong D*
> *I'm super blessed to have met you and your wonderful family. You are in my prayers.*

## Community Support
### *By Karen Turnbull — May 7, 2013*

Throughout all of this Mike and I have been amazed at the outpouring of support our family, friends and community has shown us. So, we felt it was important to share with everyone what is happening this weekend at New Song Anthem Church. At 1:00 PM this Saturday the 11th, there will be an unbelievable display of talent performing in honor of Mike! The fabulous musicians of Las Vegas have pulled together their talent, time and energy to put together a two-hour music concert complete with food and drink afterwards! We have even heard that the famous Rich Little will make a guest appearance! The amazing pastors at New Song along with our friends Danny and January have been working like mad to make this happen. We are humbled by all of this and do not know how we could ever repay the kindness and generosity that has been shown to us. So ... if you are looking for a great way to spend your Saturday please come celebrate with us at this unbelievable event. It is going to be AWESOME! We would love to see you there!

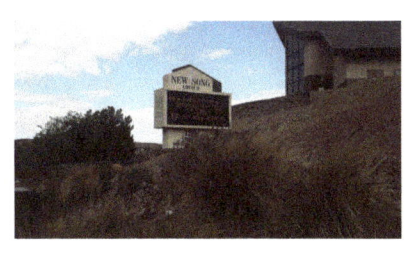

### *Jennifer S*
*Hi, Mike and Karen. Just wanted to let you know that my thoughts are with you and that I am wishing you the best. Wish I could be there with you this weekend.*

### *Megan H*
*Mike and Karen, Jim and I do wish we could be there to support this! What a wonderful and amazing thing Danny and our community is doing! As I keep saying ... I am not surprised. Vegas has some of the most caring people in the world. Enjoy the entertainment and embrace the love coming your way! Can't wait to meet you one day! Many blessings!*

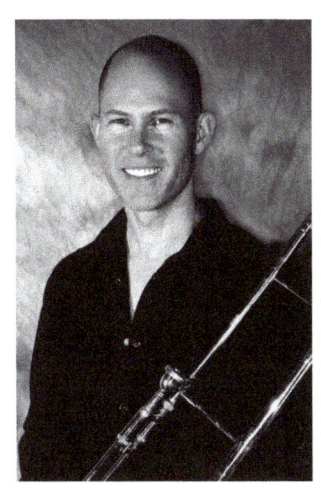

## Event Details
*By Danny Falcone — May 9, 2013*

Mike Turnbull, trombonist with Donny & Marie Osmond, was diagnosed with stage IV thyroid and tracheal cancer. Mike has undergone a radical procedure and has been unable to return to work. Please come out and support this benefit to help a most wonderful man and his family recover from a most trying time. The line up of entertainment is beyond spectacular.

# Amazing Event!

*By Karen Turnbull — May 13, 2013*

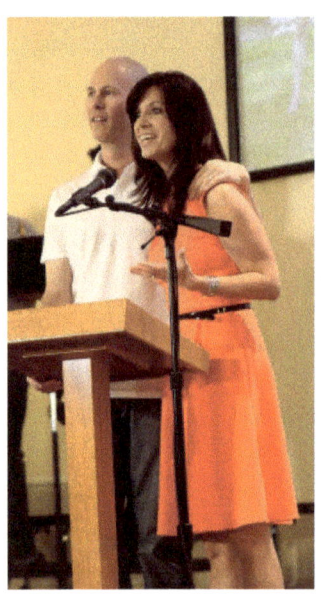

Wow! Words cannot even come close to describing the awesome event that took place yesterday! Mike and I are so humbled by the outpouring of support that has come our way. New Song Church was packed and the talent in the room was awesome! It truly was a celebration! Danny and January Falcone outdid themselves making this happen! Not only have the two of them been there for us throughout this ordeal, they managed to pull the community together for this unbelievable event. We know how hard they worked and how little sleep they got these past weeks! You two are amazing (you could open an event planning business!). The list of talent went on and on and each act was its own unique gift. My face hurt from smiling so much! And the food … Las Vegas caterers Sara and Rodney donated their time and talent and it was seriously some of the best food I have ever tasted! (Unfortunately, Mike was unable to taste it due to iodine levels so we will have to hire them to do a dinner for us when this is all over!) The love and support in the room was unbelievable. I know the main reason behind this was to help us through a financially difficult time but it did so much more. It renewed us and reminded us that we are not alone in this journey. We are surrounded by loving, kind and generous people. We do not know how we can ever repay or properly thank everyone who has helped us. To everyone who was there I hope you enjoyed it as much as we did. For those of you who gave your time, talent and energy … you rock! We are amazed by your talents and humbled that you gave them for this event. To everyone who donated and couldn't be there your generosity is so touching.

Thank you everyone!

> **Brenda M**
> *TJ and I really enjoyed all the talented singers and musicians and Mr. Rich Little at Mike's benefit fundraiser! But we really liked hearing*

*Mike, Karen, family and friends talk about the amazing miracle that had occurred with the surgery and healing! Mike you are truly blessed with an amazing wife and family. It was a pleasure meeting your wife! Mike, you looked great and humbled with all the caring people around you! You go, Toxic Avenger ... lol! I can't wait to see you at work again alongside your buddy Gil! Continuing Prayers for All!*

**Bethany B**
*Chris and his parents have not stopped talking about what an UNBELIEVABLE day Saturday was. I am so excited for you both that you got to experience the abundance of support this community has to offer you. I hope the faith and love of all those people can continue to carry you through your amazing journey to recovery!!*

## Back to Work

*By Michael Turnbull — May 16, 2013*

Last night (and tonight) I went in and played the show, just over six weeks after my surgery. It went surprisingly well, considering I play a wind instrument and my windpipe was just replumbed. I took a few things down an octave and played approximately 80% of normal volume, but my sound was decent and I didn't need to lay out at all. I didn't feel any extra strain, just muscle soreness which I already had from trying to regain range of motion.

Everyone at work was extremely welcoming and so happy to see me, which was great. Donny & Marie were both thrilled and surprised, and they and everyone else cautioned me to take it easy (as Karen, my mom and my surgeon already had!). Just the simple act of going to work made me feel normal again. I am so grateful for the ability to do this for a living, and I felt real joy to be making music again.

Next week I will begin I-131 (radioactive iodine) treatments, so I will be quarantined and unable to work for a couple more weeks. I figured I'd sneak a week's worth of income in while I had the chance.

**Randy C**
*Great news, Mike! Congrats. I'm so happy for you getting back this soon! You continue to amaze. A wonderful event this weekend. The music was extraordinary and the sentiments expressed heartfelt and sincere. Best to you, Karen and the boys as you go through your treatment. Do you need me to pick you up a toxic avenger suit?*

*Dene R*
*Hey, Mike. I just get "goose bumps" every time I read your updates ... wow ... what a miracle you are in so many ways! It's so awesome to see all the great, kind people who are on your side! Keep the faith and I pray God's continued blessings for you and your family.*

*Nandita S*
*Hey, Mike! I'm so glad that you are able to play again. Amazing! I hope the week of creativity helps sustain you through your iodine treatment quarantine. I am in awe of you. You are a rock star!*

# Iodine

*By Karen Turnbull — May 22, 2013*

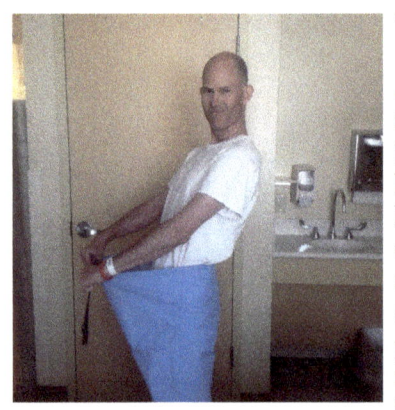

Mike was admitted to Sunrise Hospital today to receive the radioactive iodine treatment. He will be there for three days in isolation while his radiation levels are at their highest. After that we have made arrangements for him to stay at a hotel since he can't be less than six feet from people for extended periods of time (more than twenty minutes.) Seeing as our little ones love their Daddy and consider him a jungle gym we thought it best to not risk it and stay apart for an extra week. We will chat via FaceTime and he is supplied with DVD's and Netflix so hopefully the time will pass quickly (at least for him). He is doing great and is ready to tackle this treatment and move on. The low iodine diet has become just a part of our life so a few more weeks will go quickly. After that, Mike has hinted at wanting a bacon double cheeseburger! Which, for those of you that know him well realize, is something he has not put in his body for probably at least twenty years! At the very least I know he will enjoy a good piece of grilled salmon! Thanks again for your thoughts, prayers and comments. Mike and I appreciate all the love and support so much.

We will keep you posted.

*Erica M*

*Hi, Mike! You are an amazing man! I am sending beautiful thoughts your way daily. Hang in there and know you have so much support surrounding you ... especially in NY :-). I love you guys! xoxo*

*Fran H*

*Karen and Mike, we are amazed at Mike's progress; it is nothing short of miraculous! We hear you'll be coming to Pittsburgh for a couple of weeks and receiving more TLC from your loving family. Enjoy the break! We'll continue to pray for your complete recovery and return to normalcy which, of course, is the new normal. (But sooooooo much better than what you were facing just weeks ago.) God bless you all.*

# The Toxic Avenger

*By Michael Turnbull — May 24, 2013*

Well, I'm still here at Sunrise Hospital, but I'm hoping to be released later today. It all depends on how toxic I am! I was pretty darn radioactive to begin with, as my nuclear medicine doctor decided to administer a higher than average dose due to the extensive metastases. Immediately after swallowing the pill, the technician (who was standing fifteen feet away from me at the door to the room) pointed a Geiger counter at me and it pegged to maximum.

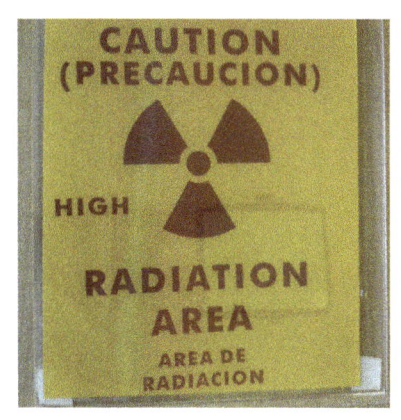

I have a lovely view of a Denny's and the Stratosphere in the background, and for some sick reason I have been torturing myself by watching the Food Network. The television chefs haven't prepared a single thing I could eat on the low iodine diet, and it all looks so appetizing that it's putting my salivary glands into overdrive. This is actually a good thing, as it squeezes the radioactive saliva out and flushes it through my system. I am supposed to consume as much fluid as possible, which will bring the levels down and hasten my departure. I've never peed so much in a two-day span in my life.

The whole experience has been easier than expected. The way various sources were speaking, we were expecting a lead-walled* room with an airlock doggie door for food delivery, the nurses to be prohibited from entering the room, and the pill to be handled with shoulder-length gloves and barbecue tongs. In reality, it is a normal hospital room (save for the bright red radioactive waste bin and the sign on the door), the nurses come and go (just not very often or for very long), and the technician handed me the pill while wearing regular latex gloves (although it was in a lead container). In fact, the gelatinous capsule had warmed and stuck to the container, so I had to pry it it out with my fingers. I guess when you are ingesting 250 mCi of I-131 it doesn't matter if you touch it. The only surprising aspect of this process was the sides of my face swelling up like a chipmunk, which I was not alerted to until just prior to ablation. If you've ever played with one of those "fat face" apps, you'll have a good idea of how I look at the moment.

So the technician just came back as I was composing this and my levels are low enough to release me! On to a hotel so I can avoid the kids for another week. Their developing thyroids are at a much greater risk from radiation exposure than adults, so I have to stay several feet away from them, an impossibility in our house.

* I found out later that the walls were indeed made of lead. They were just covered with drywall so you couldn't tell.

> *Megan H*
> Wow ... Maybe you will be able to leap tall buildings and develop x-ray vision! Oh, wait! You already ARE one of those Super Men! What a trip! I am sure the hardest thing will be the time away from your young 'uns. We are thinking of you and your family constantly and we know that YOU know that WE KNOW!! Lots of love and healing vibes!
>
> *Laurence A*
> Spiderman got his super powers from a radiation dose, no? You're on your way, brother. Lol. You're so amazing, Mike. Keep on!
>
> *Frank S*
> So you actually peed more than when we did that pub crawl in Dublin? Good Lord!

# Hotel

*By Karen Turnbull — May 25, 2013*

I was able to see Mike yesterday at the hotel and he looks amazing! The swelling is completely gone and his spirits are up. The boys, my niece Megan and I went to the hotel yesterday to stock it with iodine-free groceries and bring linens and pillows from home. The medical technicians told us he was fine to sleep on the hotel linens but we thought we would just be a little extra cautious. His room overlooks the pool and so he was able to watch the boys swim and wave to us. This seemed to help ease Evan's mind to know where Daddy was staying and that he is doing great. I was able to chat with him in the hotel room and get caught up with how he was doing. (We just stayed on opposite sides of the room.) He has lots of movies and books and will hopefully get some good rest. The room is perfect. Big thanks to my mom and dad for hooking us up with points! He has a full kitchen, living space, desk and bed. So hopefully it will make the week more comfortable. He is only about twenty minutes from us so we can go swim and visit from afar during the week. Oh, and the other good news is his thyroid medicine has been changed to just once a day!

Yippee!

> *Melin F*
> *Keep up the good work. You guys are amazing. I'm so proud of how you handle each and every step. My heart goes out to you and I continue to pray for all of you!!!!*
>
> *Jeanine C*
> *Following your journey ... in awe of your strength, humor and positivity ... thrilled for the fabulous progress ... sending love and prayers to the Turnbull family daily.*

# Beach Bound!

*By Karen Turnbull — Jun 13, 2013*

Last Thursday Mike had a follow-up appointment with Dr. Wang, his surgeon. We are very happy to report that he doesn't want to see Mike for three months! This is wonderful news and means that he is healing beautifully! On Friday we saw Dr. Toy, the radiologist.

His feeling is that because of how aggressive the cancer was and as he put it, "A cancer cell strong enough to eat through a hard cartilage wall," it is in Mike's best interest to proceed with the external beam radiation. Dr. Toy feels confident that he can be aggressive enough for it to work, yet it should be mild enough to not cause any long-term side effects. Short-term effects may be hoarseness, laryngitis and a sunburn feeling. These shouldn't last too long and will hopefully only be a slight annoyance. Dr. Toy is impressed with how well Mike has handled surgery and the iodine treatment. He says he is in this for the cure and the external beam radiation should hopefully be the last step in keeping this gone for good. This is all scheduled to start the end of August.

We then went on to see Dr. Obara, the oncologist. He too was impressed with how well Mike has handled everything and feels he is doing well. He does want to continue to check his thyroglobulin levels and make sure his medication is at the right level. So we will continue to see him to monitor Mike's blood work.

Mike has returned to work for two weeks and is playing his trombone with a new appreciation for the gift he has been given. Dr. Wang and his wife Dr. Barber, who assisted on the surgery, attended the show last Saturday and got to see their awesome work up on stage performing! How do you thank someone who quite literally saved Mike's life? We have no idea, but we thought getting them into the show might at least be a small thank you.

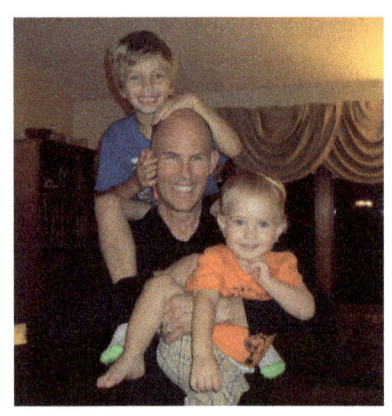

Next week we will head to Hilton Head, South Carolina for a celebratory week at the beach with my sister Marianne and her family and my brother Mike and his family! We are so excited to have this much needed family time. The boys have been so patient during Mike's healing and the idea of riding bikes, building sand castles, swimming and playing with Daddy is better than any Christmas gift ever! As for me, when I see our children wrap their arms around Daddy's neck with its new scar I am brought to tears! That scar is a reminder to us that life is a precious gift and we have to treasure every moment because you just never know what may happen. Thank you again to everyone for the prayers, love and support. Unfortunately, we are not the only ones battling this monster called cancer. To our friends fighting the fight we love you and pray for you daily.

Stay strong!

> *Sandy B*
> *Been following your fantastic progress, Mike. So glad to see you are getting better and stronger every day. Enjoy the sun, sand, family and a few beverages. Cheers.*
>
> *Jennifer O*
> *We are so happy to read your last entry. This is fantastic news!! I just finished twenty-five radiation treatments a couple weeks ago and I feel great!! You will do very well, Michael, because you are healthy, have a great support system and a positive attitude. Feel free to call me ~ we are both members of the "C" club. Enjoy every minute! Lots of Love oxoxooxoxoxox*
>
> *Megan H*
> *Three cheers for the Turnbull Family and their fearless, trombone-wielding knight in shining brass!! Karen, your query about how to thank a doctor, or team of doctors, for their role in keeping Mike with us is deep. I think you are right that he relished seeing/hearing Mike up there doing his thing at D&M. I believe their reward is seeing people like Mike successfully climb the mountain, using their tools and skill set and brain power. Their desire to beat down the monster has to be all-consuming and as much a passion for them as music is to our husbands. Thank God for people so driven to make other people well! Thank you for your constant support and love. I so look forward to the day our families finally meet! It will be a grand celebration. Enjoy Hilton Head ... family and the beach. I can think of no better combination. Much love.*

## Radiation Has Begun
*By Karen Turnbull — Sep 11, 2013*

I know it has been quite some time since our last post. I am happy to say it is because we had a wonderful summer off from treatments with no news to report! (Other than that we had a great summer full of wonderful family time!)

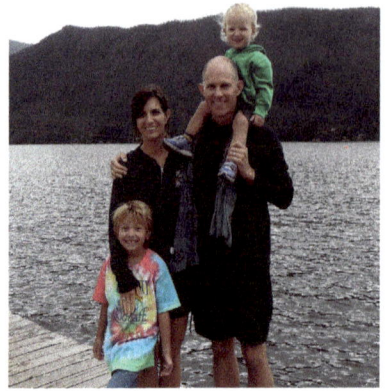

Mike's last appointment with his surgeon (last Thursday) was great. He is healing beautifully both on the outside and on the inside. Dr. Wang did a scope to check out the inside of his trachea and it looked as if nothing had ever been done. His vocal cords are working perfectly and there is no visible scarring. (He puts it up on a screen in the office so we can see!). Mike has returned to work and is feeling great. Because he is feeling so good it has been a little difficult to begin this next stage of treatment.

We met with Dr. Toy a few weeks ago and asked if the external beam radiation was necessary. His response put it into perspective ... if thyroid cancers were considered the cat family, typical thyroid cancer would be like a common house cat. Mike's cancer is more like a lion. Do we dare take the risk of letting the lion out of his cage? We decided "no!" The concern is that if his cancer were to make a comeback (which we are sure it will not!) it would most likely resurface at the trachea. The problem with this is that Dr. Wang already removed four and a half centimeters of trachea, which means there is no room for a second chance with surgery other than a complete tracheotomy. Could we take our chances? Yes, but we are not willing to do that. Our doctors are in this for a complete cure, as are we.

So, this past Monday, Mike began external beam radiation treatments. This will consist of about ten minutes a day of radiation for the next six weeks, five days a week. I will let Mike fill you in on the exact details of the treatment. He has mentioned it feels like something out of a Star Trek movie. The side effects should be minimal but could include fatigue, skin irritation similar to a sunburn, heartburn, laryngitis or a feeling of bronchitis. All of these would just be temporary and if he feels them at all, it shouldn't be until the last few weeks of treatment.

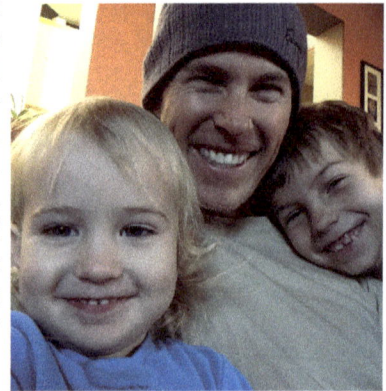

The bonus in all of this is that the radiation office is very close to my job, so we have been able to see each other every day for lunch! Making lemonade out of lemons! Nothing brightens my workday more than seeing him outside my studio door! As brief as it is, seeing him strong and healthy powers me through the day. He continues to inspire me every day with his strength and positivity.

Thanks for the continued prayers, love and energy. We feel it and are so grateful.

### Frank S
*It sounds like you guys are making the right call going through with the radiation. Enjoy those lunches! I miss you both!*

### Jean T
*Karen, thank you for keeping us all up to date. I'm a friend of Mike's mom and know how heavy this has all been for all of you. The picture of the four of you in Grand Lake this summer is wonderful! Stay strong and know there are folks you don't even know praying for you.*

### David N
*Such a blessing it is to pass Mike as he enters the backstage door to his dressing room at the Donny & Marie show each night. To watch him perform and play his trombone, doing what he loves, as he always has, as if nothing ever happened, as if nothing ever changed ... but it has changed. And we are, all of us that know Mike and are aware of his journey, a little bit closer to our Spiritual Being. Hey ... thanks for that, Mike!*

### Shari B
*My dearest Mike and Karen, you are such an inspiration to everyone in how we live our daily lives. You are some of the dearest people I know and we love you so very much!*

### Katey J
*Thinking about you all as you walk these next steps in your journey. Keep making lemonade. We are all blessed by your amazing spirits!*

# Half Way!

*By Karen Turnbull — Oct 1, 2013*

Today Mike completed fifteen of his thirty radiation treatments! It feels good to know we can start counting down from here! Overall he has been doing amazing. He has been really good about applying aloe to the area several times a day (thanks Suzanne for the tip) and his neck is only slightly pink. The biggest side effect began last week. Basically he has described it as stabbing razor blades every time he swallows! So far he is managing it and is even continuing to play (he is at a gig right now!). They gave him a prescription blend that is supposed to help numb the pain. So far, though, it has numbed his lips to the point he couldn't feel his horn. His throat still hurt and his tongue was numb, which caused him to have no taste for the food he was trying to swallow and it was still painful to swallow.

Through all of this Mike has never complained and he just takes one day at a time, staying confident that this will soon all be over. During the week he is feeling pretty tired come 3:00 PM but I am not sure if that is strictly from the radiation. After all, he wakes every morning at 6:30 AM to get the kids dressed and fed and Evan off to school. Then he heads out for his treatment and returns home to take care of William until I get home from work. And, he still plays his show at night so I think he is quite justified in needing a 3:00 PM nap!!!! Despite all this he smiles, laughs and makes us smile and laugh all day.

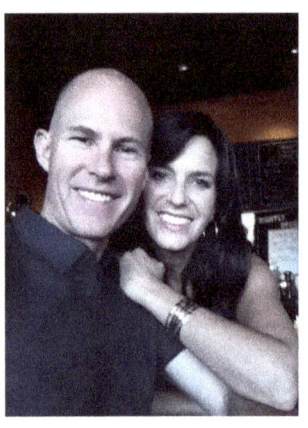

We celebrated our eleventh wedding anniversary on Saturday! Our vows hold new meaning for us as we look back on this past year, but even with the cards we have recently been dealt there is nowhere I would rather be than by Mike's side. He continues to be the best daddy to our boys and the most amazing husband. He insisted on taking me to dinner for our anniversary even though he probably would have rather stayed home and had a smoothie and a nap. We celebrate every day and treasure every moment together.

Thanks for the continued love, support and prayers. We both appreciate it so much.

*Nandita S*
*Sending lots of love and good vibes in the final stretch. I am amazed by the grace with which you have all handled this incredible challenge, though not surprised. Love you all so much!*

*Issa F*
*I can't believe you are gigging through this! Wow! Music is a healer, though, that's for sure. You and your family are certainly in my prayers! Hang in there!*

*Dave W*
*Thinking about you a lot as you go through this, Mike. Hang tough! Shared your story with Joy last week. Her and Nancy both send their love and prayers. You are an inspiration to me. Hope the next fifteen days goes by quickly for you!*

*Michael M*
*Mike, just want to tell you I think of you often, and wish you a speedy and permanent recovery. I miss playing with you and hanging out. That is a lovely photo of you and your family.*

*Sara O*
*It was so good to see all of you while visiting my daughter and family this past week. So thankful they have you guys for not just neighbors but extended family. It blessed my heart to see how well Mike is doing. You are sure right, Karen ... Mike is a wonderful daddy and husband. So glad I've had the opportunity to know all of you. Love & hugs.*

*Lisa L*
*Happy belated anniversary to both of you. Love the new photo on the site. Mike is constantly in my prayers. Kudos to Mike to keep doing what he loves.*

# Happy Early Christmas!

*By Karen Turnbull — Nov 5, 2013*

First off, I apologize for the delay in getting this written. Somehow the days turn to weeks and here we are. Anyways, to get everyone updated Mike has officially finished his six weeks of radiation! As has been his usual style throughout this entire ordeal, he has done amazing! He had a nice sunburn on his neck for a while, which then turned to a really nice looking lizard pattern, but it has healed beautifully and in a few more weeks it should be completely back to normal. The razor blade feeling in his throat subsided and the internal scope that Dr. Wang performed last week showed zero damage to the vocal cords! Thank you God (and Dr. Toy!).

During all this Mike played every show and even added in a few extra gigs here and there. I don't know how he did it all but he was determined to keep playing and maintain as much normalcy as possible. Also, the oncologist has been carefully watching Mike with weekly blood draws. His white blood cell count has been at a critically low level for a few months. They believe it is related to the iodine treatment and, from old blood records that we pulled from five years ago, his baseline seems to be on the lower end of normal. So while no one seemed overly concerned, it was still enough of a red flag that it had to be monitored. Today we saw the oncologist to check his blood work and see how everything looked. His counts are up and things look good! Music to our ears ... "I don't need to see you till next year." Woo hoo!!! The weekly appointments have been our new "normal." I honestly never even thought we could celebrate the holidays without running to doctor visits. Now next year technically means January, which is only two months away, but I will gladly take it!

For now we celebrate and thank God for all He has blessed us with! Thursday is Mike's birthday. I know it would mean so much to him to hear from all of you who have been supporting him, reading our posts, praying for him and keeping him in your thoughts. He really is a very special man and despite the challenges this year has brought, he has found a way to smile and laugh through it all. I know it is pretty obvious but I have to say it anyways- I love him with all my heart and can't imagine being anywhere but by his side.

So, with that, I wish you all an early very Merry Christmas! I am ready to celebrate!

> *Vince V*
> *You guys are amazing! Happy Birthday, Mike. I'm in awe of how you are attacking this head-on, and that you're still playing. Keep it up, and know that you're an inspiration for everyone to live well and enjoy every moment.*
>
> *Brian M*
> *Go Mike! F..k Cancer! A very joyous birthday to you.*

*Nandita S*
Happy early birthday, Mike! I'm so happy to hear about the progress of your treatment and that you can be doctor-free for the rest of the year! You have been in my thoughts all year. I can't believe how much has happened since I visited in January. You are a hero among heroes. Enjoy the holiday season! With love.

*Hayley M*
WAHOO! It's a Christmas Miracle! What fabulous news for you ALL. I can't begin to imagine what you have both been through whilst keeping everything normal at home. Brilliant news. Congrats to Mike and Love to you all. Have a VERY Happy Birthday, Happy Thanksgiving and an especially "Merry Christmas!" Cheers! Lots of love. Miss you all very much. xxx

*Bethany B*
Chris and I could not be more happy for your family! What an amazing sigh of relief you all can take for the next few months. You have continued to be in our thoughts and prayers and we wish you all the best as we head into this holiday season. Hugs from Arizona for each of you!

*Cathy M*
We are endlessly grateful for this wonderful news! Mike, you and your family have shown us how to live this year. You've been the ultimate inspiration. We all send you our warmest wishes and lots of love for a very Happy Birthday!

*Kathy T*
Happy Birthday, darling son. Love you so much. Mom

*Issa F*
Congratulations and Happy Birthday! Wow, to think at one point you probably thought you wouldn't see this birthday! And ya did! Mike, you have such a fantastic sense of humor, I'm sure it has sustained you and your family more than you know! Cheers!

*Doug M*
Hey Mike, it's your friend Doug from the Royal Viking Sun! Really have been thinking of you a lot this past year and saying lots of prayers for you and your family. Such a great human being you are ... this world needs your spirit around for a long time yet. So keep your head up on this journey, and know you are never alone. Have

*a Happy Birthday, and may this year bring you peace and joy. I sound like a greeting card, but I really mean it! (caw ... caw ... those are bird noises.)*

# Happy Thanksgiving!
*By Karen Turnbull — Nov 28, 2013*

This Thanksgiving has a whole new meaning! My list of thanks this year is huge and I felt it was important to share it with all of you who have traveled this journey with us. So here it goes ...

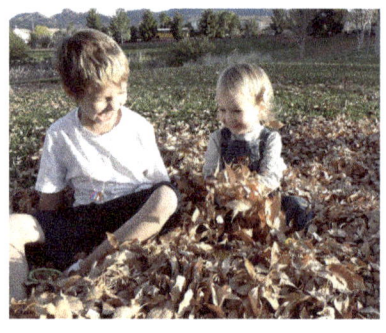

This Thanksgiving I am thankful for my amazing husband, who has battled cancer, never complained, never even thought about giving up and has tackled every day with a smile. My children; I can't even type this without tearing up, they bring such joy into our lives every single day. My parents for loving me and supporting us through everything. My siblings; it is amazing how the years go by and I think back to Thanksgivings and Christmases past and laughter fills my heart as I remember turkey tournament ping-pong matches, Kris Kringle, trips to the cottage and Seven Springs, sled riding, etc. I have the best family ever!!! Marianne, my most amazing sister and angel here on earth; I really don't know what I would do without you. You pick me up when I am down, you listen to me ramble and cry when I am scared, you love my children as if they were your own. Thank you for all the flights out to Vegas to help us. I am so blessed to have you as my sister and friend! My brother-in-law Mark; I will never ever forget what you did for me on that horribly long day, March 30th, 2013. I don't know how I would have gotten through if it weren't for your amazing strength. For those ten hours during Mike's surgery you were there with me for whatever I needed. Somehow having you there made me stronger and I am forever grateful! My sister-in-laws Ellen and Adrienne; your encouraging messages, emails and texts all helped me so much. Thank you for your prayers, love and support. They helped power me. My unbelievable and beautiful nieces, Melissa, Michelle, Megan, Jill and Ali; you guys are amazing! You never once questioned that Mike would beat this. Your pure belief in him was felt across the miles. You are amazing young women! And Megan, you flew out here twice to help with the kids! Thank you for helping set up Mike's radioactive iodine camp with me and for helping me recover from my hernia surgery (even if you making me laugh made me cry in pain, I am still grateful!). My sweet little nephew Gabe; my boys have the best time playing with you. I love you and your sweet giggles that melt my heart. Mike's mom, Kathy, and sister Wendy; I know how hard this has been on you. Thank you for all your love and support, for flying (or driving twelve hours!) here to be with us, help with the kids and share your love. I am so lucky to have you! Mike's grandma Louise, or GG to the boys; you have been so kind and full of love for all of us, you are an amazing woman and I am so grateful to have you in our lives. To all of our aunts, uncles and cousins, I know you have all been sending prayers, love, healing thoughts and energy our way. We have felt it!

Our friends, near and far; you have all been amazing with your support. I know what a shock this was to everyone. Thank you for loving us and supporting us. Tammy, January and Devonee ... I am speechless! You dropped everything to help us! Thank you for loving our children and taking care of them as we bounced around to doctor appointments. You removed the added stress of worrying about them because we knew they were in great hands, and I cannot even begin to express what a gift that was! January and Danny; WOW, talk about going above and beyond! The benefit concert that you put together for us was one of the most remarkable events I have ever attended. I can't believe you made it all happen! Thank you for all the time and energy you spent bringing the community together to help us. The love we experienced that day helped power us through these past months. To all the remarkable musicians that came together to perform at the benefit, we were truly blown away! Thank you doesn't even begin to express what we feel about all of you. Your gifts and talents are truly amazing and the fact that you freely gave them to help us is just too much. We will always remember and be grateful for what you did for our family.

Our community; you brought groceries, donated money and sent prayers and love to us. Thank you. My administration and co-workers at LVA; thank you for your support and prayers. It truly touches my heart when a fellow teacher sees me in the hall and asks me, "How is your husband?" I appreciate your thoughts so much and I am so grateful to have been able to take the time I needed to be with Mike through this process. The cast of Donny & Marie; I know you were all pulling for Mike. Thank you for the cards, donations, visits, love and laughter!

The amazing pastors of New Song Church; you accepted us in with open arms and helped pick us up when we felt at our lowest. You drove across town on Holy Saturday to pray with us before surgery. I will never forget the feeling of calm that came over me as we held hands around Mike's bed and listened to Pastor Marta's amazing words. That gift will stay with me forever! The Cancer Families group; although I wish it was under different circumstances, I am so glad we met and became friends; our Sunday night sessions brought so much healing to us, and for our children to be able to talk and play and try to make some sense of all of this - wow! What a blessing!

Frank S, what a crazy turn of fate that you were here for a gig the exact weekend of the surgery! I am so glad you were!!!! The Tom Jones gang; you wrote, called and visited! You made it a priority to let Mike know you loved him. Amazing! Frank L, I love you! Thank you for flying out here to celebrate with us! That was a forty-eight-hour visit I will treasure forever! Suzanne; your meditations brought light and peace to us! Annie and Ande; your healing basket was amazing! Kathy, your healing energy work was felt across the miles! To everyone who sent us healing love, energy, prayers and thoughts we couldn't have done it without you.

Our amazing team of doctors; for two people who don't even like to take Tylenol, you brought us through this crazy journey safely. Dr. Wang and Dr. Toy; in my heart, I know you saved Mike's life. Both of you said to us at our first visit that you were in this for the cure. I am extremely grateful that we found ourselves in your hands.

If there is anyone I have forgotten to mention please know that I am grateful for you, too! This year has been a crazy blur but in it have been remarkable gifts. This Thanksgiving I feel truly blessed and I am so grateful to God for guiding us through all of this. My faith has always been strong, but when I have been surrounded by so many amazing acts of kindness I can't help but feel a renewed sense of strength. I don't know why we were dealt this hand but I do know that we were given everything we needed to play and win.

Thank you everyone. We love you! Happy Thanksgiving!

> ### Sara O
> *Happy Thanksgiving to all of you! As always, I love reading the updates. Thank you, Karen, for a very blessed one on this special Thanksgiving. Hope to see you after Christmas on our visit to your special neighbors. Love and hugs to all of you.*

*Melin F*
*On this Thanksgiving I am grateful for all the people who helped you both on this journey ... I send my love and continue to send healing thoughts. Karen, what a wonderful tribute you wrote ... I am awed by you. Mike, what a good job you did and to the boys, Bravo Zulu ... good job in nautical terms.*

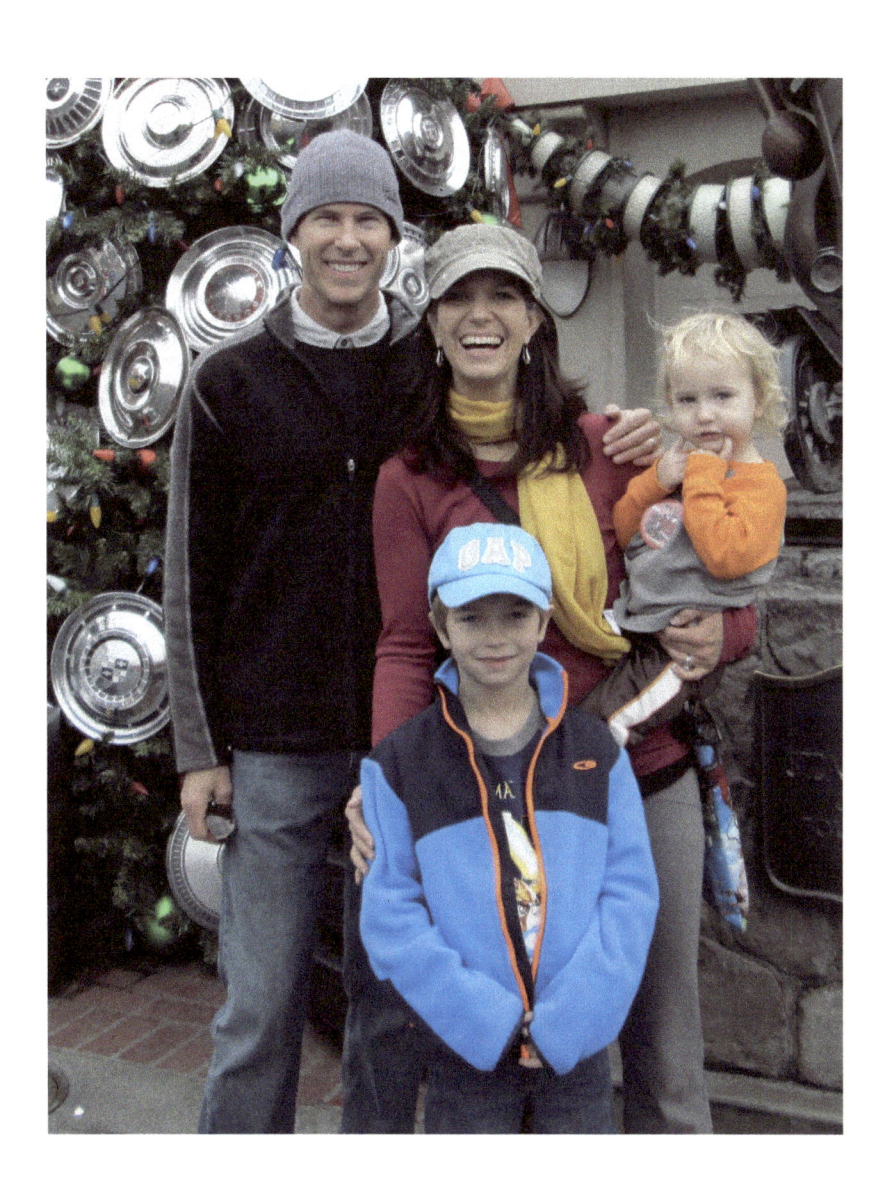

# CHAPTER TWO

# Dark Skies Ahead
## 2014

## Hallelujah!

*By Karen Turnbull — Feb 11, 2014*

Miracles do happen! Today we received the news we have been praying for ... no signs of cancer! Mike had his Iodine-123 scan last Wednesday and Thursday to see if there was any remaining thyroid tissue/signs of cancer. The results came back negative!!! We are so happy and extremely grateful. We are feeling very blessed right now as we celebrate this victory. Last night at dinner our six-year old son Evan decided to teach his two-year old brother William about miracles. Out of the blue he said, "William, do you have any miracles that you want to thank God for?" Mike and I just looked at each other with stunned faces. Mike asked Evan if he knew what a miracle was and if he had any he was thankful for. Evan very calmly said, "You being ok after your big neck surgery." Wow! What more can I say? Thank you everyone for all your love, support and prayers!

> *Dave Ro*
> This is the best news EVER! I can feel your amazing spirits all the way across the country right now. I'm so happy and so thrilled that you shared this. GOD BLESS!
>
> *Dene R*
> YES, Miracles!! Blessings! Grace! What more can be said ... thank you Lord for this family and for taking good care of them ... please know how special you all are!! Sending love from Texas!
>
> *Sharon H*
> I believe angels have always been watching over you ... I am so happy for all of you and I love you all so very much ... xoxo

*Vince V*
*That is a miracle. You guys are amazing. I'm so happy to hear Mike is doing so well. It's amazing how you included the kids in so they gain understanding. Forget about any one holiday, I say "Happy Every Day!" We send all of our love and gratitude your way!!!*

*Dan C*
*Awesome news! We are happy for everyone in the Turnbull family!*

*Anne-Corinne B*
*Hooray, hooray! We are so grateful for your fabulous news! And, thank you for sharing about miracles. We have told your story to friends and such joy has brought tears of happiness and confirmation of love. You have blessed us. Sending cheers!*

*Ron J*
*Hi, Mike. My best to you and your family. I hope you continue to feel better.*

# One Year

*By Michael Turnbull — Apr 14, 2014*

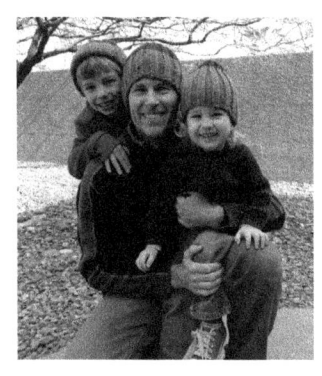

Hello. Amazingly, it has been one year since I underwent a ridiculous and unexpected surgery to have thyroid cancer removed from a good portion of my neck. March 30th (two weeks ago today) marked the one-year anniversary of that crazy event. I intended to post a triumphant synopsis of the past year in celebration of another year of life. There are a few reasons I didn't get to it.

A) As I think I mentioned before, Turnbull is Scottish for procrastination.

B) At the benefit concert our good friends the Falcones organized and hosted for us last spring, Karen and I got up to say a few words. After Karen's beautiful speech, where she so eloquently summarized our situation and emotional state for the audience, my first words were, "I got nuthin'." Since she has more than adequately kept you all abreast of our adventure, I figured I'd just stay out of it.

C) Unfortunately, the cancer has recurred. Just two months ago, as you may recall, Karen posted an entry describing our elation at the fact that the results of an I-123 (radioactive iodine) scan I had recently received came back clean. In other words, no remaining thyroid cells and therefore no cancer. One month later, after having routine lab work (blood tests) done, I received a phone call informing me my thyroglobulin levels had increased to the point that I would need to have a PET scan immediately. From what I understand, thyroglobulin is a protein detectable in the blood that should not exist without a thyroid gland or thyroid cells present in the body. It can be used as a tumor marker for well-differentiated follicular thyroid cancer. This is the marker my surgeon, Dr. Wang, has been most interested in monitoring. Apparently, the I-131 (heavy duty radioactive iodine) treatment I received almost a year ago was not completely successful. The initial scan showed uptake in the thyroid tissue, and the post-treatment scan showed no residual tissue, but it looks like a few rogue cells got loose. This was definitely not a result of too little iodine, as according to Dr. Toy, my radiation oncologist, the nuclear medicine doctor administered the highest dose allowable by law in North America. He determined that I had much to gain and little to lose, and was young and healthy enough to handle it. Unfortunately, in a few cases the rare and aggressive form of follicular thyroid cancer my body decided to harbor (Hürthle Cell Carcinoma) does not always respond to radioactive iodine ablation. Such is the roller coaster of cancer treatment.

The past two weeks, I have undergone a barrage of diagnostic tests, including a PET scan (as I mentioned), a couple of CT scans, a couple of biopsies and plenty of blood tests. The scans revealed hot spots, or nodes or lesions, in my neck as well as my chest. Thankfully, the lymph node biopsy I had last Monday (performed by the same extremely skilled doctor who did the initial biopsies last year) yielded a negative result. Most likely, the lymph nodes that seemed affected on the scans were lighting up due to a routine cold. However, I also had a CT-guided sternal biopsy performed last Friday, and we are currently awaiting the results. The scans revealed invasion of the manubrium, which is the part of the sternum that connects to the clavicle. The sternal biopsy was basically a bone marrow biopsy.

Tomorrow I will meet with Dr. Toy to determine a further course of treatment. It looks like at this point another major surgery is not the most viable option. Judging by the pain level resulting from the manubrial biopsy (only local anesthetic, lidocaine if I recall correctly), I can only imagine how much pain having the bone completely removed would cause. I know childbirth, kidney stones and neurological pain are far worse, but I have to admit I'm a bit relieved as far as that goes. Most likely the area will be blasted with external beam radiation, as that seemed to be effective in preventing recurrence at the tracheal resection site. So that's the latest. We'll give you more info when we have it. With continued gratitude for your love, support and prayers.

### Bethany B
*Our hearts broke when we read this. We are so thankful for the time you have had between treatments and pray that time has given you the strength and courage to take on this fight again. You have always been and will continue to be in our thoughts and prayers. Big hugs to each one of you! XOXO*

### Laurence A
*Keep on, Mike. I love you to pieces!*

### Arthur F
*Love you, Mike.*

### Christina P
*Sending all the love and kick-cancer-in-the-ass vibes we have plus more! Your community of love and support is right behind you. If you needed it, there would be hundreds of us at your door on a moments notice. Remember that and hold us near to your hearts.*

### Sharon H
*I will never stop praying for perfect health for you, Mike. It is my mantra ... it is my prayer ... I love you ... I love Karen, and oh, how I love those boys ... sending you beams of light.*

### Margaret H
*Many prayers lifted up. Much love to you all.*

### Cynthia E
*Oh Mike, I am sorry to hear of the news, but I know you and your family are very strong. Nothing prepares us for the unexpected. All I know is that we are blessed to know you and your family and I've always thought you and your wife are the best parents. Life throws so many things at us, but I know that there is a plan, somewhere, somehow, and I will definitely ask God what his plan is with us all!*

### Jodie M
*Cancer picked the wrong dad! I know good news will come. Stay strong! xoxo*

*Darelle H*

*Mike and Karen, as always we will keep good thoughts going in your direction. Added strength and love and friendship will always be yours from all of us who are lucky enough to call you friend. Stay strong. I send love to you both.*

*Andrea H*

*So very sorry to hear but glad your great doctors are keeping a good eye on you. Know you are surrounded by truly wonderful family and friends ... just want you to know all of you are in our thoughts and prayers.*

*Dave Ro*

*I can't imagine how emotionally spent you must be from all of this. I have no doubt that this is just another hurdle on your way to the finish line. You will win! Let's just hope this is the last hurdle. I think about you guys often and want you to know that I will continue to send good vibes your way.*

# Update

*By Karen Turnbull — Jun 1, 2014*

Hi everyone! This update is way overdue and for that I apologize. Not quite sure where the time is going but it is going very fast. First off, we are good! Really good. Mike is as amazing as ever and although the past sixteeen months has been a roller coaster ride he is stronger than ever. We recently got to celebrate our niece Melissa's wedding, and hearing the vows brought new meaning to the words "in sickness and in health".

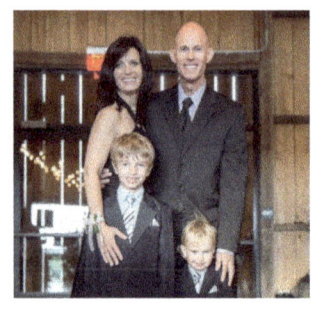

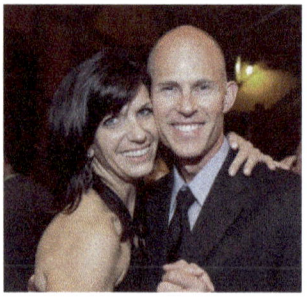

The last post filled you all in with the news that the cancer had shown back up. This time it was located in the manubrium (the upper portion of the sternum) and was about two centimeters. Dr. Toy, Mike's radiation oncologist, decided to hit it fast and hard. So Mike had five treatments to the area about a month ago. His body handled it very well with virtually no side effects. Not even the typical radiation sun burn; even Dr. Toy was shocked by this.

Since then we have been living, laughing and focusing on all the healthy cells rather than on the cancer cells. (Which is partially why we haven't posted anything.) Mike goes tomorrow for the first follow-up blood work since the treatments. We needed to give it some time. On Thursday we meet with Dr. Obara to find out the results. We are hoping for close to zero readings of the thyroglobulin level. This will tell us the treatment did indeed work and that his body is clear of any other thyroid cells. Then we basically live life under a watchful eye with regular blood work and scans. Since his particular cell type is so aggressive, it could come back but we don't know for sure if it will or when.

So, we just have to stay strong and live. This black cloud we now live with will probably always be lurking over our shoulder but we can either try to run from the storm or dance in the rain. So, our mantra has become "we are dancing in the rain" and loving life. Thank you all so much for your continued care, concern, thoughts, love and prayers.

Much love to you all.

> **Megan H**
> *Fantastic news! Keep dancing ... Love is your umbrella!*
>
> **Brian M**
> *Thanks for the update! As Steph and I both live with our own little black "C" clouds we have adopted the same policy. Maybe that's why the Seattle weather doesn't faze us? Hugs all around and hope I get back to Vegas to visit you soon. Dance on ...*
>
> **Frank S**
> *Thanks for the update. I'm happy for the good news! It really seems like you guys are blessed with a great medical team, and your healthy attitude along with Mike being such a stubborn #!\*# is probably doing wondrous things, too! I love you guys!*

*Kim B*
Your family is always in my prayers. Will pray extra this week. I love dancing in the rain. It's good for your spirit. God is good ... all the time.

*Karen K*
Karen, I read this with tears in my eyes and so much love in my heart. I can hear that great laugh of yours and see the way Mike looks at you when you do! God is with you, that is for sure. Your positive thoughts are an inspiration and proof that with love and faith, we can get through anything. Looking forward to more updates with good news.

*Jeanine C*
Love your whole family! You are inspiring, amazing and beautiful. Good energy, prayers and love to all of you. xx

*Erica M*
I'm dancing in New York for you guys! In the rain, in my apartment, on Broadway and in my thoughts. I love you both and think of you more than you know. Sending strength and Love always.

*Andrea L*
Remarkable - the mantra to live by. You are both an inspiration. I am overwhelmed by your positive energy and am sending more. Love you.

*Heather L*
I love your beautiful attitude and completely agree! A positive attitude is everything. We are thinking of all of you. Sending lots of positive thoughts for healthy cells and great results!!

*Rocco B*
Karen and Mike, our prayers are with you both. Karen, thank you for keeping all of us updated. Your care is that of an angel. May God bless you. Mike, I have never met any one person that handles matters of this magnitude, or simply matters at hand, quite like you do. You are not only an amazing person for what you are doing for your family but an inspiration, that life does not stop! Those who hinder your space will have to deal with something much greater than the cancer that you are beating! Thank you so much for your friendship and your courage. You truly are a breath of fresh air. Love to you both.

*Katey J*
*Hugs to you all and keep dancing in the rain!*

*January F*
*We love you, Turnbulls! Prayers and hugs nightly from us!!!!*

*Brenda M*
*I love the attitude. It is inspiring! Keeping you all in prayer! Always looking up!*

*Pam Ra*
*Mike and Karen, please know I have been thinking about you and I am sorry I have not been in touch. Of course Mike did not have the typical radiation sunburn - he is not "typical" now, is he?! Go Mike, go miracles, and go Turnbulls! I love you guys.*

## Feeling Good

*By Karen Turnbull — Jun 5, 2014*

So today's appointment went well! Mike's blood work came back showing really low thyroglobulin levels. When this resurfaced, his level was 70.5. Today it was 2.5! Great news! Also his platelet levels look good and white blood cell count is coming up. Happy summer!

*Betty S*
*So happy to hear the good news!!!! Prayers are being answered!!!!!!*

*Ivy W*
*YESSSSSS!!!*

## Had to Share

*By Karen Turnbull — Jun 6, 2014*

So at 3:00 PM today Dr. Toy called us personally to tell us he saw the blood results and was more than pleased! He said he expected the numbers to be lower but not this low! He joked and told me that he would guess they might be the lowest thyroglobulin levels in town. He then spoke to Mike and asked him how he was and if the treatments had "hurt him too bad." When Mike told him he had no side effects Dr. Toy said, "That is remarkable!" Mike and I both feel like this added confirmation was what we needed to breathe a little easier and celebrate a little more. The next step will be a PET scan and blood work at the end of July. Here's to praying that this has been kicked for good! Love to you all.

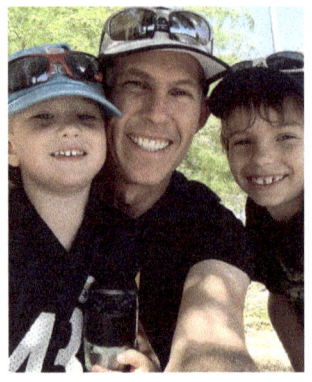

*Mark S*
*Way to go, Mike. You're better than this nasty disease. You go, dude.*

*Annie W*
*I love you both and am so thrilled to read this awesome news. Continue healing! Xoxo*

*Christina P*
*Great, great, great news! Continue to enjoy every minute and we will continue to send every bit of positive healing energy your way. The Turnbull Warriors are fierce and you continue to inspire and motivate us! Many, many, many loves and hugs coming your way.*

## Blocked Tear Duct

*By Karen Turnbull — Oct 11, 2014*

Hi all! Things have been pretty smooth lately. Life has been good and our home is filled with lots of love and laughter. Mike's blood work has been pretty good. His thyroglobulin level at last check was 2.8 (which is slightly higher than the check before this one). We want this number as close to zero as possible. It had spiked to 70 last March, which is how the recurrence in his sternum was found. The lowest it has been since this all started is 2.0, so it is being watched closely. His white blood cells are still running on the low side but it seems like his baseline runs a little low so no one seems to be overly concerned. That being said, if they do not come up in the next few months we may be looking at a bone marrow biopsy to rule anything else out. We have known this could be coming but we would love to not have to go through this painful test.

The biggest update is that Mike developed a blocked tear duct. A CT scan came back negative which proved it was NOT a new tumor causing the blockage. After doing some online searching, Mike and Dr. Toy found some studies that showed a direct correlation between radioactive iodine and blocked tear ducts about one year after treatment. So we are going with that as the probable cause. He is in surgery right now as I type this sitting in the waiting room. The amazing part of all this is that just seconds before he was wheeled into surgery he had me laughing so hard my stomach hurt. He was just being his usual self which is all it takes to make me smile and laugh. I told him to behave himself in there so the doctor could do his job. Hopefully he listened. I will let you know when he is out and how everything went.

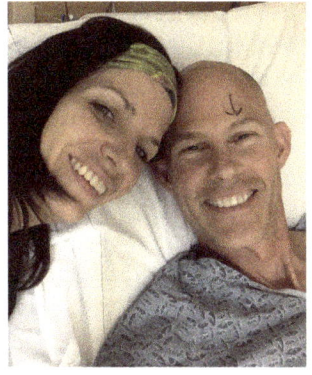

As always prayers, thoughts, energy are all appreciated.

### David N
*Good morning, Karen. Though I rarely have much time to chat with Mike at work, I watch him performing onstage and note how healthy and happy he has been and how great he seems to love each moment playing his trombone with his buds in the band. He is a shining spirit and hero to us at the Donny & Marie show and I hope to see him at the show on Tuesday. (Those other cats that fill in for him from time to time just ain't got his chops!!). Much love and healing thoughts to you, Mike and the family from the Donny & Marie cast and crew!*

## Out of Surgery
*By Karen Turnbull — Oct 11, 2014*

He is done. I'm just waiting to see him. Doctor said it went great. Now lots of ice to help him recover. Thanks all!

### Mariana R
*We send you our love!!!! Keep strong!*

### Rosita P
*Soooo happy for you, Michael. On behalf of "la banda que manda" LATIN ALL STARS ORCHESTRA, prayers and good energy ... missing you a lot. God keep blessing you dear.*

*Shari B*
*Karen, thank you so much for keeping us updated and reminding us of Mike's amazing sense of humor and incredible attitude! I'm so happy that all went well with Mike's surgery! We love all of you so very, very much!*

*Janna R*
*I was thinking of you guys the other day when the girls went out and danced in the rain, literally. We hope all is well and everyone is feeling good.*

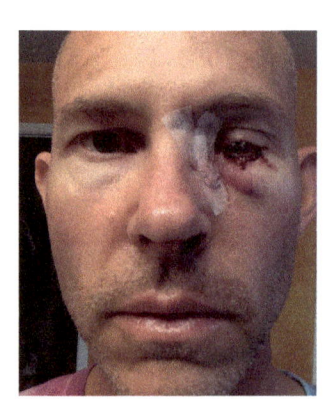

## Hospital Visit

*By Karen Turnbull — Nov 8, 2014*

Well, just when life seems to be going along nicely we are again reminded how precious every day is. Yesterday, November 7th was Mike's forty-seventh birthday. At 6:00 AM his alarm went off to get the kids up and ready for school. I was downstairs getting my things together before heading out to teach. I ran upstairs to wish him a happy birthday and found him lying on the floor, definitely not ok. He was dizzy, nauseous and his right leg and fingers were numb. He said it felt like when you lose circulation and get "pins and needles." Every time he tried to sit up or stand he became violently nauseous. He was unable to stand without holding on to me or the counter and even that was difficult. The dizziness was too much, and coupled with the violent need to vomit he was a wreck.

I quickly called in to work to say I would not be in to teach and then got the kids next door to my amazing neighbor Tammy, who took the kids and sent me home to get Mike to the ER. I got him down the stairs by having him slide on his butt and then lean on me to get in the car. The car ride was rough for Mike but we made it to Sunrise Hospital, where we were quickly put through triage and began tests. Mike had an EKG, chest x-ray and a CT of the brain. So then we waited for results. During our wait Mike was only able to lie down as every time he even slightly sat up the need to vomit would return. The CT showed a lesion of some sort in the brain. Of course given his history we both began to freak out just a little.

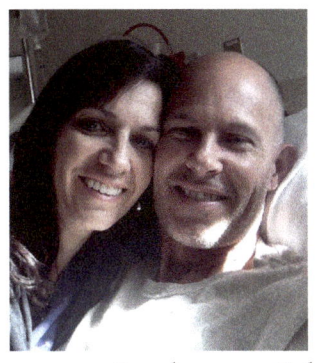

I immediately called our "team" of doctors: Wang, Obara and Toy. Dr. Wang called me back from his conference in Chicago and asked to be kept in the loop. An MRI was ordered to get a better picture, they admitted Mike and here we still sit waiting for the neurologist to give us details. Mike did have a routine PET scan on Thursday and that came back negative. We are feeling pretty good that it is NOT cancer, but Dr. Obara said this morning when he visited Mike that the only way to rule it out 100% would be to biopsy it. However, that does not appear to be a good idea due to its placement in the brain, so we continue to wait to see what it is and what we do.

The good news is Mike is much better than yesterday. He is able to eat and is not nauseous anymore. Walking is still a little tough as he is still numb on the right side. He says he feels like he is coming out of anesthesia, like he is in a fog and moving in slow motion. He is talking fine and knows everything that is going on. So far we have heard that it could have been a minor stroke, or a cluster of blood vessels that started to bleed slightly (bleeding the size of a pin head) that maybe he has had forever, and of course the last scenario is a tumor which could be cancerous or not. We don't know much more than that. Hoping the neurologist comes by very soon to tell us what it is and what we do. Praying we are through the worst of it and he will begin to heal, recover and be back to his crazy self very soon.

While we have been here our amazing friends have come to the rescue and immediately made plans to keep the kids busy and happy. This included their first sleepover at their friends' house! Thank you so much! Friends came to visit and kept me company the entire hour Mike was getting the MRI. They even brought birthday balloons and some great pics of Penelope Cruz to make him smile :-) and Pastor Marta came to visit and pray both yesterday and today. Mike's mom just flew in so we are surrounded by love. I promise to update as soon as I know any more.

As always prayers, thoughts, energy and meditations are all welcome!

> **Kelsey P**
> We love you! Keep fighting.
>
> **Suzanne P**
> Karen, my heart goes out to all of you. I will be praying, meditating and sending healing energy towards Mike. And a lot, lot of love.
>
> **Cindi R**
> He's a fighter, that boy. Hope you get some positive answers soon. Praying that God would surround you with his peace and healing.
>
> **Lisa L**
> So glad you updated this. All of us at work were worried about you guys. I will keep the prayers coming. Tell Mike we are all praying for him and that he is such a trooper. Much love.
>
> **Cathy M**
> I am heartbroken to hear this. As always, Mike is in my heart, thoughts and prayers along with the whole family. May he be blessed with a good outcome. I'm grateful to hear that some of his symptoms have subsided. Tell him are holding him in a big embrace and sending prayers to the heavens on his behalf. Much love.
>
> **Dawn K**
> Oh, no. This is not what I wanted to hear when I saw the journal update. I'll keep Mike in my thoughts and am sending good energy his way. Thanks for letting all of us know and as always, I am thankful for you being Mike's amazing support. Love you all!
>
> **Katey J**
> Thanks for the update, Karen. Sorry to hear about this turn of events! We will be praying for all involved in Mike's care and that he is back to his fun silly self soon. Please let Matt and I know if you need anything!!! Give Mike a hug from us too!

*January F*

We had a blast at our sleepover!!!! We want many more when you and Mike are out on date nights and not in the hospital!!!!! Xoxo See you guys tomorrow!

*Edward E*

Our Prayers are always with you, Mike and Karen. You and your family are so special and wonderful. All the best to all of you.

*Kathy A*

Always sending positive vibes and love. Happy Birthday, Mike!! You got this! I love you both with all of my heart ... xoxoxo

# Latest News

*By Karen Turnbull — Nov 9, 2014*

Ok, here goes ... Doctor called it a cavernoma, which is basically a cluster of funny vessels. It is small and circular with clean edges. Does not give any indication of being cancerous! The next step is to do a femoral catheter angiogram. They will go through the femoral artery to take pictures of this cavernoma located in the brainstem. Obviously we are scared. The risk is if we do nothing could this happen again, possibly worse? We will know more in the morning when we talk to the team of doctors.

I am doing okay and so is Mike. I have been in touch with Dr. Wang and he gave us some valuable input. Once we have more information it may be that it is something that will heal on its own and we don't have to do anything. Or they may be able to fix it through the angiogram procedure. Believe me, I know it's a lot of information to take in.

Thank you all for you love, support and prayers. Please keep them coming.

*Mark S*

Thank you so much for the update. Your strength through this is astounding. Much love to you all.

*Marianne M*

Karen and Mike, it is so hard for us not to be with you right now. We are, of course, sending warm hugs, positive thoughts and many, many prayers that this is just a minor bump in the road. Our love to you and the boys.

*Ellen So*
Thanks for updating through this difficult process. We are all sending positive energy your way. Love you all.

*Jeneane H*
Hope you are being your strong self. Know I am thinking of you. Praying.

*Beth G*
Thank you for the updates, but please take this time to be with Mike and the kids. That time is priceless. We are all thinking of you and wishing you all the best from near and far. We all know that Mike never gives up without a fight. Sending my love.

*Karine Z*
Karen, the fact that you have the strength to type and keep us posted is incredible. Thank you. Wish I was there to hold your hand. We love you, Mike and Karen!

*Kim B*
Oh my, Karen. You two have been through so much. My prayers are with you both. Good health for Mike and strength for you. I will put a prayer request through my church. You can never have enough people praying for you. Big hugs are wrapped around you and the family.

# Home

*By Karen Turnbull — Nov 10, 2014*

Mike is home. He was released last night. The doctors decided that the angiogram would not necessarily give them more information than the scans. Unfortunately we do not have any answers. The latest news we have received is that the lesion has characteristics of both a cavernoma and of a tumor. Because of the placement in the brain stem it cannot be easily reached, so surgery at this time is not an option. We have been advised to follow up with our oncologist and get another PET scan that focuses more closely on the brain. Also, we are to see a neurosurgeon in two weeks for a repeat MRI to see if the lesion looks the same or different. So we are in limbo. We know something is in his brain that bled and caused his stroke-like symptoms but we don't know what exactly it is.

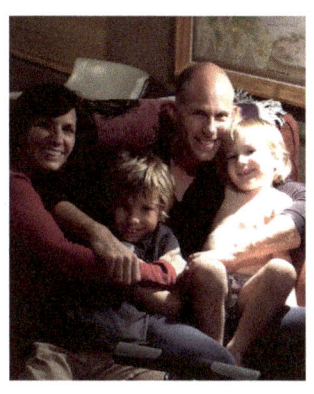

As to how he is feeling, he is definitely better than Friday when this mess started. He is walking more upright, although he is still a little dizzy. His strength seems a little better but definitely not 100%. Spiritwise we are both frustrated and to be honest, a little angry. I look at this man who came into my life and made me see life in a whole new way. He can make me smile and laugh like no one else can. He is the most gentle and kind soul I could ever ask to spend my days and nights with. I just cannot believe that he has to deal with yet another obstacle of this size. It is not fair. I have always believed God brought him into my life and brought us together. I just can't understand why things like this happen to anyone, let alone him. I know we will get through this. I know that Mike is stronger than whatever it is we are dealing with. It is just so hard to not be able to fix whatever it is that is going on. I keep praying for clarity. For there to be some light in this situation that gives us a path of direction. So please, continue to hold this amazing man in your hearts and prayers. We are in the land of waiting which can just be so hard.

Thank you all for your comments, love and prayers!

### *Magally L*
*I am sending my prayers and love your way. He does have that magical way of making people laugh and smile. I am praying for his health and all of your spirit.*

### *Karen K*
*Oh, sweet Karen & Mike. Your love is and always has been so special. We will hold you in our thoughts and our prayers. xoxoxo*

### *Sandy B*
*Dear Mike and Karen, you are correct. You and Mike are stronger than what's being thrown at you. You both are an inspiration to us all, showing us what love and faith can conquer. In our thoughts and prayers.*

### *Megan H*
*Karen and Mike, it is not fair. Period. Anger about the situation is warranted (I am frustrated and angry for you, too). There is no rational explanation for why good people suffer. It will make*

*you insane trying to figure it out and sap much needed energy. There is only hope ... and the ability to rise above the irrational. To embrace the amazing human spirit in the face of the staggering fear you are being forced to handle as you have done so beautifully in the past. You and Mike WILL get through this. And then this, too, will be in the past. Sending you so much love and support to carry on through this new struggle. Your family is in our hearts and in our thoughts.*

### Dave Ro
*My heart continuously goes out to both of you. I KNOW that you will get through this and your love will be the medicine to make that happen. Love to you both!*

### Suzanne P
*I understand your anger and frustration!!! I agree, when I look at you, Mike, and your two boys, I can't begin to fathom why this has happened. I am angry, too! I have you in my prayers, meditations and my heart. Together we will get this, just like you both did for me. I wish I could hug you.*

### Sara I
*Your love for one another will get you through these trying times and your faith will guide you both through the darkness and into the light. Love and prayers for you both and your beautiful family.*

### Nate K
*If I've said it once, I'll say it again. I'm not worried about a thing. Mike is the strongest person I've ever met in my life. To someone of his resolve, this is nothing more than a brief inconvenience on the path to greatness. I know Mike will smash this to pieces as he has everything else, and emerge a more glorious version of himself.*

### Lisa L
*Frustrating seems like an understatement. I know that you guys were not expecting that this would be, as you say, "your new reality". Just know that you have lots of people sending love and prayers your way to Mike with his health, you for strength and the kids for day-to-day joy. Yes, I will definitely keep praying!*

### Erica M
*You have a bond that can withstand anything! You are surrounded by love of all kinds and you WILL get through this. I love you both*

*dearly and I will continue to send love your way. If there is anything in the world I can do to help please let me know. Keep the faith.*

### Darelle H
*Karen and Mike, your anger and frustration is completely warranted. It is not fair and that is all there is to it. None of us understands why such lovely people have to go through such bulls\*\*#. I am angry, too. And I know there are many people who share your frustration and anger as well as your joy, love and hope. We will try to abide the former and live in the latter. Love to you both.*

### Frank S
*The waiting game has got to be terribly frustrating! I hope you two get some answers as soon as possible. And like you said, Karen- "Mike is stronger than whatever it is." I truly believe that! I love you both.*

### Michael M
*Karen, just know you and Mike are in my thoughts often. I really hope the doctors can figure out how to rid Mike of this. You're right, it isn't fair.*

### Curt M
*You are right - it is definitely not fair. People like Mike should not have to go through this kind of stuff. We are all sending positive energy his way.*

### Lou G
*Anger and fear, frustration and helplessness are the hardest, and the instant, inevitable human response to life. The not-knowing-what-will-come-next, worrisome, terrifying parts of the days when the sun shines and birds sing and all should be beautiful, but we are in the darkest moments. We aren't supposed to go through any of this 'til we are much farther down the road. Not 'til we are seventy-nine, or eighty-seven, but not at forty-two, or forty-seven. You are blessed to have each other, and to be surrounded by love and hope. Your spirit will grow, love will flourish, strength enough to heal and mend is within you and you have faith, courage and hope. But some days, I know so well, you will just want to sit on the steps and hold your head. That's part of the strength and hope holding you together while you think you are coming unglued- the most human parts, the parts that make us better and stronger and heal us. With you in prayers and healing thoughts, and I always see Mike, sitting in the*

car, with a laugh and a smile, looking at your son with love in his eye. Always. Love to you all.

**Sharon H**
I will continue to pray with you, Karen. Mike is an extraordinary and beautiful man. I am angry too, but I truly believe prayer is a powerful game changer. Hold on my beautiful family and know that there are many holding you up in prayer!!

**Janna R**
Glad you guys are home, not glad you have no answers. Frustration is probably an understatement. Our thoughts and prayers are with you. I will pray for some joy to find you in this madness. Hugs to all.

**Dan S**
Karen and Mike, we will continue to hope and pray and wait right along with you over these next couple of weeks. We love you!!!

**Adrienne S**
Sending Prayers, Love, Hope & Hugs. xoxoxooxoxoxo

**Joan F**
A candle is lit for all of you! You have a special place in our thoughts and prayers, and a special place in our hearts!!

**Betsy A**
Karen, I'm so sad to hear you are now faced with more challenges. I, as you know, can relate to the frustration and helplessness you speak of, but you will get through this. Mike is a FIGHTER and so are you! I'm here if you need to vent! And as always, I will pray!

## Latest

*By Karen Turnbull — Nov 17, 2014*

Mike is doing pretty well, although he is still feeling the effects of his latest ordeal. He had another PET scan of his brain on Thursday and it showed no metabolic uptake. So for our purposes right now they are saying that this is not cancer. The thought is that it is a pontine cavernoma, which is basically a cluster of vessels in the left pons area of the brain which is located deep in the brain stem. This area of the brain is hard to reach so it cannot be biopsied or, to our understanding, even treated. We are scheduled to see the neurosurgeon on Tuesday, December 2nd after another MRI to compare to the first one. They want to check and see how it looks after having had some time to heal. Maybe it will miraculously disappear? One can hope, right?

As to how he is feeling, things are definitely better than a week ago. He is able to move much better and no longer has to shuffle his leg. He is stepping with more even pressure and if you didn't know what had happened you would think nothing was different. The dizziness is still there but not nearly as bad. He attempted to drive today but that seemed to trigger some dizziness so he came home. He also played his horn tonight. That, he said, was a challenge but he was able to do it. A new development has been some tingling and numbness in his lips. As a dancer I know the power of "muscle memory." Thank God his is strong! Even if he can't feel everything 100%, his muscles know what they need to do and his amazing musical ears know how to find the sounds. He wants to work tomorrow so I will drive him in and pray that all goes well. As for our spirits, honestly, we are doing ok. The anger at all this has calmed down (at least for now) and we are navigating through this latest obstacle. We laugh often and we are still celebrating all we have. It helps that we have two of the sweetest and funniest boys to fill our days with love and laughter. One moment and one day at a time. I promise to keep you posted.

Much love.

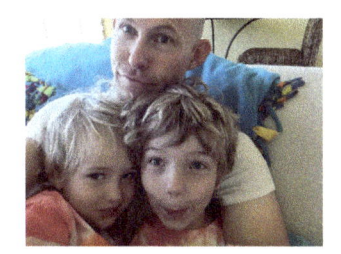

*Nate K*
*Mike, you inspire me man. Deeply. Keep up the great vibes. Hitomi and I are sending positive energy your way.*

*Tom E*
*A day can be a lifetime if you really live it. You two must know that far better than most. I pray you love and live one hundred thousand lifetimes together.*

*Nandita S*
Hang in there, Karen and Mike! I know you two do everything with a spirit of fun and generosity, and I hope all that you put out comes back to you a millionfold. With so much love.

*Birgit D*
Never lose hope and keep your faith. Praying for Mike and your beautiful family.

*Cindi R*
Hugs and prayers from Michigan for peace in strength and joy in the midst of the storm. And complete healing.

*Heather L*
Karen, it breaks my heart to see your family endure so many ordeals. Each time, you find the strength to get through it and you will get through this, too. Miracles do happen, especially with so many people praying for your family. Sending positive thoughts your way!

*Sonny H*
Hey Mike, glad to hear you're playing the horn! You, Scann and I gotta record our version of "Peanut Vendor."

*David N*
Karen, thank you for delivering our precious cargo [Mike] to the backstage door tonight, if he's up for it! He'll be so welcomed back with open arms by his family and friends at the Donny & Marie show!! See you at the theater, Mike!!

*Kim B*
Karen, I pray for you. This makes me so sad that such good people have to go through this. Big hugs around you and your family. And yes, your children are such a blessing. They can brighten up the hardest times.

*Cathy M*
I am endlessly inspired by your strength and perseverance. Please know I am with you in these struggles and admire your strong will in overcoming these dramatic obstacles. I have every faith that you will emerge victorious and applaud you for the courage you show every step of the way. Always praying for you all.

*Mike G*
*Oh, Karen ... sending so much love to you and your wonderful family! xo xo xo xo*

# Emotional Roller Coaster

*By Karen Turnbull — Dec 3, 2014*

I knew when I met Mike that he was a special and rare find. I am continuing to learn just how special and rare he is. Since my last post he had been doing great. He still had tingling down his right side and experienced moments of dizziness but for the most part he was functioning. He could take care of the kids, get them to school, drive and work. He wasn't 100% but he was improving every day.

On Wednesday of last week, he was scheduled for a follow-up MRI. The scheduler made the appointment for him at Sunrise Hospital because that is where he received the first MRI on November 7th. The day before, Mike called to see if there were any special instructions and was told the MRI had been cancelled. Turns out insurance would not cover an outpatient MRI at Sunrise and he needed to go to Desert Radiology instead. With it being Thanksgiving week there were no available appointments until this Thursday. So he scheduled the Thursday appointment and I tried to remain positive that this would give his brain an extra week to heal and the results would be good.

We also had an appointment to see Dr. Toy. This had been a regularly scheduled follow-up but we were both anxious to get his take on everything. At that time Dr. Toy felt pretty confident in calling this a cavernoma and suggested we seek many opinions from some very smart neuro people, possibly even looking to get help from out of state. So I made some calls and planned on picking up and delivering his scans to doctors on Monday, December 1st.

Thanksgiving was great! We celebrated with our friends and truly felt thankful for the many blessings we had. Friday was equally good and then came Saturday. Mike went downhill. He felt more dizzy, the tingling sensation was spreading and he just felt off. Sunday things got worse. On Monday he was even worse. Symptoms included dizziness, nausea, numbing on his face, difficulty chewing, blurred and double vision. I immediately called Dr. Toy and he advised me to get Mike back to Sunrise Hospital for another MRI. We went to the ER and waited for the MRI scan and then for results. Finally last night at around 6:30 the

ER doctor came in to tell us the results. What he told us we definitely did not see coming. The lesion on Mike's brain has doubled in size in just three and a half weeks. On top of that it looked like it had bled more. The increase in size, bleeding and swelling of the area is the cause of how awful he had been feeling for the past three days. They strongly believed this was a metastatic lesion. In other words ... cancer.

I think at that point we both fell into a state of shock. I remember pacing the small room, crying, cursing and shaking. We sat with each other and stared blankly at the gray walls. The doctor ordered steroids to bring down the swelling and said they would be admitting him. I then came home to try to retain some sort of normal for the boys. (They had spent the day having fun with the awesome team of Tammy, January and Devonee). That is when reality hit and I fell apart. My beautiful friend Jen came over and cried with me. It was exactly what I needed at that moment.

Today was a new day. I got the kids to school and headed in to see Mike. He finally got moved out of the ER room (where he spent the night) into a nice, quiet room. Doctors came and went, all basically saying the same thing. Considering the new MRI, no one believed this to be a cavernoma. All signs now pointed to cancer. I know all of this sounds really bad, and it is, but tonight I received the answers I have been praying for. Dr. Toy called me to share with me what he had spent all day figuring out. He managed to find one rare case study from Japan of a patient with thyroid cancer that later presented with what all the doctors believed to be a cavernoma. After removal and dissection it was clear that it was not a cavernoma, but metastatic thyroid cancer in the brain. Mike is now the second case. Like I said, very special and rare.

The good news in all this craziness is there is now a plan. Dr. Toy is on it and will treat Mike immediately. Probably this week. He is figuring out the best and safest way, probably Gamma Knife radiation. I hung up the phone and felt a wave of relief. Answers finally! It is super tricky and really scary but we will get through this. Mike has beat it before and will again. Of that I am sure. I don't know any more details but will keep you all posted.

I have to say that our support system continues to overwhelm us. My amazing mother-in-law flew out here to help when all this blew up three weeks ago. I can't even imagine how hard this is for her and yet she is always there for whatever we need. Thank you! Tomorrow my sister and brother-in-law are flying in to be with us and care for the kids while we get through this next phase. Unbelievable kindness is constantly falling into our hands and I don't know how we would get by without all the support. My team of friends here, you are family away from family and I love you all!

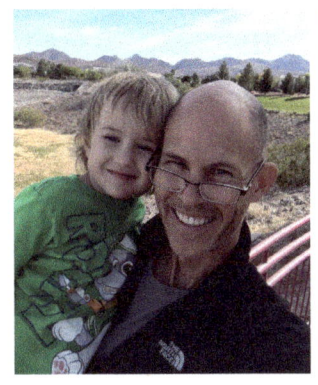

In spite of all this I continue to thank God for this amazing, special and rare man I am honored to call my husband. If I had to choose between a desert island by myself or a hospital room with him I would choose him every time. Mike, I know you will read this at some point so for the record I love you more every day!

Good night and keep the prayers coming. I know they work!

### Sara I
*Positive thoughts and prayers to you and your family during this difficult time, especially with the holidays! Please know we are here for you always, big or small ... really anything day or night! Love and Prayers.*

### Pat C
*There is a call to arms to pray for our brother Michael and his family. Karen, whatever we can do to help, the Caddick family is in.*

### Jayme R
*Karen- prayers, prayers and prayers to you, Mike and the boys!!!!*

### Sara O
*Karen, yes, Mike is amazing, but so are you!!! So thankful you have each other and the love and support of family and sooo many other people. God Has brought you guys through so much and He will continue to do so. Thankful you do have some answers now and that a plan of action can begin. Lifting all of you up to The Father in prayer and believing that once again His healing will happen! Love & hugs.*

### Birgit D
*So saddened to read this. My love to you and Mike. You are one strong couple and will get through this once again. My thoughts and prayers are with Mike and your family.*

*Estelle T*
Sending love and prayers your way. Keep dancing in the rain!

*Andrea L*
I was just looking through photos from last year at this time, when we were able to spend an entire perfect day with your family. We were in awe of Mike's strength and the love exuding from your family. When Mike beats this phase we will come out again. Until then we continue to keep him at the top of our nightly prayer list. Sending love, strength and determination to fight from Florida. We love you.

*Ellen Sn*
My heart is tearing apart for both of you. I will keep you in my prayers. Stay strong.

*Jessica S*
I'm in disbelief with all that you have been through. I'm praying for all of you.

*JoLayne G*
This old dance friend will be praying for Mike, you and your boys often. I have not met him, but I can tell through your words how special he is. I pray for strength, healing, peace that passes understanding and faith. Praise God you have a doctor who seems to be going the extra mile. When you dance you do it one step at a time, and in this that is all you can do as well. Keep on taking those steps and keep dancing in the rain!

*Cathy M*
We've always considered Mike to be special and rare! He is an extraordinary man in many ways. He is a beacon of light and hope in the face of these terrible obstacles and we know he will again vanquish this dark moment. Always in our thoughts, prayers and hearts.

*Fernanda G*
Sending prayers and well-wishes. Please let me know if you need anything. I have been keeping up with your journals and you are very brave. My heart goes out to you. May God guide your family and keep giving you strength in these tough times and with his help, God willing, you shall persevere.

*Karen P*

*Karen, not only is Mike a rare and special person, you are just as rare and special. Our hearts go out to both of you right now. We will continue to send prayers and healing thoughts. Much love.*

*Brian M*

*Karen, the strength and grace you and Mike have displayed through this whole ordeal is a marvel. I am holding Mike close in my thoughts and sending you all love.*

*Abby A*

*We love you both so much. Thank you for keeping us up to date and we are sending hugs, prayers and healing light your way.*

*Pam S*

*We continue to think of you throughout the day and send you our love. You are the bravest and kindest people we know. Thank you for keeping us posted.*

*Angela W*

*Mike and Karen, you sweet, loving, strong people. We love you guys! Sending you love! We miss you! xo You are both incredibly unique and AMAZING!*

*Doreen L*

*I think of Psalm 91:11 and pray that He will give his angels charge of you to guard you in all your ways, and that He will extend His healing hand over you. ASAP would be nice, too.*

*Debbie M*

*We love you guys and are so sorry you are dealing with this again. We are here for anything you need.*

*Cindi R*

*Hi, Karen and Mike. I'm just reading this now. As I sit in my office with tears on my face. So hard to understand. I echo the thoughts and prayers of everyone below. You are loved and supported from all around the country. Cherish each other, stay strong and let the doctors do their thing.*

*Vince V*
Sending you all the best wishes. It's amazing the resolve you both have, and how definite answers give you hope where most would cower. Stay positive, keep your love in the forefront, and lean on everyone around you. Please let us know if we can help with anything.

*John M*
Karen, we're praying for you and Mike and the kids. Mike and I hung around at UNC back in the day and, while I haven't had a chance to meet you, your courage and confidence are motivating and inspiring to me! I'm so glad Mike has a good one like you next to him through all of this!

# Home
### By Karen Turnbull — Dec 3, 2014

I realized this morning that I left out an important detail. Mike is home. He was released from the hospital last night. He is on an oral steroid medicine to help keep the swelling down. Unfortunately today is really bad. He is not feeling well at all and even the slightest movement makes him feel worse. He is not up for visitors so please just surround him in your thoughts, your hearts, your energy, your prayers. I can't stress enough how in need of prayers we are.

*Megan A*
Love you, Karen. I have been sending up prayers for you all day.

# Christmas Fairies
### By Karen Turnbull — Dec 3, 2014

Tonight the "Christmas fairies" left this at our door. This is now the third surprise goody bag left during the past week! I don't know who you are but thank you!!!!

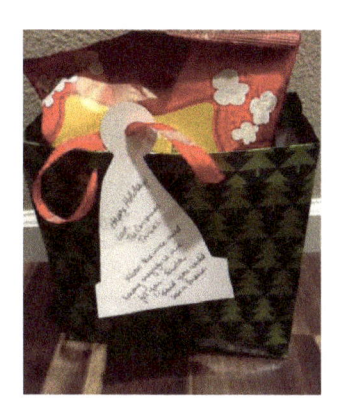

***Nancy W***
*Hi, Mike! I am keeping you in my thoughts and grateful that you have such an amazing family and medical team. Hang tough! Much love and life.*

***Kristine K***
*So sweet. I love the Christmas fairy! I took care of your class today. We all bowed our heads in prayer in honor of you and your beautiful, loving, generous family. Speaking his name aloud we prayed for Mike with vigor.*

***Heather L***
*That is wonderful!! It is little acts of kindness that truly warm your heart.*

## One Moment at a Time

*By Karen Turnbull — Dec 5, 2014*

I know everyone has anxiously been waiting to hear an update. Thank you for being patient with us as we process everything and figure out the next step. Thank you everyone for your responses, emails, texts and phone calls. Mike and I feel your love surrounding us and continue to be amazed by the outpouring of love and support. Thank you everyone who has brought us food, cookies for the kids, cards, healing energy work and love. We appreciate every one of you and you definitely help us find light in these days which can feel a little dark.

These past few days have been the hardest we have endured yet. Unfortunately, Mike's symptoms have gotten worse. He is basically tingly on his entire face as well as down the right side of his body. The dizziness hits with even the slightest movement and walking is more than challenging. His vision is blurred and double except for close range with reading glasses. So, at least he is able to pass the time playing games on his phone. I never thought I would be grateful for video game apps but if it provides entertainment and passes the time during these difficult days then yes, I am grateful! He has been eating well due to the generous friends who have brought us food! Thank you!!

As for what happens next it has been a back and forth game with doctors, Sunrise Hospital and insurance. During the course of all this we discovered Dr. Toy was no longer on our plan. I think it is finally worked out and here is the game plan: On Tuesday I will take Mike in to see a neurosurgeon working with Dr. Toy. This is simply a formality to get insurance on board with what needs to happen. He will order another MRI to be done most likely Thursday morning. This new MRI will then be reviewed by Dr. Toy, the neurosurgeon and an unbelievable team that Dr. Toy has worked all week putting together. From my understanding, Dr. Toy was not satisfied with the neurophysicists here in town for Mike's particular case, so he is flying someone in from California. He has also been working with his mentor in Japan! So, in short Mike has a team from around the world working to make this happen and be successful.

The actual Gamma Knife radiation treatment is scheduled for Thursday at Sunrise Hospital. Not only has Dr. Toy put together the best team, he has also had to jump through hoops to get everything cleared through insurance companies to make this happen. When he was dropped from Mike's primary insurance, I spoke to him about wanting to find a way to pay him and he simply said, "This is a zero. You need to not worry. I get paid enough for other things that I do." Did I mention that I love this doctor?!?! So, Thursday is the magic day! It is outpatient and Mike will come home that day. How he will feel or how long recovery will be we do not know. It really doesn't matter because at this point we need to be completely present in this moment. So that is what we are doing. We are breathing and taking each day moment by moment. Some moments are better than others. We are focusing on how healthy his body is and that it is just one small spot in his brain that is making him feel bad. The rest of him is healthy and strong.

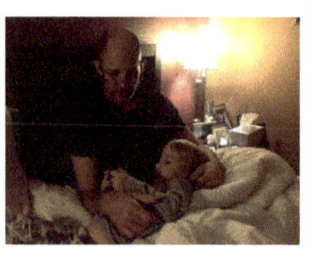

The kids are handling things pretty well. They are giving him love and snuggles and praying for everything to get better soon. I am hanging in there. I am not going to sugarcoat. It is hard, sometimes really hard. I am trying to juggle being a good mom, wife and nurse. I pray that I am doing ok. Thank God for my sister Marianne and brother-in-law Mark for taking care of me these past few days. They make sure I stop and eat and that I rest with Mike. The kids are happy they are here too. I know we will be ok. We couldn't have a better team, of that I am sure. Everyone is asking what they can do and the best thing truly is to keep the prayers coming! I believe Dr. Toy and his team can do this! I believe Mike can and will recover! I believe this season will pass and life will be full again! I pray for the strength to get us through this difficult time. I pray that Dr. Toy and his team are guided every step of the way. And, I pray many prayers of gratitude. Even in these tough moments we are surrounded by so much love and beauty. I am and will be forever grateful for the kindness of the human spirit. My goal is to keep Mike as comfortable as possible and with as little stress as possible. So, if you find his phone is off or he doesn't reply to a message it is because I have taken it away so he can rest. He is not really up for visitors because he is just too tired. His sweet nature makes him want to talk and share stories but it is really just too much.

So, for now send your love and know that he feels it. And so do I!

> *Abby A*
> *You are warriors ... Beautiful, kind souls ... Wish we were there to hug you ... Sending prayers, light and healing.*
>
> *Randy C*
> *Yay, Dr. Toy!! Thanks for the update, again, Karen, as I so badly want to know how Mike is doing. I know you two are fighting hard, and we are all praying hard for both of you and the kids. Lots of love.*
>
> *Ellen So*
> *Thanks for taking the time to write this. It must be so difficult with everything going on but you always find a way to let everyone know what is happening. Love to you all. Prayers are always being sent.*
>
> *Jenny F*
> *Can't stop thinking about all of you. I always knew Mike was lucky to have you in his life! You are an amazing mom, wife and human!! I'm in awe of you, truly, and sending prayers for one of the dearest guys I've ever had the pleasure of meeting. xo*

*Trish T*
And every moment you stop to take a breath is every minute we are praying.

*Julie Y*
Sending so much love and prayers. That's an unbelievable team! I'll get our prayer teams on it in the Bay Area, Karen. Much Love.

*Jeanine C*
In awe of all of your strength. You are doing way better than an okay job, Karen, you are amazing. So is Mike and so are Evan and William. Appreciate your beautifully worded updates. Keeps us with you every step. Much love, light and peace to all of you.

*Kristine K*
Much love to Mike. What a beautiful love you have for each other. You and Mike are very brave and I admire you both. You are loved.

*Curt M*
Karen, thank you so much for these updates. We were all talking about Mike today at the session. I am so glad the doctor is taking care of the money thing with you guys - what an incredible benefit. I haven't called since I spoke to Mike ten days ago or so because you mentioned he is not up to it, but please know we are all thinking about him constantly. Let us know if you need anything. We are here for you guys.

*Tammy C*
So thankful for Dr. Toy! What a blessing! Our family loves you all and are continuing to pray and send lots of love! Will be so glad when Thursday gets here and Mike can begin his journey to wellness!!

*Karen K*
You are such a light of inspiration, Karen! Oh, how I wish I could do more, but I know firsthand what prayers can do. So many of us are keeping you all constantly in our thoughts and prayers. I'm so sad that it's been so long since I've seen you both, but I can picture so many wonderful memories where I witnessed your love for one another. xo

*Clare T*
Thank you for taking the time to update everyone. What an incredible team you make. Your strength and love will help you through these challenging times. Dr. Toy sounds amazing and what a blessing to have such an amazing team on your side. I shall hold you in my

*thoughts this week and going forward and send you love and hugs. You are doing an incredible job. xxx*

### Matt J
*I deeply appreciate the updates. More prayers from the Johnsons. What a marvelous physician you have. Godspeed to all of those who are on the treatment team.*

### Nellie S
*Dr. Toy sounds amazing! I pray for him, I pray for you and Mike and the kids. Lots and lots of hugs.*

### Devonee M
*I love the picture of Mike snuggling his boy! What a precious family! We love you all so very much!*

### Jeff L
*You are constantly in our thoughts. Sending love to you, Mike and the kids. So happy you are blessed with such an incredible doctor, too!*

### Gailyn A
*Karen, your courage and grateful spirit are an inspiration. We are praying for Mike every day! And Thank God for Dr. Toy!*

### Tina B
*Karen, I continue to send my love and blessings. Stay strong and trust in your faith! Love to all.*

### Hayley M
*Hi, Karen. Well, it certainly sounds like you have found your angel in Dr. Toy. We will as always be keeping you all in our prayers and will be thinking of you and Mike Thursday. I can't begin to imagine how you are keeping it all together right now. You are a strong woman. Much love to you all.*

### Magally L
*My love to you and the family. Thank you for taking such loving care of my sweet friend who I miss making music with. Please give my love and hugs to Miguelito. You guys are always in my prayers.*

### Katie C
*Always praying and thinking of Mike and your family. You are so strong, Karen!*

*Dan S*
Karen, thank you for taking time to write and post these updates! We continue to send prayers and positive energy as we all take one day at a time with you. Much love.

*Katey J*
Dear Karen, thank you so much for the updates you provide all of us who love and care for you and Mike and your family. We continue to pray and be grateful for God's love and blessings even in challenging times. We lift you all up and pray for the medical team assembled for Mike's surgery this Thursday. Love and hugs and hope you continue to feel the embrace of all those who love you.

*Birgit P*
Many good thoughts are coming your way from Minnesota. I am writing this with tears in my eyes, though. I'm so happy for these amazing doctors that are helping you guys.

*Catherine J*
Sending all our love and we'll be rooting for you all on Thursday!!!! You both are amazing, Karen and Mike - strong, centered in spirit, grounded in and surrounded by love. Xoxoxo's from the three of us!

*Melin F*
What a gift to have such an amazing team of doctors, family and friends to help you and Mike. We are sending love and prayers and have asked for prayers from our extended family. Know you are in our thoughts and on Thursday, even more so.

*Cathy M*
Forever in our hearts, always in our prayers, present in our every thought. You two are the finest example of devotion, strength and purity of purpose. We have every faith that your extraordinary team and Mike's strong, healthy body, mind and spirit will emerge victorious on Thursday and the days ahead will be blessed with healing. We love you all.

*Mary F*
I appreciate the updates, Karen. Your family is truly one of the strongest, kindest and most loved families I've ever known. Sending tons of love and prayers!

*Keith N*
*You all are in our prayers. God is strong. God is faithful. God can do this. We love you guys and will be with you in spirit on Thursday.*

## Untitled
*By Karen Turnbull — Dec 7, 2014*

The Christmas fairies struck again last night! Brought drinks for the family!

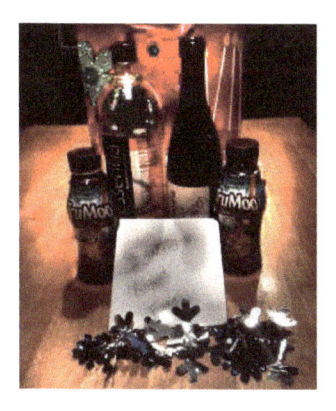

*Karen Mc*
*Karen, you all continue to be in our thoughts and prayers.*

## The Stars Have Aligned
*By Karen Turnbull — Dec 10, 2014*

Today I received a phone call saying the stars have aligned and everything is set for tomorrow! This phone call came after exactly twenty-four hours of stress and chaos. Yesterday morning we had an appointment with the local neurosurgeon. This was presented to us as simply a formality. This was to establish us as a patient in his office so that insurance would cover Mike's procedure. We thought we would be in and out. This was not the case! We sat in the office for four hours. Of those four hours probably twenty minutes were spent with the doctor. That being said, he was on call and did get interrupted to deal with emergency situations. We were calm and patient and understood and also thanked him for taking us on as his case and helping us through this. The frustration really occurred when we spoke with the assistant and were told that there was "no way this procedure would happen on Thursday!" As you can imagine my wall broke down and I trembled and cried in her office. This couldn't be happening! According to her, it was very difficult to schedule the three surgeons to be at the same place at the same time as well as to schedule the machine. This was a different story than we had been told. In our mind everything was set and this was just the final step.

I came home and immediately called the mastermind of all of this, Dr. Toy. This man spent more time with me on the phone than we had spent with the neurosurgeon. He assured me that all three doctors were lined up and ready to go. He also had three backup plans in case this did not happen! He told me that he had spoken to three administrators at Sunrise Hospital, two at Culinary Health Fund and two at Teachers Health Trust (our two insurance companies). He was on it and was doing everything possible to make this happen! I then called the representative from our insurance company that had been in touch with me. I told her about the holdup. She assured me she could get everything authorized in a day. Within an hour she called back to tell me she had done it and we were approved to go, so now we just needed a machine to be available.

I spent the night in much of a daze and I have to say my amazing husband held it together better than I did. Last night's emotions ran from anger, frustration and sadness to utter disbelief. It just didn't make sense to me that if three doctors were already cleared to do this procedure and all felt it was an urgent case, then why could it be held up by an insurance and scheduling glitch? As of this morning we still had not received a final answer. I then decided to check on things myself. I called the assistant who was supposed to be making everything come together. She told me she now needed a letter of authorization and that the number was not enough. I hung up and called the insurance representative I had spoken to, Lori. She had never heard of needing such a letter. After getting phone number contacts to her I patiently waited. About an hour later she called me back and we were a go! Everything has been approved and scheduled!

So, tomorrow morning at 5:00 AM we will check in to Sunrise Hospital. Mike will be admitted as if it were a regular surgery. They will do all the normal pre-op protocol. At 7:00 AM someone from the Gamma Knife center will come and get Mike. They will then wheel him to the center where he will have the procedure. This will involve him having four bolts put into his head so that he can be secured into a frame. The precision must be 100% accurate. Then he will receive an MRI which will guide the three doctors treating him. Our team consists of Dr. Toy, the neurosurgeon and the neurophysicist who is being flown in from California. The actual procedure will involve two hundred beams of radiation at a very low dose entering his brain. These beams will then intersect at the exact point and location of the tumor. When all these low beams intersect it will be a very high dose frequency to kill these cancerous cells. We do not know how long or what recovery will look like. Honestly, it doesn't matter. At least as of tomorrow every day will be a step in the right direction. Please, if there has ever been a time when you have held us in your thoughts, your prayers, your energy, your love and your light, tomorrow is the day we need it most.

Thank you all for your love and support. We will get through this one breath at a time. Much love.

### Tiffany P
*Praying for Mike and his team of doctors. Sending you all much love and light! Our thoughts are with you always. We love you.*

### Pam S
*You have more good Karma available for this than anyone, anywhere. Our thoughts are with you.*

### Doreen L
*I was going to text to ask you what time the surgery was to happen so I could pray at that particular time, so I really appreciate your update! Karen, I know Mike is going through the physical/mental/emotional pain - I also care so much about what you are going through. I know staying strong is good, but so is breaking down and crying, screaming (in the garage, maybe?). I can tell you have good friends who are there for you - if you need one more who's had experience with "stuff," let me know. Know that my prayers are with your family and with Mike specifically tomorrow.*

### Darelle H
*Every beat of our hearts go to you and Mike. You are loved.*

### Andrea L
*Not a day or night goes by that Mike is not at the top of my prayers. I pray so hard - please God- keep the Turnbull family safe. I know our God is good Karen. I will not stop. Blessings and love to you all.*

*Beth S*

Breathe ... one breath at a time. You are a rock, Karen ... all our love and prayers coming your way tomorrow (and every day after). Go get 'em!!!!!

*Mike S*

Mike, Karen ... you are always in our thoughts, hearts, prayers. We love you guys so much and we will continue to pray for you and this amazing team! Sending big hugs for Evan and William, too!

*JoLayne G*

I can hardly believe people going through so much have to go through such rigarmarole. Way to go being proactive and pushing people. Lord God, the Great Physician, please put your healing hands on Mike. Guide the hands of the surgeons. Make them steady and sure. Lead them in wisdom and discernment as to what needs to be done. Give everyone involved good rest tonight and a peaceful and calm morning. Comfort Karen and Mike and their boys. Take away any anxiety and help them to leave it in your sure, powerful, strong and loving hands. Give them everything they need during this time. In Jesus's name I pray, Amen.

*Beth L*

Wonderful news, Karen! Sending love, prayer, light and every bit of healing energy I can to you guys. Thanks so much for the wonderful updates. Stay strong.

*Stacia F*

Oh, Karen ... the words won't come for me, but the prayers are there for you. Know that!

*Cathy M*

Standing beside you in body, mind and spirit. Across the miles I'm sending you my love, thoughts and prayers with every fiber of my being. Godspeed to Dr. Toy and the magnificent team. Rest assured, Mike, tomorrow will have you on the path to healing and wellness. Karen, you are the finest example of a strong and loving woman that I know of. You and Mike are an inspiration to us all. Love & hugs.

*Kristine K*

Much love and support to you and Mike. May you come through this with renewed strength, wisdom and love. My thoughts and prayers to you, sweet Karen, resilient Mike and your two beautiful children, Evan and William. xxo

*Shelley De*
*Karen, you are a pillar of true hope. Mike will do well and the unbelievable team of doctors will make it happen. This is the time for miracles. Thoughts, prayers, positive vibes and constant streams of hugs are being sent your way. You will be in our never-ending thoughts tomorrow. God is with you both.*

*Megan H*
*One breath at a time ... Good advice for all of us. All of our light, love, hope and wishes with you, Mike and your boys. Hold each other tight and stay positive. Looking forward to hearing good news. Xoxo*

*Brenda M*
*Prayers, positive thoughts, hugs, you got it! I'm so thankful Mike has you in his corner, Karen! Your strength, patience and fortitude to make calls, go to appointments and all the while keeping us informed! May God continue to bless you and to keep shining through all of this!*

*Monique E*
*I'll be praying for you all all day! Stay strong as I know you are. Love your way!*

## Let's Do This!

*By Karen Turnbull — Dec 11, 2014*

This sign greeted us as we pulled out to head to the hospital! Thank you!!!

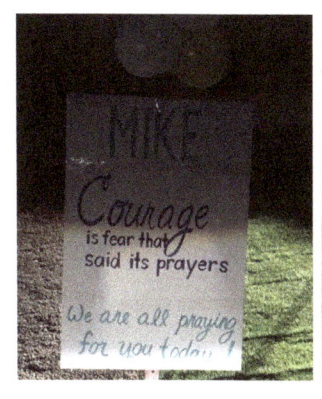

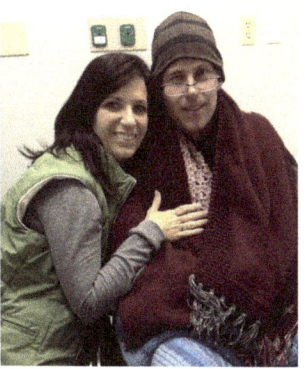

*Jayme R*
Prayers are surrounding you all. You are not alone in this. God has provided an army of prayer warriors and we will be armed and praying today!

*Suzanne P*
I love it!!!! Mike and Karen, I am sending my love to surround you and prayers for healing and strength. They said this morning that all of the planets are lined up today for positive energy. They said it is a very special day and to expect the unexpected! I have so much love for you. Yes, lets do it!

*Karen K*
We went to bed praying and woke up praying. God is with you and your very skilled team of doctors. So much love to you. So much faith that Mike will come through this. xo

*Betty S*
KAREN - God Bless your many, many families you have away from home. Mike, Karen, Evan and William you are always in our thoughts and prayers. Mom & Dad

*Cindy E*
The boy's long-lost cousins and their parents sent a circle of love and prayers your way at 7:00 AM. We will continue praying all day. You are so courageous and your medical team is amazing. Lots of love.

*Sara I*
Beautiful Message. We'll be thinking of you both all day and saying prayers continuously!!! Love you both.

*Joey F*
Come on my friend. All of us are pulling for you!!!

*Christina P*
Sending all the prayers and love we have. Time to kick some more cancer ass!

# Here We Go!

*By Karen Turnbull — Dec 11, 2014*

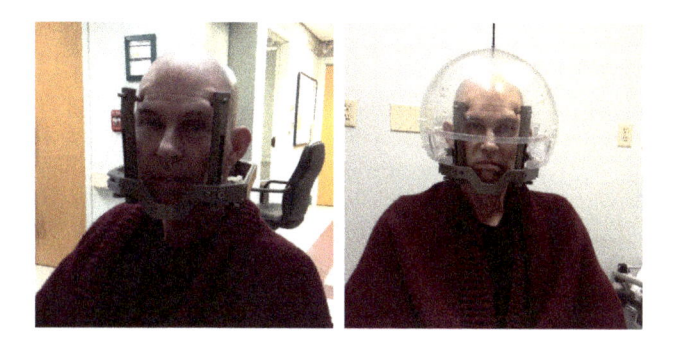

Mike just got wheeled in to begin the radiation process. Everyone here has been phenomenal! The nurses at the Gamma Knife center have quickly become like family. Their kindness and support has been unbelievable. Our team has gone above and beyond. The neurosurgeon was excellent this morning. He is the one that actually attached the frame to Mike's head. As you can see in the picture this frame is bolted into his skull. The other end will then be attached to the machine so that there is no movement at all. This will make the precision spot-on. The MRI this morning was more thorough than any he has ever received. It did show that the tumor has grown one more millimeter, but it also showed that it is just the one location. No new tumors have developed. This is a great thing! So now we wait. It will be about ninety minutes. Dr. Toy and the neurophysicist will administer many small doses to target the spot. They are both very optimistic that this will do what it needs to do. The other thought is that hopefully his recovery will happen as quickly as the decline did. Keep prayers coming.

> **Jordan B**
> *Faith, prayer, and love being sent your way. Be strong, Mike (and Karen)!*
>
> **Christie P**
> *Sending positive thoughts and prayers your way. Xoxo*

*Rosita P*
*I will keep praying for Mike. He's a wonderful human being. The entire band Latin All-Stars Orchestra send their best vibes and energy. God bless you.*

*Andrea L*
*Prayers sent for Mike and for the doctors to do what is planned with precision and full success. Please Lord give the doctors the strength to make it a perfect surgery. Not one second has gone by that you haven't been on my mind today. Thank you for posting these updates. I hope you feel the love coming from far. Xox always.*

*Fernanda G*
*You guys are constantly on our minds. My mom is here and we were just saying how we wish everything will be ok. We're praying and hoping for the best. May God be with all of you, doctors included, continuing to give you strength and guidance. Keep the faith.*

*Susan V*
*The doctors are amazing ... such a blessing ... keep the faith ... prayers for you both!*

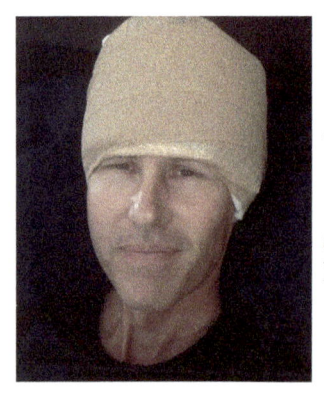

# Home

*By Karen Turnbull — Dec 11, 2014*

We are home. Mike feels pretty beat up but he's doing ok. Now we pray the treatment worked and his beautiful brain begins to heal. Keep the prayers coming! Thank you!!!!!

*Avi H*
*You are all an inspiration!!!!*

*January F*
*Awesome ... I love you, Turnbulls! P.S. He already has a healing glow ... are you seeing this as well? There's a difference ... a big one. Amazing.*

*Miguel R*
Glad he's home. Wishing his beautiful brain heals quickly!

*Angela W*
Welcome home, Mike! Been thinking about all of you and sending love your way. You are all incredible!! Miss you!

*Dan S*
Mike, so happy you're home!!! Rest up!!! I have no doubt you'll be back to your old self soon!! Sounds like one amazing team that took care of you today!

*Colleen S*
Praying ALL day!! We'll keep them coming!!!

*Elizabeth H*
Prayers being offered up here in WV for Mike and Karen and their precious family. We will continue to keep you in our hearts and prayers in the days to come. May God bless you and keep you as the apple of His eye.

*John M*
Go Mike! Praying for the best for you. I'm glad you've got such a great wife to support you through this.

*Hayley M*
My Goodness, I can't believe you have had to go through all this. We think about you both often and please know our prayers are with Mike for a speedy recovery and with you, Karen, for your strength. It's lovely to see you have such a support system with your family and marvelous friends around you. Much love to you all. Awaiting your next post!

*Shelley Dr*
The most beautiful brain, for sure. Loving thoughts and prayers sent your way. Thanks so much for the updates, Karen. The two of you are incredibly beautiful together. Love, Shelley, Kevin and Anjah

*Jen F*
We are praying for you all. May Mike's healing be quick and perfect, may Karen continue to find support, strength and rest, may the boys feel the love surrounding them and may Our Savior provide the peace that only He can give during these times. We send love and hugs from two thousand miles away and will continue to pray as you navigate the weeks ahead.

# One Week Post Gamma Knife

*By Karen Turnbull — Dec 19, 2014*

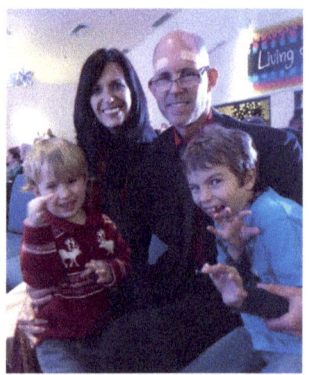

I have been putting off writing this because I kept hoping for something positive to write. Unfortunately there has been no positive change yet. In fact in the past few days things have gotten worse. Mike's symptoms have increased. His vision is worse and his right side is pretty much completely numb. The good news is he has been sleeping a little bit more. Our appointment with the neurosurgeon the other day did not give us a whole lot of information. The sites from the Gamma Knife brace in his head have healed well and that is great. As for his symptoms, it sounds like it's just going to take some time. We see Dr. Toy Monday morning. I am hoping that he is able to at least give us some information. As we have been dealing with Mike feeling worse these past few days I have been praying for some sort of understanding. What I have come up with is this: his tumor was treated aggressively. Keeping this in mind, I have to believe that what we are seeing are simply some side effects from the treatment. Deep down I know we were all praying for a miraculous quick recovery. I do believe miracles are surrounding us and will continue to come our way, but this time we may just have to wait a little longer. With the increase in symptoms has come an increase in frustration. Mike has been truly amazing! But he is tired, frustrated, and although he won't say it, I think he is scared. I know I am. Please continue your prayers for health and healing. Mike is healing from this thing called cancer. He needs our constant love and light surrounding him. I know he can conquer this, it's just going to take some time.

Much love.

>  *Marianne M*
>  *Praying every minute and wishing that we could be there with you! We love you so very much. Stay strong.*
>
>  *Cindy E*
>  *Constant prayers for healing and continued strength for you both. We love you!*

*Laura H*
*If anyone can pull through this, it's Mike. I have no doubt. Please tell him his Disney All-American College Band family is thinking of him!!!*

*Cathy M*
*Sorry to hear Mike is suffering. He has a formidable opponent but not one that is stronger than all the collective love, support, strength and prayers that surround him in his struggle. Mike is such an extraordinary man and deserves only the best. We hold him and all his family in our hearts. Keep fighting the good fight and we will be right there with you. Stay in the light and may each day hold some improvement. Much love, Cathy, John & Paige*

*Jacqueline S*
*As always, thanks for the update and as always, love and prayers coming your way. xx*

*Edward E*
*You are in our thoughts and prayers, Mike and Karen. We wish only the best for you. All of our love to you both. Lots of love.*

*Trish T*
*Karen, with such grace you write this. You all certainly are in our daily thoughts and prayers. Kick cancer's ass, Mike.*

*Heide F*
*Hello, Karen. Sometimes no answer is the best one to have. I know we all are waiting for some positive developments, but sometimes, especially now, there is very little to say and the situation gets scary, seemingly endless and we feel helpless. I am pretty sure all of this will pass, it will just take a little longer. May you find peace, strength and hope from the eyes of your sons. When times get rough I seek the company of my children and it works like a charm. They are our guardian angels. Sending wonderful healing thoughts over. Much Luv.*

*Nandita S*
*Continuing to send love and healing thoughts to Mike and strength to you for the Herculean effort you have made. You inspire me with your love.*

*Brenda M*
*Praying for Mike's healing and health! God has His arms tightly around you both. Hold on to His love! Please give Mike a fist bump from me!*

*Kathy A*
*You both have all of my love, always ... xoxoxo*

*Michelle R*
*Thinking of you and wishing you miracles and strength and answers and hope and healing and togetherness.*

*Carol B*
*Can't say enough prayers for you strong and beautiful people.*

*Ken P*
*Hi Mike, just heard the news from Laura about your situation. Just wanted to let you know you are in my thoughts and prayers. Remember- if you can make it through playing trombone in ninety degree heat with stifling humidity while wearing a red, white and blue polyester jumpsuit, you can get through anything. Be well, my friend. Ken (1989 Disney Band)*

*John M*
*Thanks for taking the time and energy for the update. It sounds like it's hard for you both right now. Hang in there. I'll continue to pray. Blessing to you.*

*Kristin U*
*Dear Mike and Karen, I've been thinking about you and sat down to look up how things have been going. You are all in my prayers, and on this Christmas Eve I'm praying for a Christmas miracle, for you to feel good, Mike, and for healing and health to surround you. Karen, I pray for you for strength as you bravely keep up all your roles as mom, teacher, wife, insurance navigator, etc. You are just as admirable and amazing as your incredible husband! With so much love and a heartful of prayers.*

# Merry Christmas

*By Karen Turnbull — Dec 25, 2014*

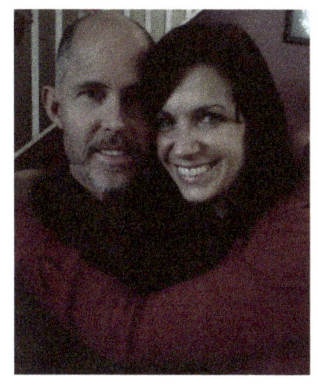

Here's hoping you all have had a blessed and wonderful Christmas. No new news to report on our end. Mike is still trying to recover. The days and nights are both difficult. His right side is still completely numb and his vision has not yet improved. We remain hopeful and strong in the thought that it is just going to take time. On a positive note, Mike came downstairs last night to enjoy our annual family Kris Kringle via FaceTime with my family in Pittsburgh. He also managed to make it to church for Christmas Eve service. I know this was not easy for him but it was beautiful to have him there with us. He also was a part of Christmas morning and tried his best to enjoy the kids. The kids had an amazing Christmas! Thanks to our wonderful friends and community who pitched in to make sure our children did not feel the effects of our situation this Christmas. I am forever grateful for the kindness that continues to be showered upon us.

On that note, my amazing niece Michelle has put together a fundraising account to help us get through these next difficult months. This was her Christmas gift to me and to Mike. We are overwhelmed by her ability to capture our story in a few paragraphs. I am sharing the link not so much to ask for donations but because so many have asked me what they can do. When faced with this question I find myself coming to a blank. I honestly don't know, so Michelle has taken it upon herself to find a way for people to help us. My way of thanking her is to share it. Thank you all so much for the love you continue to show us.

Keep the prayers coming! Merry Christmas!

> *Ivy W*
> Merry Christmas! I'm sending LOVE & LIGHT your way! Xo
>
> *Cathy M*
> Sending all our love and support to you on this blessed Christmas night.

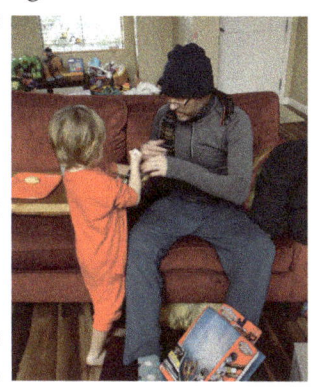

*It is snowing hard here and our prayer is that for every snowflake that falls your family will be blessed and Mike will be healed. God bless Michelle for the fundraiser. It is good to know there is some small way we can help in this dreadful situation. We love you Mike and hope that your symptoms diminish and that you will be comfortable again. Our hearts are with you all.*

### Kenny A
*I love you guys so much! I think about you every day and hold you and your family in my heart. Things will get better, I know it! Give Mike a great big hug from me. Stay strong Karen, Mike's gonna get better. He's so blessed to have you by his side.*

### Fernanda G
*Merry Christmas to your beautiful family! May God be with you in these trying times. Keep on keeping the faith :)*

### Carol B
*Merry Christmas Mike, Karen, Evan and William. Prayers every day for healing from Conifer Mountain, where there is close to a foot of Christmas snow!*

### Kim M
*Merry Christmas, Karen, to you and your family. We continue to pray for all of you!!*

## Christmas Morning 2014
*By Michelle Moulden — December 25, 2014*

A lot of you have been asking what's been going on with my family, so here it is. This year, we are all wishing for a Christmas Miracle. I decided that this year my Christmas gift to my Aunt Karen, Uncle Mike and my cousins Evan and William, would be a little bit of hope and a whole lot of love. I know this isn't the same as perfect health, but I am praying this makes a huge difference in the coming year.

For those of you who have been fighting right alongside with us, we can't thank you enough. Your endless love, support and prayers have been unwavering in this difficult time. We love you all.

Please consider supporting Team Turnbull this Christmas. We could all use your love and support! Merry Christmas to your family, from ours!

I've been thinking about this for weeks. Trying to come up with the right words, the right thing to say or do, some way to help or cope, and I've been at a total loss. Today, I found my solution. A lot of you have been asking what has been going on with my family, so here is our story. For those of you who are already aware of our situation, here is the absolute best way to help, along with your continued prayers.

March 2013, my Uncle Mike was diagnosed with Stage IV Hürthle Cell Carcinoma, which invaded his tracheal cartilage. To give some perspective to this particular disease, there are four main types of thyroid cancer and this one is a distinct type that makes up only 3% of all thyroid cancers. In only around 10% of those cases does it invade the lymph nodes, and in only a handful of those does it affect the trachea. So, to say that this was a rare, complicated and downright scary circumstance would be quite the understatement. However, in typical Mike fashion, he managed to come out of it even stronger than before. In fact, just six weeks after having a radical neck surgery (we're talking complete reconstruction of his trachea/neck area), he was back to playing his trombone with Donny & Marie. After a long road to recovery, filled with hormone injections, strict diets, iodine treatments and quite a bit of radiation, Mike was cleared of all cancer by February 2014. He truly is incredible.

June 2014 we had another scare. The cancer had come back. Luckily, the doctors were able to hit it quickly with some radiation and things seemed to head in a better direction.

Fast forward to November 7th, which also happened to be Mike's forty-seventh birthday. Karen found Mike collapsed on the floor, nauseous, dizzy and numb. Some birthday present, right? After a myriad of tests and quite a few insurance issues, we soon found out that Mike has brain cancer. But, again in typical Mike fashion, it isn't just any type of brain cancer. Not only is the cancer in an inoperable area of the brain (his brain stem to be exact), but there is only ONE other case study where a patient with thyroid cancer later presents with metastatic thyroid cancer in the brain. This makes Mike the SECOND case where this has ever happened, which means we really have no idea what the road to potential recovery will even look like. Mike's, in fact, is even more complicated and rare in that the tumor is located in the brain stem, whereas the only other case was in an operable area of the brain. The doctors performed a Gamma Knife procedure just two weeks ago, in the hopes that the radiation would be able to break apart the cancer cells, kill them, and get them out of Mike's body. Since the area of the brain where the cancer is located is completely inoperable, this is really our only hope for any sort of treatment. Unfortunately, two weeks post-op and we don't have good news to report. In fact, things have gotten worse.

Mike is completely numb on the right side of his body, which means he can't walk on his own, eat on his own, or even go to the bathroom on his own. Mike is also suffering from severe double vision, which means that even if he could walk on his own, he wouldn't be able to get from point A to point B easily and it is also causing debilitating headaches. He also has a constant ringing in his ears, to the point where he can't sleep, and without sleep, it's hard to heal the body. This incredible, strong-willed, independent man went from conditioning for a triathlon to practically immobile in a matter of weeks. He is unable to take care of his own kids, let alone himself. However, the thing is, this isn't just about Mike. This is so much bigger than Mike. WE are Team Turnbull. WE are in this together. WE are fighting this awful disease. Unfortunately, it's his body that has to take the hardest hits.

However, that doesn't make this any easier on anyone else. For those of you who know Karen and Mike, you know that money is the last thing on their mind, and always has been. Karen still to this day doesn't know how to balance a checkbook! They're both firm believers in the philosophy that love is all you need, and they practice what they preach every single day. And you know what? When your best friend is battling every single day for his life, I can't help but think there is no better way to live life - enjoying every single moment you have together, good or bad. However, the more rational side of me also realizes that fighting for your life comes at a high price …

It goes without saying that Mike is unable to work, and with no immediate family in the area, Karen is on her own to manage the household. She has the ability to go on Family Medical Leave, however it is unpaid, which leaves them with no income for the foreseeable future. Since Mike is unable to take care of himself or the kids, someone has to be home to do both; it is literally a full time job taking care of two kids and an immobile husband fighting brain cancer. There has to be a better solution, and I think this could be it.

A lot of you have been asking us how you can help. You can help by spreading the word. You can tell others of Team Turnbull's battle. You can donate money so that Karen will have the opportunity to stay at home and take care of her family. You can donate money so that the boys (ages three and seven) are able to have some sort of normalcy in their lives. I know it's a lot to ask, and there are so many worthy causes out there that it can be hard to choose where to put your time and money. But I'm begging you to choose us. If you've ever met anyone in my family, you know that we love hard. We love harder than most. But with that love comes great pain, and nothing pains us more than to see one of our own go through something so horrific and not be able to help. This is our opportunity, and we're asking you to join us!

We want nothing more than for Mike to overcome this battle, except for Karen to be right by his side while he does it. Please consider supporting Team Turnbull during this excruciatingly difficult time.

## New Year's Eve

*By Karen Turnbull — Dec 31, 2014*

I am sitting in the Neuro ICU looking at the famous Las Vegas Stratosphere from Mike's room at Sunrise Hospital. We came in yesterday because Mike had developed some new symptoms. He felt as if he was on a carnival ride because the room was spinning. Also I noticed that the left side of his face was not moving. When he smiles only the right side goes up. When I called the neurosurgeon's office I was advised to bring him straight into the ER, so here we sit again. A CT scan was done yesterday which showed that the spot in his brainstem measures quite a bit larger. Almost three centimeters. However the hope, prayer and focus is that it is just angry from the Gamma Knife treatment. We are currently waiting for an MRI to give more clarification. Another neurosurgeon came in this morning to talk to us. She was wonderful. She spent a lot of time with us and gave us a lot of information. Her hope, and ours, is that it truly is just inflammation from the treatment. So now we wait.

It is quiet in this wing and the nurses have been wonderful. Mike is able to rest peacefully, so that is good. He is able to talk and is eating well, so I am grateful for that. In the meantime it is snowing at home (but not at the hospital yet). Our kids are at their friends' house playing in the healing snow from Heaven! I refuse to think anything else but that our miracle is on its way!

Please keep the prayers strong!!!! Much love and here is to HEALTH, happiness and love in the new year!

*Kristin U*
I believe in miracles with snow, too!! Tell Mike he is in our prayers. LOVE to you all.

*Liese W*
Praying diligently along with the healing snow in Vegas and the beautiful refreshing sunshine in New Orleans, that the inflammation is taken down and continuing healing IS occurring on the New Year's Eve. Love, Laughter and Healing Light flowing through Mike every moment.

*Ro K*
Our prayers for healing for Mike and strength for your family in the new year.

*Michelle B*
Karen, you are the strongest woman I know! I hope the door closing on 2014 will open to a new year of blessings and health. We are continuing our prayer vigil for Mike, you and the boys.

*Katey J*
We continue to pray for you, Mike and Karen and children and so many others involved in your immediate surroundings, be they family, friends, doctors or nurses! We know that God is faithful and has the ultimate plan. We specifically pray for the swelling/inflammation to be reduced and return Mike to perfect condition! Love from Katey, Matt, Aaron and Corinne

*Estelle T*
Thinking of you and praying for hope and healing as you enter the new year.

*Melin F*
Aren't kids wonderful ... playing in the snow!! Evan is so tall and I can see the joy on his face. My heart goes out to you both and my prayers are strong for your miracle.

*Karen P*
Our prayers are with you. We are holding you close to our hearts. Your children are lovely and we are so glad they can be children and play a bit with each other. God Bless all of you.

*Sara I*

*The Lord never gives us more than we can handle and miracles happen every day! Keep the faith as we continue to keep the prayers coming your way! You're stronger than you know!! Much love to All of You. Please let us know if you need some gourmet meals versus hospital food. Love from our family.*

*Tim L*

*We are praying every day, Karen. You, Mike and the kids are on the prayer chain. Praying for total healing and a Miracle for Mike. Please give him a hug for me!!*

*Hope M*

*Dearest Karen and Mike- Herman, Logan and I have you plugged in BIG TIME in our prayers. We love you and wish we were closer so that we could give you a big group hug. We are in awe of your spirit and we are so grateful for all of those incredible people that surround you. Here's to a new year filled with health and family time.*

*Tara F*

*Praying for Mike on this New Year's Day for a healthy recovery and sending love to you and the kids. Xxxxxxx*

*Jodie M*

*I miss our crazy Henderson snow days! Much love to you, Mike and the kids! You're always in our thoughts and prayers! xoxo*

CHAPTER THREE

# The Storm Intensifies
## 2015

## UCLA Bound

*By Karen Turnbull — Jan 1, 2015*

Last night I went home from the hospital and felt completely defeated. We had been told that the MRI still left them with questions. Yes, the lesion looked bigger. Yes, there appeared to be new bleeding. Yes, there was swelling. What were we to do about it? That was the big question that had no answers. We were told that it might be time to seek a second opinion from somewhere like UCLA. How to get there was the question. Would insurance cover it? Would any doctors get us in? Or did we have to drive there and walk into the ER much like we did here. The thought of taking Mike on a four and a half hour drive to LA in his condition was heartbreaking. And then to think of sitting for another day in the ER while we waited to maybe get a room and be seen was more than I could begin to comprehend.

I think that last night was the darkest I had ever felt. I was broken and I cried harder than I think I have ever cried before. Through the tears I prayed. I prayed, screamed and asked God to please give us some answers. Some sort of direction. I just didn't know where to go. I had written to Dr. Wang, our original doctor who did Mike's thyroid surgery. I asked him if he had any suggestions as to who we should see. I also wrote to Dr. Toy's assistant. Dr. Toy is currently out of the country so I asked her if she would email him for me.

This morning I came back to the hospital with no clearer vision as to what to do. I spoke with my amazing friend Kathy and expressed to her my need for some sort of sign. Something to guide us in what to do. Something to give me a glimmer of hope to hold on to. The amazing thing is within minutes of talking to her we received our answer. I received a text from Dr. Wang. He had spoken to Dr. Toy and Dr. Obara. All three were in agreement that UCLA was where we should head. Then the neurosurgeon came in to speak to us. She was in agreement that the new MRI did show change, but she was holding on to the hope that this was all just part of the healing. To her it made sense to think that three weeks post intense Gamma Knife treatment the area would be inflamed and angry, so if she can hold on to that hope, I can too. It is still possible that this will all resolve. She also was in agreement that seeking a second opinion and possibly some other options for care would be a good idea. She felt that if they could work the paperwork and get insurance on board they could set up a direct transport. Finally it felt like we were getting answers and things were falling into place.

Shortly thereafter we were told that insurance was indeed on board and we would be transported by plane to UCLA. They were not sure if this would happen today, being it was New Year's Day, or tomorrow, but at least we knew it was in the works to happen. I went home and packed a bag and talked to the boys. That was actually the hardest part. Sweet little Evan. I cannot even imagine what it must feel like for a seven-year-old to first try to understand why Daddy can't get out of bed and now to try to understand why Mommy has to fly with him to some other hospital. Why is this happening to our family? That I will never be able to answer.

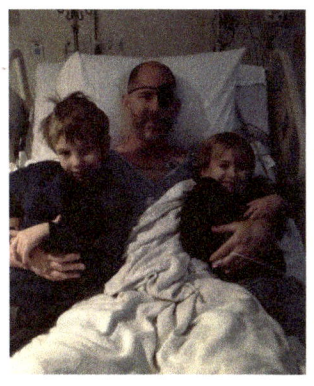

After many tears and long hugs we managed to pull ourselves together. I brought Evan and William to see Daddy at the hospital. I think this was healing for everyone involved! Mike's face lit up when he saw our beautiful boys, and our boys faces lit up too. Mike's mom, Kathy, flew in tonight. She will stay at our house to care for the boys and will have assistance from our many wonderful angel friends and neighbors. The gratitude I feel towards everyone who helps us so much every single day is overwhelming. I will never know how to thank everyone enough. Also, the miracle of my niece Michelle's gofundme account is more of a blessing than I realized it would be.

I do not know how long we will be at UCLA. While we are there our insurance will cover Mike's care but I am on my own for my lodging and expenses. Thanks to the amazing, generous donations from so many I do not have to worry about how to pay for everything. Again, my gratitude is beyond anything words can express. So, it looks like tomorrow we will make our trip to UCLA. My prayer is that there is someone there who can help. Whether it be that more advanced screening techniques can tell us this is all part of the healing process and time will heal these wounds, or that there is some study or treatment that can be done to help speed the process and alleviate Mike's symptoms.

It is a new year and new miracles are around the corner! I am not giving up hope and after today my faith is renewed. Thank you God for answering my prayer and giving us direction. We are at peace with this decision and feel at least we are now doing something. Thank you everyone for all of your love and support.

As always, keep the prayers coming! I know they are working! Much love and Happy New Year!

### Miles P
*Mike, you have been in my thoughts and prayers over the past few days. It has been years, but I remember having the good fortune of being around you like it was yesterday. I know the traits that have made you a great husband, father and friend are also the traits that will get you through this difficult time. Get well soon!*

### Randy C
*Words fail me, but looking at the faces of your three boys together is definitely healing for me. Godspeed to UCLA and bring Mike back better and soon.*

### Jason M
*Praying for your family. Blessings, light and love to you both on this journey.*

### Nancy R
*Continued prayers for Mike's recovery and for your strength. You are an AMAZING woman, Karen.*

### Judy E
*It saddens us knowing what a struggle this is for your entire family. We too are praying for clear answers to guide you and the boys and heal Mike's body. God bless all of you!*

### Birgit D
*I am saddened by the struggles your family is facing. My continued prayers for all of you. You are a very strong woman, Karen.*

*Betty S*
Karen, your strength and courage has always been a part of you. With God's help ... we are all in this together. Karen, Mike, Evan, William. We Love You --- Mom & Dad

*Katie C*
Thinking of you guys always. Love and healing thoughts.

*Issa F*
I think about and pray for your family every day. Thank you, Karen, for taking the time to write these posts even through your pain to keep all us old friends up to date. There is a lot of love coming at you from Colorado!

*Sharon H*
Oh, Karen! I stand in agreement with you! I am hopeful that the gamma treatment has made that lesion angry as hell!!! Good!!! Go!!! Get!!! I want to come see you and Mike and help out in any and every way I can. I love you both so much.

*Matt J*
Hi, Mike ... You may not get this right away. You have been on my mind continually every day. I deeply miss your presence at rehearsals. We have a Boneheads rehearsal at Curt's this weekend, but it just won't be the same. Katey and I have been following Karen's CaringBridge updates. You may already be at UCLA by now, perhaps not. If enroute here's to a smooth flight, my brother. Godspeed!! Love and steadfast fervent prayers for you, Karen and the boys.

*Lisa L*
Mike, you continue to be in our thoughts and prayers. Karen, whenever you just need to talk, vent or have someone listen, then I'm your girl. Prayers, positive thoughts and love to you.

*Kim M*
Constantly thinking of all of you, Karen. Thankful the power of prayer has brought the next steps for Mike and praying that UCLA will have answers.

*Alicia B*
I have no words. All I feel is inspired by your strength. We'll keep praying, you keep fighting.

# No Room at the Inn

*By Karen Turnbull — Jan 3, 2015*

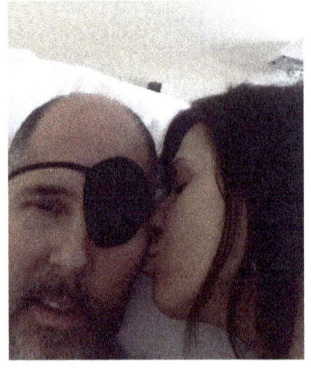

We are still waiting for a bed/room to become available at UCLA. Otherwise, everything is set. So, here we sit and wait but there are worse places we could be. The nurses have been wonderful and Mike and I are just hanging out. He is eating well and resting. It tires him out to talk too much so we are just quietly "being" together. I was able to go home to the boys last night so that was good. One less night apart is a good thing. Hopefully we will get transported today. We are both ready to take the next step.

Love to you all and keep the prayers coming.

### Marianne M
*You are constantly in our thoughts and prayers. We love you so much and know that good things will happen when you get to UCLA. Stay strong. God's love and protection is with you both!*

### Megan H
*Hang in there. The downside of UCLA is both oncology and neurology are small wards and beds are always full. The upside ... they are small wards and the care you will receive is remarkable. So glad you have more time with the kids ... you need and deserve the fuel they will give the both of you. We are with you.*

### Ellen Sn
*This is just a little setback. I know Mike knows how to rock and roll!!! So start the music!!!! Keeping you all in my thoughts!!!!*

### Betty S
*Prayers and thoughts are constantly wth you both!! Just wish you were not so far away!! Love, Mom & Dad*

# 6:00 Flight!!!!

*By Karen Turnbull — Jan 6, 2015*

Medical transport is here! We are on our way! Miracles are about one hour away!!! Prayers prayers prayers!!!!!!

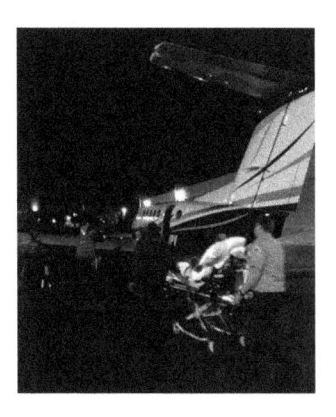

*Elena S*
Tonight at dinner we prayed specifically for favor in getting a spot/bed at UCLA asap. Praise God! Continuing to pray for healing and the best care possible. Love to you!!! GO MIKE!!!

*Charles D*
Thinking of you guys and sending all the positive thoughts we can. Small anecdote: turns out we have a mutual friend and she and I were discussing how amazing you and Mike both are! Small world ... thought you both would enjoy hearing that :) Please send Mike my best wishes!!!!

*Suzanne P*
I see you flying on the wings of angels. Sending you love and healing.

*Tom E*
Way to hang in there, Mike and Karen. I'm praying for your procedures, Mike. Karen, you are one of world's greatest all-time cheerleaders. God bless you guys!

*Abby A*
Love & light & hugs 'n kisses ... Stay strong you warriors ... We love you.

*Cathy M*
*Healing miracles await you! Blessings on you both for providing us with real-life heroes and an endless source of inspiration! Continued strength as we send more prayers, love and admiration.*

# We Made It

*By Karen Turnbull — Jan 7, 2015*

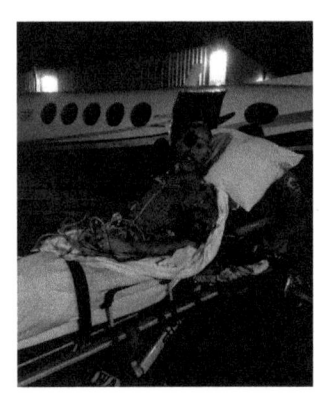

This was Mike before they loaded him onto the plane. Flight was safe and smooth. Walking down the hallway to the Neuro ICU felt more like walking down a museum hallway. It is beautiful here. The nurses are getting him settled and already labs have been drawn, neurologist has been in and MRI's are being evaluated. Also he has just received a medicine that specifically reduces swelling in the brain. A tiny little pill that will help "dry out" the excessive fluid that has caused so much turmoil. I am so grateful to be here!!!!! THANK YOU GOD!!!!

Thank you for all the prayers! Please continue them ... I know they are working!!!!

*Nathan T*
*Good news! We will keep the positive thoughts coming! Love to you all!*

*Annie W*
*I love you both and am sending prayers, love and energy your way!*

*Darren K*
*Wow, so glad to hear things are now at least moving forward towards some relief for Mike. We're on high alert here in Colorado for all your updates, Karen. Thanks for posting so many updates with lots of info. Let us know if we can help in any way.*

# What a Ride!
*By Karen Turnbull — Jan 8, 2015*

I have often compared the ups and downs of these last (almost) two years to being stuck on a roller coaster that we never got in line for. Well, the ride continues. It turns out that after three different teams (of about ten doctors each) have reviewed, discussed and collaborated ... we have a plan. Shockingly enough this lesion in Mike's brainstem looks in fact to be a cavernoma as first thought and NOT a recurrence of his cancer!!! The confusion has been that it is something that none of our team in Las Vegas had seen before. Its location, its bleeding and swelling all confused things. Plus, with Mike's past history of cancer, it just seemed more likely to be that. After serious testing, the group here feels confident that it is not cancer. Our other problem in Las Vegas was that no neurosurgeons wanted anything to do with this as it was just too risky. They did not have a comfort level with a case this complex. I am grateful that they knew their limitations and when all they could do failed they got us here.

The care we have received has been unbelievable! I keep saying that I feel like I'm in an episode of Grey's Anatomy! The teams of doctors here are hungry to not only help but to continue to learn. I am inspired by all those that we have encountered. It would be easy to start to think that we have done things wrong or done things that didn't need to be done. I am choosing not to think that way. I am choosing to believe everything that was done was done at the right time with the information that we had. And now we have new information. We have tried other things and now it is time to try this.

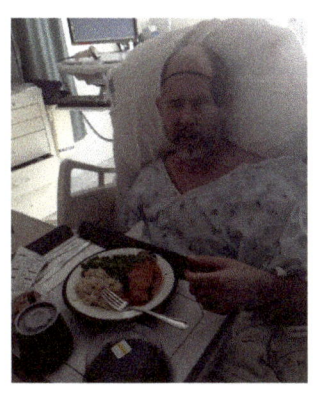

At 10:00 last night a calm, confident and well-informed gentle giant entered our room. Dr. Neil Martin is the head of neurosurgery here at UCLA. He is as high up on the chain as we could possibly go. He is nationally known and we have been informed that only he and one other doctor at Johns Hopkins are skilled enough to do this particular surgery. He was AMAZING!!!! Mike's situation is bad but he has actually seen and brought people through worse! He wants to monitor Mike for about a week, then do surgery. If Mike gets worse he will move it up but the hope is swelling and bleeding will calm down some, making

surgery slightly easier. Right now the consistency of the blood around Mike's lesion is like pudding. The hope is that in a week, it will become more liquid-like and easier to remove. It is a complicated, intricate and risky surgery. He would not recommend surgery at all unless there was no other option. In Mike's case there appears to be no other option. But ... Dr. Martin feels he can do it! When he looked me in the eyes and told me that this is not cancer and that we are in a better position than we thought we were, I knew, with every cell in my body, that he would do everything he could to bring us through this.

The surgery itself will be very long. Possibly longer than Mike's original thyroid surgery. When Dr. Martin asked Mike if he was in good health before this happened Mike smiled his half smile, chuckled slightly and said, "I was training for a triathlon." His response was, "Perfect, you were training for surgery. That will work in your favor." Recovery will be hard and long and he will be worse directly after surgery. However, Dr. Martin feels that six months from now there is a high likelihood that Mike will be better than now. As far as how much these deficits will be permanent only time will tell. Recovery could be 25%, 50%, 95%. I know I am not alone in believing that Mike will shock us all with his recovery! It is all so overwhelming but Mike and I trust Dr. Martin, his team and UCLA. We believe in his confidence, calmness and kindness.

Hopefully, I have done an okay job at relaying all this information to everyone. I am sure there are things that I missed. As things progress or we have an exact surgery date, I will let everyone know. Until then, keep sending loving thoughts, energy and prayers. I do believe that this is the miracle we have all been praying for. Pray that Mike stays strong and focused on his successful recovery. It is a long road ahead but with the support around us I know Mike (and me and our amazing boys) can do it. Thank you all so much. You will never know how much your comments, love and prayers have kept us inspired and focused!

Thank you, keep the prayers coming and we love you!

> *Dave W*
> *Keep hanging tough! Thoughts, prayers an much love from us and all of your Denver/UNC musician friends!!!*

> *Karina B*
> *Phenomenal!!!!!!! Can't wait for Mike to compete in this "marathon" and come out VICTORIOUS!!!!! xoxo*

*Tim L*

*Sitting here reading this update with my wife ... Not a dry eye at this point!! So glad to hear this positive news and we know it will only get better from here ... Prayer works!! Blessings.*

*Betty S*

*Stay Strong, Karen! We know you have made the right decisions and choices along this rocky road. God has guided you along the way, and he is not finished yet. Mike, Karen, Evan, William - Our love and prayers. Mom & Dad*

*Birgit P*

*That's good news! Karen, Mike has the best wife ever and the two of you will get through this. Hugs and positive thoughts from the Popes.*

*Doreen L*

*So wonderful to read your upbeat update! So informative and positive, yet realistic as well. So happy for you and know many are sharing tears of joy with you as we read this. Praise God and keep the miracles coming, Lord!*

*Kathy M*

*We continue to keep you in prayer. No looking back ... only forward, knowing that God is with you every step of the way.*

*Kathryn L*

*Karen - you are an inspiration! Keep looking forward - good things to come. You and Mike made the best decisions based on the information you had at hand. GOOD JOB! You can't do better than that. We're sending positive thoughts your way. Say hi to Mike from Mark and me.*

*Rocco B*

*Karen, thank you for your post. Not a day goes by where Mike, yourself and your children aren't being thought of and prayed for. We are thankful that Mike is getting the best of care. He deserves it!!! You both truly deserve life and well-being! Our prayers are with you all! Mike, you made it as a professional trombonist. If you could do that, I'm pretty sure that you'll handle this one. We are rooting for you, pal! May God bless you all.*

*Jeanine C*
This is great news. Mike will keep showing us how amazing he is. So glad you have the UCLA team around you. Sending love and prayers to you all. xx

*Betsy A*
We'll keep praying!!!! Mike can do anything with you by his side and his two beautiful boys to look ahead at! Love to you!

*Edward E*
This is amazing news!!! Go get 'em, Mike!! What a great cheerleader you have!! Xo

*Nancy R*
You are truly an inspiration to me, Karen. AMAZING. Many prayers.

*Karen P*
You have found the right man (other than the wonderful one you married) to get you through this. I can feel it in the words I see on the screen. All our hopes and prayers are on you through this. Thank you so much for the updates.

*Dan S*
Wow!! I am sooo happy you got to where you needed to be at UCLA and are in the best possible hands! Continuing with the positive energy and support! Love you guys!!!

*Andrea L*
I am in tears. I know that this is the prayer you have been asking for. I feel that you are in good hands there. Mike will be healed. Our prayers will be answered. We love you. Have not stopped and will not stop praying. Xox

*Kathy L*
Your message is so full of JOY!! There are angels surrounding you, Mike and the kids !!

*Sharon H*
Hallelujah! Hallelujah! Hallelujah!!!!!!!!!!!!!!!!!!!

*Dave Ro*
Now THIS is a Happy New Year's story. Keep the faith, keep the

hope, keep the love. You both and your boys are an inspiration in courage and perseverance. Peace & love!!!

### Ellen F
Kim and I send our prayers and fervent hope that Mike's healing is underway. Karen, you are a strong woman and supporter and caregiver. Blessings to you and your kids and your neighbors helping you on this journey. God is good!

### Beth S
Such great news, Karen!!!! There is your first miracle. Your first silver lining of many! Prayers of speedy healing and a safe surgery one step at a time :). Breathe.

### Christine E
I believe in miracles and it is my belief your miracle will happen. I love you both so much and all my prayers are with you.

### Jean T
Karen - A few years after this is all very successfully over, you two can gather these CaringBridge entries together and put it all into a book. Title could be: Never, NEVER! Give Up. Thoughts and prayers continue.

### Sam Ba
Our prayers are with you, Mike and Karen. May our Lord guide your steps, guard your path and continue to hold you in this storm.

### Jenna L
After reading your posts of Mike's battle with cancer and cavernoma, the scripture "All things are possible with God" keeps coming into my mind. You are in our thoughts and prayers and we are believing for complete healing for Mike! You are on our prayer chain at our church and will be lifted up in prayer as you face this surgery and recovery. May God give you His strength, peace and grace each moment.

# Holding Strong

*By Karen Turnbull — Jan 12, 2015*

I wanted to let everyone know how things are going here at UCLA. Right now we are in a holding pattern. Mike is out of the ICU and in a lovely room on the Neuro floor. It is quite large and big enough for me to stay with him. I did take a break for a few days and stayed at a hotel to get some solid nights sleep and some very hot, long showers. Overall, I think Mike is doing quite well, although he doesn't necessarily think so. It is very difficult for him to move and because of the steroids and the high level of sodium, his body is very swollen. The sodium is used to help remove some of the fluid from the brain but the side effect is the body itself retains fluid. He has not been in much pain until last night, when his knee and ankle on his good side, the left, started hurting. Eventually we got him positioned more comfortably and some pain meds kicked in. The PET scan last week did show a few small clots in his lungs so they had to put a filter in to protect him from any further clots moving towards the lungs or brain. Basically this is preventative and can eventually be removed. Physical Therapy has come by a few times and gotten him moving a little but it is really challenging.

The plan at this point is surgery either Friday or Saturday. The procedure will take approximately fifteen hours, possibly more. The reason it might be Saturday is that the top team members (anesthesiologists, assistants, etc.) might be tied up with other procedures Friday. So, if having the "A" team in place means waiting a day that is ok by us. It was described to us that the spot they are working on is about the size of his thumb. They will work in half millimeter sections to remove as much as possible and not nick any nerves. It is intricate and scary. Somehow, though, Mike and I are currently pretty calm and even finding moments of laughter.

We have had some lovely visits from family and friends in the area which has helped pass a little time. Visits are hard and need to be kept short but I know he does appreciate the love. Thank you for all your comments on here. I read them to Mike and he is always touched to know people are thinking of him and sending love and prayers. We don't know too much about the after-surgery plan. Definitely a few days in

ICU, then some time in the regular Neuro rooms. We still don't know if rehab will be done at home or start in a live-in facility. We will cross that bridge when we get to it. I will post again as things progress and surgery day gets closer. Thank you everyone! It is amazing to know that the love, support and prayers has followed us to UCLA.

As always, please keep them coming!

> *Darelle H*
> *Okay, thank you for the update. Breathe, rest when you can and let those genius doctors do their thing when they will. Grace to you both and big hugs and prayers as always. We are with you.*
>
> *Andrea L*
> *Been waiting anxiously for an update. This journal that you so eloquently write is so special on so many levels. Mike is so lucky to have you by his side. It is good to know that you can feel the love and prayers coming from far. We never stop here. Love you.*
>
> *Jordan B*
> *Stay strong, Mike and Karen! Thinking about you daily here in St. Louis. Prayers and positive thoughts being sent your way!*
>
> *Pat C*
> *Feel the love. Our prayers are relentless. We believe a complete healing is in order.*
>
> *Karen Mi*
> *Vegas is with you! Our family sends love and prayers! :-)*
>
> *Judy E*
> *You are both amazing and a living testimony of faith and God's love. God is using you to touch lives, to encourage others and to put life into perspective. We pray that God guides the hands of the entire team, that you both make believers of all those around you and that God continues to lift you up and holds you in His hands throughout this journey. YOU are truly vessels of HIS love.*
>
> *Brandon T*
> *All of your trombone brothers are pulling for you. Stay strong, Mike!*

*Karen P*
Mike and Karen, you both are an inspiration. Your positive attitude in this incredibly bad situation is just admirable. We don't know how you do it. We are sending lots and lots of love and prayers and healing thoughts from the high country of Colorado. You can do this!

*Laurence A*
Hey, Mike. So many people here love you and we're all pulling for you. You are strong like bull! Oxox

*Roxane G*
Mike and Karen, you both are in our prayers. Keep fighting hard. I'm so glad you are getting such great care at UCLA! God bless.

*Beth L*
Love, light and prayers for you all. Mike, you're a strong guy, and your family and friends are so firmly in your corner. You are going to win this fight! Lots of love to you all. Let me know if I can do anything for you.

*Sharon H*
You are in the best of hands with Dr. Martin ... the very best of hands. Holding you in deep, abiding prayer.

*Kathy A*
I love you both so much! You are in great hands ... sending healing energy, prayers and tons of love. xoxo

*Robin C*
Thinking of you and holding you in my heart and my prayers. Sending love and hugs. The boys were great at God's Kids Thursday night. Evan is so good with his little brother. Karen, your sister sounds just like you.

*Cindy E*
Lots of love and prayers coming from our family. We were dancing in the rain yesterday after church, saying a prayer for your family.

*Joni S*
You know that we are here for you and of course continuing to pray and send positive thoughts. Please let me know if there is anything we can do here in Vegas. You both continue to inspire me with your strength and love. xoxo

*James M*
*Thanks for the updates, Karen. Mike and your family continue to be in our daily prayers. We are praying for strength and comfort for all of you. You are a very strong woman and Mike is truly a fighter! Keep looking up! Blessings.*

*Jennifer M*
*Always thinking of you and your family. Stay strong. We are praying every day.*

*Debra L*
*Our family constantly has you in our thoughts and prayers. My hundred and one year-old friend prays for you both, too. She even gets down on her knees for you and that is no easy task at one hundred and one! Let us know if we can help.*

*Doug M*
*I love that you share all of this with us. Thank you both. What an amazing team. We should all be so blessed to have a partner in life like you two have. Love and prayers coming your way.*

*Sara I*
*Love you both so much! I truly believe when God closes one door he opens another! UCLA is your new door and we truly believe this is your miracle and where you're supposed to be. We're here for you all! Positive prayers and much love coming your way each and every day!!!*

*Pam Ro*
*We are thinking about and praying for you. Let Mike know that Cruz wrote a story about him today. It is titled "The Healthy Dinosaur." It ends with the nurse running in, saying, "Good news, Good news, Good news! Your cancer is gone and you can go home now." Mike the Dinosaur skips home playing his trombone. From Cruz's mouth to God's ears we are praying for this ending.*

*Lynne E*
*I admire both you and Mike for your courage, faith and positive attitudes. We send prayers and love your way and to the rest of your family and the friends that support you. May 2015 bring healing and give you and Mike the strength that will take you through the coming rehab. You are in our thoughts and prayers daily. Thank you for the time that you take to keep us up to date. I love when you talk*

*about Mike's smile ... what a dear man you have as your partner and he is so lucky to have you as his wife. A match made in heaven, some would say.*

### Franz C
*Prayers and best wishes for you, Mike and the family! Glad he's getting physical therapy. I'll be all over it when he's ready for home PT, too!*

### Darci P
*Karen and Mike, we're so glad you are at UCLA and getting the miraculous care Mike needs. Sending hugs and prayers.*

### Joey F
*Hey Mike, just like at the D&M Show ... I am in your corner. I hope you know my little family thinks the world of you and yours. Lets get to the part where we are hanging by the pool, having a cocktail, watching the boys do their best to break everything in site ... deal?*

### Marc H
*Hi Karen (and Mike). You don't know me, but my dear friend Sharon told me all about you and your beautiful family, and Mike's journey, and I was humbled to hear about this brave warrior, Mike Turnbull! I just have to share that you are in the right place. UCLA and Dr. Neil Martin saved the life of a dear friend of mine a few years back as he and his team performed a nineteen-hour surgery that truly TRULY saved her life ... simple and true. She's a walking miracle, and quite happy to talk to either of you. It could be inspiring for you to talk to her. Keep the faith and march forward knowing that you are S A F E and blessed to be under Dr. Martin's care. You'll all be in my thoughts and prayers as I follow your incredible journey!*

### Suzanne P
*I loved reading the post by Marc H. Although I don't know anything about Dr. Martin, I also felt that you were in the right place with the right doctors after reading your last entry. Marc H's post was a sign from the universe that everything will be ok. Not easy, but ok. You have the right team! Mike, keep your eyes on the goal and the finish line. Your body will get the message and follow suit just like it did when you were training it for the marathons. Continue meditating and visualizing your cells getting healthier and healthier when they reproduce. I used to visualize PAC-MAN going through and taking*

*out whatever didn't belong or wasn't healthy for my body. I would also visualize my cells laughing and having a party when they were recovering and reproducing. Do whatever works for you and speaks to your body. Laugh, even if it is in silence. It is the healthiest thing you can do for your body. Mike, you got this. You have been training for it your whole life. I am standing at the finish line cheering for you and sending you tons of love and encouragement to keep a steady pace. This April is my ten-year mark and I wouldn't be here to encourage you if it weren't for you and Karen loving and encouraging me. Keep thanking your body for being so strong. So much love to you, too, Karen. Mike couldn't have picked a better partner to have on his team for life. P.S. Those long hot showers are the best, aren't they?*

## Getting Close

*By Karen Turnbull — Jan 15, 2015*

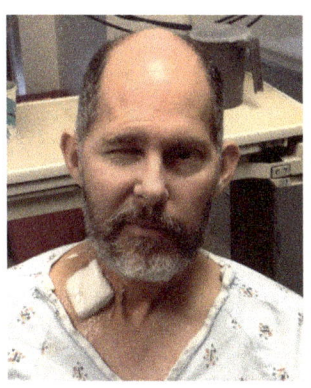

This morning the doctors came in and told us that from now on, starting at midnight, Mike will not be allowed to eat. This is so that he is prepared and able to go to surgery at any time. Once the nurses hear that the doctors cannot take him into surgery he will be allowed to order food. The good news is that means we're getting close. Mike could go at any time. The bad news is he can't eat and seeing as he can't do much else, eating has become the joy of his days. Luckily, the food here has been awesome and he has been eating like a champ. So, since he can't eat, can't see and can't move, he is sleeping. Which is good, as he definitely needs his rest for the long journey ahead.

The biggest concern (other than the fact that he has a bleeding lesion in his brain stem) is that he had some clots develop in his lungs. They inserted a filter to prevent any more from moving to the lungs or brain. The other concern is that his platelet level keeps dropping. They are pretty sure this is due to the mass in his brain literally eating them up, but they will have to monitor the level closely and he is receiving transfusions almost daily. This amazing man definitely has a lot going on and the teams of doctors on hand are watching very closely.

While we wait I have begun to make some new friends. These new friends have come to me at the exact time I need them, because they have their own amazing, miraculous and beautiful success stories. One is a woman named Doriana. I had a wonderful talk with her yesterday when she reached out to us to share her story. She found herself in the hands of Dr. Martin just a few years ago. Dr. Martin performed an eighteen-hour surgery that saved her life. Hearing her story was amazing. So many similarities to Mike and she too found herself in this miraculous facility in the hands of this incredible man. And last night I had the opportunity to chat with Mike's nurse, Amy. Her daughter was born here and had her first of seven brain surgeries at the age of just seven days old. I can't even imagine! This tiny baby fought all the odds and is now nine years old! To hear Amy talk of the surgeons here was such a gift. On top of that, her aunt was also saved by Dr. Martin. So in one day, two strong women with their own horrific stories came to me. They may never know how sharing their stories has helped me, but I will be forever grateful.

For now, while Mike rests, I continue to pray. I make sure to get outside at least twice a day and take a walk and breathe in the sunshine. I think the waiting is the hardest part, but at least while I wait amazing people have come into my life to help keep me focused on the miracle ahead.

I will let you all know as things progress and as always keep the prayers coming!

> *Matt J*
> *Thank you so much for sharing these stories with us. I sent Mike a text message via his cell phone. Perhaps you could read it to him when he is awake. Mike ... the next time we hang out you get to pig out anywhere you want, and the tab's on me!*
>
> *Lance P*
> *Positive thoughts, positive thoughts, positive thoughts ... and keep on keepin' on! Thank you for these updates.*
>
> *Jennifer A*
> *Sending lots of prayers, Karen!!!!*
>
> *Sara I*
> *One day, sooner than you think, you too will be on the other end of Mike's miracle story, helping someone who once was in your shoes. Stay strong, stay focused and know you are loved, my friend! There*

is light at the end of the tunnel for you and your beautiful family!! Love you All! Sending you All Positive Prayers ~ The Ignacio Family

### Katey J
Angels come in all kinds of ways and it sounds like the people you encountered were messengers from God. We continue to pray for you all for patience through the waiting and for comfort for you and your entire family. Lots of love.

### Megan A
I love you, friend.

### Heather W
Keeping the prayers coming!!!!!!! You guys are so amazing and I know that your continued strength and positivity will carry you through the next step. So good to know that Mike is in the hands of great doctors!

### Kathy M
So glad God has sent you wonderful angels to encourage you just when you need them. You and Mike and his medical team remain in our prayers!

### Heather L
I am so happy you found some support at the hospital. So many times people are so focused and concerned about the person who is sick (and rightfully so), but they tend to forget the toll it takes on the caregiver. You are such a strong person, Karen. Please know that we are praying for Mike, you and your beautiful children.

### Alicia B
God puts the right people in your life at the exact moment you need them ... he's amazing. Sending prayers.

### Beth B
Love and Light your way!!!

# Not Today

*By Karen Turnbull — Jan 15, 2015*

Well, it will not be today. The good news ... Mike was able to get his omelet before they stopped serving breakfast. Positive thoughts ...

*Curt M*
I, and the whole music community here, think about you every day. I am so sorry you are having to go through this. You don't deserve it. But he is fiercely strong and determined. Thank you for keeping us in the loop.

*Shelley De*
Thank you for keeping us posted. Hoping for the same miracle as the others who shared with you. So glad there are others to reach out and give you positive inspiration. Michael and you are amazing and God will reward you for your bravery and strength. Remember, many are with you. Hugs and prayers.

# Blueberry Pancakes

*By Karen Turnbull — Jan 16, 2015*

No surgery today. Blueberry pancakes for breakfast.

*Darren K*
Sounds like an awesome trade! I'll take that any day.

# SUNDAY!!!!!

*By Karen Turnbull — Jan 16, 2015*

Official word from Dr. Martin himself ... Sunday! He stopped by tonight (in the exact ten minutes I stepped out to get tea) to talk to Mike. The word is Mike is on the schedule for Sunday. It will be long and intricate but he is prepared to take the time needed, so just one more day and then we start the next phase of healing. Prayers, prayers, prayers!!!!

**Curt M**
So glad you are there and have the best there is. Mike deserves nothing less. Give him a hug from all the Boneheads!

**Hope M**
Our family LOVES Team Turnbull!!!!!! Prayers and love to you both.

**Sam Ba**
We are praying for you and the medical team. May the Holy Spirit surround you all and bring strength and healing. The God of angel armies is on your side!

**Laura T**
We're all thinking of you and sending our love and positive energy. One of my friends sent this in response to my email asking everyone for their prayers and positive vibes. My prayer for Mike: God guide the hand of the surgeon ... give to him wisdom of experience, breadth of knowledge and expert skills ... let Mike's pain be bearable ... and his recovery speedy and complete!

**Liese W**
Praying. IT IS THE LORD'S Day!!! I know the doctor is truly connecting the perfect time. Love you both. Sending soft hands and healing touch to all who are in the operating room and those who are there in recovery! Love and Light to you and Mike.

**Sandy B**
Many prayers for a successful operation and a quick recovery. If any one can beat this it is you, Mikey. Go Team Turnbull!!!!!

# Cancelled
*By Karen Turnbull — Jan 18, 2015*

I can't even speak right now. I will write more in a little. Short story- there is an infection somewhere. They need to control that before surgery. I don't know more than that.

**Devonee M**
Oh, Karen. I am so sorry this is delaying. We are praying for you. For strength. For wisdom for the doctors. For some sense of peace while you wait. We love you so very much.

*Antonette L*
Thinking and praying for you guys and the surgeons who will take care of Mike. XOXO

*Trish T*
In God's time we all heal. Don't lose hope. Don't stray from faith. "Be strong and let your heart take courage, all you who hope in the LORD." (Psalm 27:24)

*Joan F*
Karen and Mike, remember this ... your spirit shines from inside and you both are bringing so much light to us that support you. That is one thing no clouds could ever hide!! God bless!!

*Sharon H*
Trust that God is in the details ... hold on ... I believe your miracle is on the way!

*Karine Z*
Oh, Karen. Holding you in our hearts. We love you dearly.

*Jeff L*
You and Mike are strong, positive, amazing people. Good things will come; the infection will be resolved and the surgery will happen. Until then, we are sending you love and strength.

*Lou G*
Praying and hoping ... cats everywhere are pulling for you all and we are all amazed that you have had to travel such a curious and hard road. The sore throat in LA, a sure and direct diagnosis, great follow-up, brilliant medical care, terrific medical teams who were available when you needed them most. Every setback has been harsh and more frightening and then, eventually, just as you needed them, more fantastic and wonderful people have come to you. Keep the faith ... we are with you. Sending love from down the road.

# Figuring it Out

*By Karen Turnbull — Jan 19, 2015*

Today was fairly busy. Lots of doctors in and out, blood tests and chest x-ray. The big question has been what caused the fever. Right now there are two thoughts. He may have aspirated some food, which caused irritation in the lungs, or it could be a build-up of some fluid in the lungs due to the many bags of IVs. The concern is that if his respiratory system is at all compromised, surgery would be even riskier than it already is. So far he has responded to the antibiotics and I'm hoping this x-ray shows it is clearing. His sodium level is holding so for now they have stopped that. The platelets held for forty-eight hours, although today they dropped again and another transfusion was needed.

I have always donated blood and not thought much of it. Now, seeing Mike as an almost daily recipient of blood products, I see it very differently. I am grateful to the people who have taken the time to donate. Right now they are a part of the miracle team. Mike is tired and feeling a little beat up and discouraged. It just seems like every step forward sends us two steps back, but we are both glad they are being so careful. So for now we wait some more. The goal is to confirm no more infection and then get this done.

Dr. Martin has mentioned that if it were up to him, he would wait a month and let the consistency of the bleeding be optimal for surgery, but he is not sure we have a month. Maybe this infection happened so that the surgery will go as well as possible.

Thank you prayer warriors! Eventually we will get there!

> *Cathy M*
> *I'm sure the events of the day require so much patience and continued courage. The care Mike is getting sounds meticulous and we're grateful to know that they leave no stone unturned in solving the puzzle. May the team be blessed with wisdom and compassion as they treat Mike. We send warm hugs and lots of love to you and Mike as you navigate each day. We are with you!*
>
> *Marc H*
> *Onward we march, steady, strong, positive and with great good hope and knowledge that prayers will be answered ... xx*
>
> *Gregory R*
> *We love you guys so much and are always here for you!!!!*
>
> *Candy P*
> *We love you! Hang in there. Sending hugs, kisses, and positive thoughts your way.*

# Best Medicine

*By Karen Turnbull — Jan 21, 2015*

Today we "danced in the rain!" My sister Marianne, Mike's mom Kathy and our two beautiful boys, Evan and William, came to visit! It was an amazing feeling to see them after two weeks apart. I have to say that if it were not for these two angel women caring for our kids I don't know what we would have done. They have kept the house and daily routine running. The boys are crazy about them and have been loved every moment of every day. Marianne and Kathy I cannot thank you enough! God has blessed us with you!

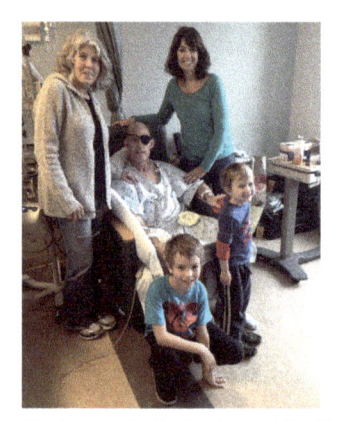

*Kathy Turnbull, Marianne Moulden*

**Les K**
Blessings, Karen! Thanks to your sister Marianne and Mike's mom Kathy for their love! Kathy is an awesome lady. Hang in there, my friends. Always praying for you and sending love and light your way:-) P.S. Thanks for the updates!

**Amy L**
XXOO I pray for you and your family daily. You are the strongest woman I know.

**Sharon H**
The most beautiful family in the whole wide world!! I love you so!!!!

**Mike S**
Love is the best medicine!

**Brook D**
Best news! Made me cry with joy. God bless those ladies!

*Melin F*
*I wait every day to hear how things are going and sometimes I open the email with trepidation ... what a wonderful day you must have had and I am thrilled that your life is full of the kind of people it is. Please give my love to Mike's mom and your sister and tell them they are always included in my prayers right along with you and Mike. The boys are beautiful and I'm sure their visit was the best medicine, as you stated. Keep the faith and know we are here for ALL of you.*

*Hayley M*
*Nothing like having two little boys around to make your day wonderful. Lovely day for all of you, I'm sure. Thinking of you all. x*

*Marie O*
*Michael and Karen ~ Our thoughts and prayers are with you and your sweet family.*

## Great Visit
### By Karen Turnbull — Jan 23, 2015

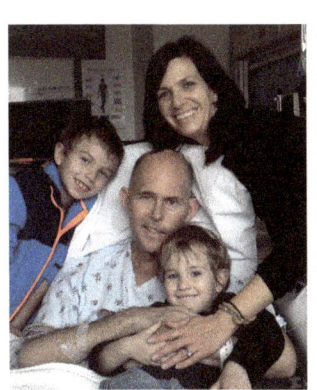

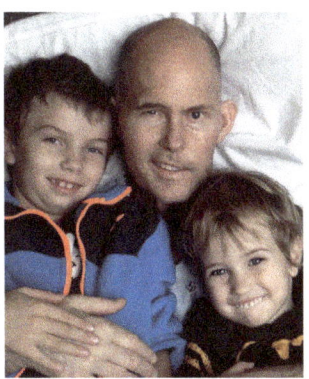

While it was hard to see the kids, my sister and Mike's mom head home today, it was amazing to have some time together. The boys got to visit with Daddy, pick lucky clovers for him, send prayers for him from the top of the Santa Monica Pier Ferris wheel and fuel him with hugs and kisses. I was able to escape for an afternoon of pure love with them and put my toes in the ocean. It was healing all the way around.

We are still on hold as we wait for the pulmonary team to give Mike the green light for surgery. Once we receive word of that, hopefully it will happen pretty quickly. Mike is holding steady. He works with PT daily and even though small, I do see improvements in his strength. His determination is as strong as ever and no matter how tired or bad he may feel he never says no to getting his workout for the day. This determination is what will fuel his recovery!

I can't believe we have been here more than two weeks already. From our first day here we have been blessed to know we are not alone and that the support behind us is great. I want to say thank you to everyone who has sent us messages, cards, donations, flowers and for the visits from friends and family: Mike's aunt Shari; his uncle Carl with wife Vicki and daughter Brie; our Tom Jones friends Les, Kevin and Hope; our New York friends Stacy (who works labor and delivery at UCLA and even did my laundry!), Nandita (who happens to be here putting up her play) and Frank (who is flying in tomorrow); new friends Doriana and Pastor Eric; and of course Mike's amazing mom Kathy, my angel sister Marianne and our beautiful boys, Evan and William. These visits, while they may be short, remind Mike and I that we are loved and not alone in this fight. Thank you everyone for all you do for us! I will let you know when we get the green light!

Much love and keep the prayers coming!

> *Karine Z*
> *You're a powerhouse family and deserve every bit of support you're getting, even more!!! We love you. Mike, you're an inspiration!!*
>
> *Robin C*
> *You are all so loved. We hold you in our hearts and constant prayers. Glad you got some cuddle time with the boys and they got to see you. I know that meant a lot to them. Remember you are always loved by so many.*
>
> *Tammy C*
> *So glad you had such a nice visit with Kathy, Marianne and the boys! Mike, although this is not the "triathlon" you were training for, I am thankful God has given you such an amazing woman to encourage you in this "race." You also have many fans out here cheering for you! I'm sure the finish line seems many miles away, but just remember ... through adversity comes redemption! Not only will you cross that finish line, you will be the winner!!!!!! Sending you both lots of love! Your fans, Brett, Tammy and Emma*

*Erica M*
*I think of you every day and I am amazed by the strength and love of your family. I keep you in my prayers and in my heart. Love you all so much. In my vision you are dancing the same way you did on your first dance at your wedding. Keep strong!*

*Gail R*
*I pray for you, Mike, and the boys every day. Thanks for keeping us posted. Hang in there!*

*John M*
*Sounds like a whole lotta sweetness during a crazy time for you guys. So glad for you that it happened and you had your hearts filled. Kids are AMAZING gifts. We're still praying, praying, praying!*

*JoLayne G*
*Your positive attitude shines through in such a difficult, and I am sure dark, time. Still praying here for full healing and for the strength to keep dancing in the rain!*

*Nathan T*
*Mike, we are still with you. Thinking about you every day. Keep up the unshakable attitude!*

## Green Light

By Karen Turnbull — Jan 23, 2015

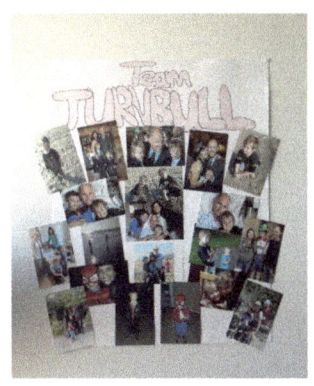

Prayer warriors unite! The hope is we are a go on Sunday! Mike is getting an MRI right now. This will be used for a fresh image for surgery. Please everyone unite in prayer that no obstacles get in our way. Mike has been amazing but frustration is setting in. This has been so hard and he is ready to take the next step. My friend Annie taught me that green is the color of hope. I have worn some token of green every day since I have been here. If you can, please wear something green this weekend and especially on Sunday. I am literally hanging on to hope!

THE STORM INTENSIFIES | 143

Thank you all. Now more than ever please keep those prayers coming! Much love!

### JoLayne G
Well, Green is always with me since it is my last name! And this Green friend will be praying hard!

### Etsuko M
Green light is great!!! You and Mike have been always on our mind, and we will be praying strongly. Hang in there!!!

### Dawn K
I also read green is the color of health. Green for Mike this weekend. Keep the faith and strength, Turnbulls. Sending love.

### Liese W
Sunday ... green ... go! HOPE! LOVE and readiness for this step. Tomorrow, the Lord's Day!

### Issa F
Well, wouldn't you know! The candle I have kept lit for you is green! Yay, happy coincidence! God is great!

### Sharon H
PRAYING!!! And yes, on Sunday, green will be the color of the day!! Standing united in prayer with all who know and love you!!

### Doreen L
You got it! Green it is! Anxious to get your next post!!!

## So Far So Good
*By Karen Turbull — Jan 24, 2015*

Mike is stable with good vitals. His platelet counts started going up and his breathing has been strong. So far we are a go. The nurses said the exact time may not be set until after midnight, probably due to traumas that may come in. I'm guessing somewhere between 7:00 and 8:00 AM. He is exhausted and sleeping peacefully right now. Thank you all for showing your support and humoring my silly request for wearing green. I just figure if all of the amazing people in our lives unite in force and wear a reminder of Mike's fight, we can be that much stronger. I will post in the morning as soon as we are a go! (Special thanks to our dear friend Frank for flying across the country to be with us!)

I am sure you know what I am going to say but ... KEEP THE PRAYERS COMING!

### *Marianne M*
*Karen, if I remember correctly Grandma Rieke's favorite color was green! With her ring on your finger, I believe she will be one of the guardian angels watching over both you and Mike. Love you both so much. I am praying!*

### *Betty S*
*The priest at Mass tonight wore green vestments!!! Dad and I just looked at each other. That has to be a good sign! Our thoughts and prayers are with you both!*

### *Hope M*
*Wearing green on Sunday ... that's Hope X 2 !!!!! We love you and are praying for all things GREAT.*

### *Rocco B*
*We are praying for a successful surgery and Mike's strength to heal. God bless the surgeons and their staff. Also praying for your strength, Karen. YES, we are all here, in mind and spirit!!!!!*

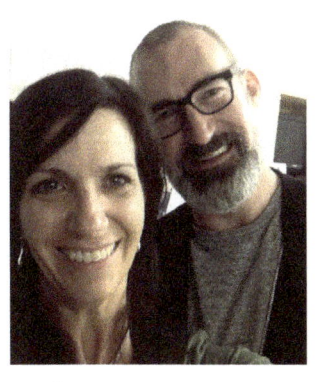

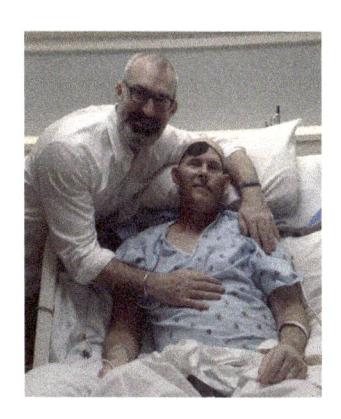

Frank Leusner

# YES!

*By Karen Turnbull — Jan 25, 2015*

Mike has been officially marked for surgery. Waiting for transport to take him to the OR. He is ready and we are both optimistic!

PRAYERS!!!!!!

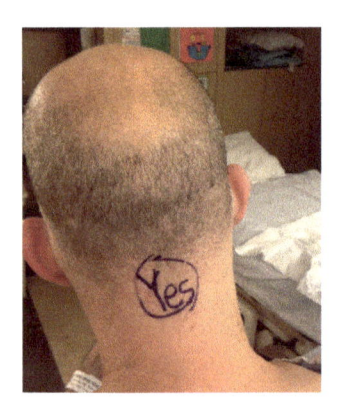

### Michelle B
*Go Team Turnbull! Kyle and I lit a candle after Mass just now for Mike and all of the surgical team that God's loving hands will guide them to success! Wearing our green and praying hard. Hugs to both of you.*

### Betty S
*We are praying!!! Wearing green & candles lit!!!*

### Karen K
*Got on our green! As did the priest at mass this morning. Candle lit at church. You are in our constant thoughts and prayers as is Dr. Martin and his team. Keep breathing, Karen! xoxo*

### Birgit D
*Praying for a successful surgery, a speedy recovery and strength for the both of you. Wearing green thinking of Mike and you.*

*Birgit P*
We are thinking of you guys and sending all of our positive thoughts your way. Green is the color in our house today!

*Suzanne P*
Karen, I have chills all over my body with anticipation of a fantastic outcome!

*Dan S*
So happy to hear!! Let's do this thing! :-) Brighter days ahead! Praying.

*Jaclyn F*
Wearing green and praying!! Stay hopeful and know that you have many, many, many people praying today and always ... some of which you don't even know!!

*Marianne M*
Your beautiful boys, Kathy and I are all wearing green! We are praying for God to give you strength throughout this day, for God to guide Dr. Martin and his surgical team and especially for Mike, that God will give him strength and guide him to a quick and speedy recovery! Love and prayers!

*Keith N*
Hope: Lord God Almighty, we direct our prayers to you on behalf of the Turnbull family. Let your face shine upon them. Grant them peace and an abundance of Grace. May the power of your redemptive love guide the doctors and support staff during this corrective procedure. Triathlon Mike, we're hanging out at the finish line cheering you on!

*Jenna L*
Wearing green and praying! Exodus 14:13-14, "Don't be afraid, just stand still and watch The Lord rescue you today. The Lord himself will fight for you. Just stay calm." Keeping you in our thoughts and prayers

*Nathan T*
All six of us Tanouyes are in green!

# It Has Begun

*By Karen Turnbull — Jan 25, 2015*

I just kissed him "see you later" and they took him back. I know everyone is already doing this but I am asking anyways ... please pray that God keeps him safe. I know they have to tell you about possible things that could happen and I believe that Mike will be just fine but it is still terrifying.

Dear God, please wrap Mike in your arms, keep him safe and hold him tight. Please guide Dr. Martin and his team of surgeons, anesthesiologists, nurses and all others who will be in the OR today. Thank you for guiding us here and providing us with the best care for this situation. Dearest Lord please be with him today for this long surgery and bring him through it safely. In your name I pray. Amen.

Keep the prayers going strong!

> ***Tammy C***
> *Beautiful prayer, Karen!! Couldn't have said it any better! Sending you hugs!! God is with you, comforting you and giving you peace! Angels are watching over you and Mike in the OR. Love you bunches!!!!*
>
> ***Karen O***
> *I look like a leprechaun! Thoughts are with you.*
>
> ***Candy P***
> *Amen. We are standing beside you.*
>
> ***Tim L***
> *Prayer for you and Mike at church right now.*
>
> ***Liz S***
> *Going to church right now!*
>
> ***Sam Ba***
> *Our prayers are with you. Pastor Tom led us in prayer for Mike and your family as we laid hands on Marianne and Mike's mom at New Song today. It was beautiful.*
>
> ***Lynne E***
> *Your prayer couldn't be more perfect so if you don't mind it will be your words I'll repeat throughout the day, with the edit that God wrap both you and Mike in his arms. Much love from both of us.*

# Safe

*By Karen Turnbull — Jan 25, 2015*

The nurse just checked in with me. Mike is safe and doing well. Dr. Martin says everything is going as planned!

*Shelley De*
Hope, faith and love are sent your way. We know Mike is safe and in good hands. He is finally getting the opportunity to become well. Team leader Karen, continue to be strong as you have a whole army of supporters behind you. Keeping you and your family in my constant thoughts.

*Issa F*
Waiting to exhale!

# Still Safe

*By Karen Turnbull — Jan 25, 2015*

Recent phone call from the OR nurse says Mike is stable and safe. Dr. Martin is still doing his thing!

Keep the prayers coming!

*Bessie D*
Have been praying all day. Thank you for all the updates, Karen.

*Monique E*
Thank you for the updates!! Praying!

*Heather W*
Praying, praying, praying! And I've done several green "costume changes" today and am attempting to wear as many shades of green as possible! :)

*Matt J*
One tiny sliver of that cavernoma at a time. One step closer to recovery. God is Great!!

# Surgery Is Over

*By Karen Turnbull — Jan 25, 2015*

Surgery is over. Dr. Martin said everything went beautifully! They got the whole thing out and Mike's brain showed electric activity right away! The only twist is that initial pathology shows it may be metastatic cancer. Full pathology results won't be in for five days. Focusing on the good news ... it is out!

Thank you everyone for all your prayers. Please keep them coming! Mike has a long road ahead of him.

> *Judy E*
> So much to be thankful for, yet so much to continue to pray for. I hope your journal becomes a book!
>
> *Matt J*
> Hallelujah ... I pray that both of you will sleep well. What an amazing surgical team!!
>
> *Doreen L*
> Wow! That was quicker than anticipated! I'm choosing to ignore the possible negative and praise the Lord for the real present positive! Of course, prayers continue for both of you and your families. Karen, hope you can get some sleep tonight.
>
> *Candy P*
> Thank you for your strength, to your doctors and for all your updates. You are all amazing.
>
> *Devonee M*
> Karen, thank you for being so faithful in your updates today. We all wore our green and prayed for Mike all day. We love you both so very much! So glad the surgery is over and was successful!
>
> *Lanie F*
> Sending more prayers. Hallelujah that they got it out!

# ICU

*By Karen Turnbull — Jan 26, 2015*

I am in the ICU with Mike. He actually opened his eyes in response to my voice! He also gave the nurse a thumbs up, wiggled his fingers and toes and also squeezed the doctors hand!!! He is on a breathing tube but they are hopeful that it can be removed tomorrow. He had a post-op CT to check the swelling and it looked good. He will have another one at 6:00 AM to watch closely for any swelling. They have him comfortably sedated but not so drugged that he can't respond. He has been through a really rough day and is pretty beat up but honestly I think he looks amazing and beautiful! It will be slow but the doctors seem optimistic that many of the deficits he experienced will begin to reverse over time. After a few months of healing we may be looking at some treatments to battle the thyroid cancer obstacle. We will cross that bridge when we come to it. For now I am celebrating a hope-filled victory! When we left Las Vegas twenty days ago we didn't know if anyone could help us. So today was absolutely a miracle.

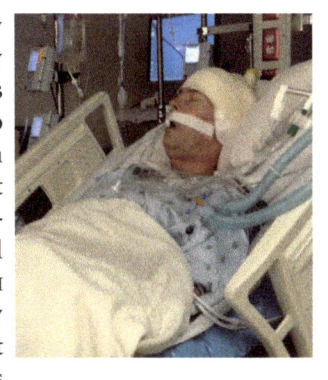

Keep the prayers coming! I know they will get him on his feet soon. And now I am going to try to sleep.

> *Megan H*
> *Yes, relief and victory will continue. Sleep well, angel.*
>
> *Marianne M*
> *Oh, Karen, I am so happy to hear this! Finally, tears of joy! Mike is one special guy with so much to live for, with you at the top of the list and the boys right behind. I love you all so very much! Sleep well!*
>
> *Jeff L*
> *Incredible, inspiring news!!! Take a deep breath, enjoy this victory and know that you are surrounded by the love of so many friends!*
>
> *Marsha R*
> *We are so very thrilled to hear the good news. We went to the Jazz Society meeting today and told everyone the news and asked that*

they all join in to wear green to support your hope and renewal. Now we pledge to keep up the prayers for total healing. We won't give up.

### Suzanne P
Awwwwwww, Karen. It brought tears to my eyes when you wrote that he opened his eyes when he heard your voice. That is the best news ever. Get some great sleep. Big, big hug.

### Ric F
Fantastic!!!!!!!

### Hayley M
What a wonderful read. So very happy that everything went well. Mike is clearly a fighter. I can't begin to think about how you have coped and held it together through all of this, Karen. We think about you both often and have you in our thoughts and prayers. Much love to you all. Get some rest.

### Liese W
Rejoicing with this news, Karen! All of you need some rest and restoring, but the healing light is shining brightly. Prayer warriors will continue to hold you all in love and joy for the first steps accomplished. Rest and reset for the next leg! Love you.

### Sharon H
On my knees in gratitude! Wonderful news!!!!!

### Jenna L
What joy! Amazing! A thumbs up from Mike is truly awesome! We continue to lift you both up in prayers and are giving thanks for the miracle you are experiencing!

### Bill B
Blessings to you and Mike! I love your comment, "He looks amazing and beautiful!" Just saying those words will heal him more than you realize.

### Kelly C
Karen, our family has been thinking about you all so much. We are so happy to read the good news this morning! Our prayers will keep coming your way! Marc, Kelly, Adam & Austin

*Jennifer P*

What a talented team of medical professionals. I am so glad Mike is in their care!!!! Sounds like he is going to recover well. Pulling for you all. Love you guys!!!

*Melin F*

I am so happy and relieved. You, Karen, have been an amazing advocate, reporter and steadfast partner through all of this. We, your extended family and friends, are amazed at your resilience and ability to remain calm and recount everything to us through this site. We will keep you and Mike in our prayers always. Bless you both ... we are with you.

*Antonette L*

Wonderful news ... sweetest of dreams to you, Karen. XO

*Ralph P*

The Las Vegas Boneheads wish you the best, always. Onward and upward!!

*Shawn M*

I marvel at your grace and strength, all of you. Sending love and prayers.

*Lynne E*

What wonderful news! Hugs to both of you. His reactions so soon after surgery are a definite indication that God and your surgeons worked a miracle. Take a good nap. I'm sure that you are exhausted. Our prayers won't stop as Mike will need them for his future rehab and complete recovery. Keep those positive vibes.

# Today 1/26/15

*By Karen Turnbull — Jan 26, 2015*

I know everyone is curious to know how today has been. To quote Mike: "This sucks." This morning they lightened his sedation to see how his responses were. This was so they could see if it was safe to remove the breathing tube. With that came some pain and confusion due to all the anesthesia. The good news is he was able to breathe just fine and after watching him closely for two hours they were able to remove the breathing tube. The bad news is the two-hour wait was awful. They had his wrists restrained so he wouldn't rip out the tube on his own, but this didn't prevent him from trying. On the plus side I was glad to see him feisty but I was also scared for him. He was pretty anxious and kept trying to sign to me. After many failed attempts I finally figured out, as he was staring at the clock, that he was asking me "how long?" and "15 minutes?" He wanted to know when they would get that stinking tube out! Finally it was out and he has been breathing steady since.

His vision is still blurry, although it may be slightly better. It is hard to tell as he is pretty out of it. The strength of his limbs is great. He is moving both arms and legs very well and it seems like he has a little more awareness of his right side. The facial drop on the left side is still there. Time will tell if that begins to improve. His left eye doesn't want to close all the way, which hopefully is just temporary, but for now it is taped shut to try to let him rest. Unfortunately he is actually hyper-aware of everything. He is in that funky drug-induced zone where things feel out of his control and he keeps thinking he is in bad shape. Believe me, I am delivering positive affirmations out the wazoo! I keep trying to reset his computer to say, "I am healthy, I am strong, I am healing."

Lastly, there is concern about his swallowing. Today when the ENT doctors did a scope they found one of his vocal cords is not functioning. He can speak, although it is a little difficult, but his swallowing is really difficult. Tomorrow they will do an X-Ray swallow test to check and see if he can control where food and drinks go. For tonight they have inserted a tube through the nose into the stomach so they can get him some nutrients and longer-lasting pain meds.

Dr. Martin warned us that things would be worse directly after surgery. I guess he was telling the truth. I keep reassuring Mike that this is temporary. I pray it is. So tonight I pray that tomorrow is a little better. I pray he passes his swallow test. Wow, the things we take for granted! I know this is a lot of information but I also know everyone is wondering how he is.

I hope this information can help focus your healing thoughts, energy, love, light and prayers. Keep it all coming!

> *Virginia H*
> *I feel for you so much, not just Mike. It is so hard to be there and unable to make it better. Mike is a fighter and you are one strong lady. I keep you and Mike in my thoughts. Keep fighting!*

*Jeneane H*
*Stay strong. I am amazed at how brave you both are. Always praying for you both. Hope Mike can find some comfort tonight. Love you*

*Megan H*
*This is an encouraging update. It HAS to be terrifying and frustrating for Mike to endure all he has endured. Triple that for the person who would give anything to take that pain and confusion away so she could make everything okay again. You are both just amazing and inspiring in your grace. I love you. Hang in there ... One step at a time.*

*JoLayne G*
*Lord, I pray his pain and anxiety will lessen and you will bring relief. I pray his swallowing will return. I pray for Karen's peace and to know what to say in difficult situations. I pray they know your presence in a very real and undeniable way. We know you know every need and entrust you to come to their aid. I thank you for being with them. Bless and keep them in your care and be with their boys at home. In your precious son's name I pray, Amen.*

*Randy C*
*I can't know what you are going through, but I do understand your frustration and Mike's. You are both doing very, very well in a very tough situation. I pray that tomorrow is better for both of you, and you can start to see the light at the end of the tunnel. God bless you both. Lots of love!*

*Michele R*
*Continued prayers of improvement and healing. Coventry misses all of you and we are here when you return!*

*Cathy M*
*Many thanks for the detailed update, Karen. Though some of it is heartbreaking, there are certainly some great victories. So grateful for Mike to be able to breathe on his own and be responding. Karen, I know you are "dancing on the head of a pin" as you witness what Mike is going through, but the comfort and love you shower him with is invaluable to his healing. Praying for a good result with the swallow test and that each day will bring Mike freedom from pain, confusion and anxiety. Holding you both in our hearts every day.*

*Nellie S*
It is temporary and it will get better. I pray for Mike to believe that and to start feeling better day by day. I pray for you to continue to be strong so you can be his rock. Lots of hugs and prayers sent your way.

*Dan S*
Thanks, Karen! Hopefully each day will be a little bit better than the one before it and they will pass fairly quickly for you both during this road to recovery. Continuing to pray!

*John M*
God bless you, Mike! We're thinking about you OFTEN and praying to the Lord for his mercy and healing grace.

*Betty S*
How do I say, "Thank You to the Army of Supporters." You are all a major part of Team Turnbull! I read your notes of true compassion being sent out to Karen and Mike. Yesterday all of you were waiting for word of the Christmas Miracle we have been praying for. Thousands of messages have been sent. Thanks Again for your Spiritual support and support to gofundme. Karen, Marianne, Kathy and Michelle, you ladies are special!!!

*Dene R*
Mike is amazing! And Karen, so are you! Keep the faith and all of your friends, family and people you do not know continue to pray!

*Nicole B*
You are an amazing caretaker! Mike is in great hands! There is definitely light at the end of the tunnel. Keep hope alive! xoxo

*Kim F*
You both are amazing. It does sound extremely promising. The brain is a remarkable organ capable of healing itself by rerouting the neurological connections. It is equally a great sign that Mike is feisty! He (and you) have too much "fight" and too much faith to let this get you down. Sending lots of love and prayers your way!

*Heather L*
Feisty is good!! Praying for a quick recovery!

*Amy K*
*We are praying for you guys! You are so strong and amazing!!!!!!!!!*

*Elizabeth H*
*Thank you, Karen, for taking the time and energy to let us know about Mike. So many people are praying and asking ... we keep praying for you all. I take you both everywhere I go in my thoughts and prayers. Love and so many prayers from West Virginia.*

*Alicia B*
*You are being so positive! Keep it going! Right after surgery is always the worst. Keep this in mind. It can only go up. Sending positive thoughts and prayers. You are all amazing fighters!!*

# Out of ICU

*By Karen Turnbull — Jan 27, 2015*

Who goes through a ten-hour brain stem surgery and moves out of ICU just forty-eight hours later? That's right ... Mike! Now, he thinks they are all crazy for thinking he is ready to move because he feels so awful, but here is today's progress: his left eye now closes all the way, he had the extra IV lines removed as well as the catheter, Physical Therapy got him sitting at the edge of the bed where he marched and kicked his legs, he momentarily was able to buzz his lips and he actually felt me touch his right arm and foot! So I would say it was a pretty busy day! The swallow test got moved to tomorrow. I think this was in hopes that some of the action may come back. He also had an MRI, which we have not heard follow-up on. Usually this means no news is good news.

The worst part of the day is that as he is working through flushing all the drugs from surgery and the pain medicines out of his body, his mental state has been confused. He had several moments of saying, "I'm scared," over and over. I kept reassuring him but he looked at me and said, "Are you lying? Are you b**s****ing me?", which made me laugh out loud, which just made him mad. I assured him that I am a horrible liar and that he was in fact doing very well. The only thing that could get him to calm down was me repeatedly telling him about the boys. Imagining their smiles, giggles, hugs and kisses thankfully did the trick. I continue to pray each day gets slightly better. He feels truly awful and his speech is pretty weak. He is also very anxious. Much of this could be due to the fact that he has had very little sleep. So as I say goodnight I pray for rest so he can be calm and heal.

Please keep those prayers coming. Things are pretty hard right now.

### *Debbie M*
*Huge progress. You guys are both amazing. You are constantly in our thoughts. Sending love.*

### *Randy C*
*Prayers coming your way to get through this tough period. So glad Mike is on the other side of the surgery. He has every right to be confused and scared. Good for you for being such a positive guide for Mike to follow. This, too, shall pass. God bless you both!*

### *Tammy C*
*So happy to hear that today was a positive day! Mike never stops amazing us with his abilitty to progress so quickly! Karen, you are doing great with your encouraging words to Mike! That's exactly what his brain needs to hear to heal. I pray for God's loving arms to embrace Mike and give him the peace that he needs to let him know that he is doing great!!! Karen, you're truly an angel sent from heaven! God knew that you had within you all that Mike needed to encourage him in his journey to wellness. Keep it up! You're both amazing!!*

### *Janna R*
*I am so glad Mike has you in his corner. You are awesome to find so much strength to encourage him. So glad for his steady improvements. Prayers and hugs from Florida.*

### *Liese W*
*You are both wrapped in love and continued rest and healing. The system flush is probably the hardest of all; many mixed sensations floating in every tissue of the body. You are a solid foundation and voice of reason. I pray a blessed day for continuing healing. Maintain the rich humor and devotion. Soon he will be talking with the kids and walking down the hallway! I wish I could bottle my student's energy and send it to Mike, but I will pray it there!!*

### *Bert V*
*What an amazing display of strength you are, Karen. Love to you both!*

*Mary Alice J*
Karen and Mike, we continue to pray to St. Anthony for both of you. Every word Mike speaks and movement he makes is truly a blessing in disguise after the surgery he has just gone through.

*Sara I*
You both are so brave and amazing! This is exciting news. You're always in our daily thoughts and prayers. We love you both so much! Keep the Faith. The best is yet to come!!!

*Cindi R*
I am sure when you are in the midst of it they seem like LONG days and small steps but reading your updates also seems very encouraging. You are right. Only forty-eight hours and he's making good progress! Continued prayers.

# Busy Day

*By Karen Turnbull — Jan 28, 2015*

Today started out pretty rough but as I am writing this Mike is (finally) peacefully sleeping. On Monday night they placed a feeding tube in Mike's nose to get him some nutrition and meds. On Tuesday afternoon it fell out. They didn't put it back in because the hope was that Mike would pass his swallow test and maybe not need it. The problems were 1) he had no nutrients other than IV fluid and 2) he couldn't get any oral medication. They gave him an IV pain medicine but within five minutes he threw up and went into another anxiety attack. This time was worse than the first. Finally I got him calmed down and he slept.

This morning he was hungry, tired and hurting. One of the resident doctors that has been working with us came in to check on him. The good news is his eyes began tracking left (which they have not done in a month) and he had more sensation in his right arm and leg. The bad news was she mentioned oncology coming in to talk to us. Up to this point Mike did not know that there was a possible link to his cancer. Given his confused and paranoid state I felt it best not to upset him more, especially since nothing had yet been confirmed. Well, this news set him off, understandably so. I explained to him that nothing was yet confirmed and one step at a time. As it turns out oncology never came by so we still don't know what they have to say. We got through the morning with a small dose of morphine. The swallow test happened at noon today and I am very happy to say he passed! So now he can eat puréed food and get oral meds crushed in applesauce. After a giant Jamba Juice smoothie and some pain meds that work for him, he is resting!

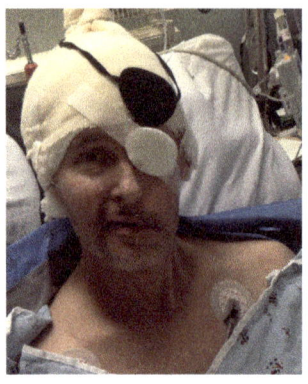

The other news is the social worker from UCLA called to tell me there is thought of discharging him, possibly as soon as Friday. We think this is a little rushed considering he is still incredibly beat up. Occupational Therapy came today with the hopes of getting him to stand. That thought was pushed aside when just sitting on the edge of the bed made him throw up (we think due to the reaction from last nights pain meds). So I am thinking Friday may be a little bit of a stretch but it is nice to know that our time here is almost over. The plan will be to move him to an acute rehab physical therapy facility. The question still remains whether that will be here in Los Angeles or at home in Las Vegas. A lot of this will depend on insurance, the best facility for his case and safe transport. Details are being worked out and I will let you know the plan. We are looking forward to the next step, but just want to be sure we get him there safely.

Keep the prayers coming!

> *Randy C*
> Well, I know it's rough, but I sure like what I'm reading! Especially Mike regaining moves he previously lost. That can only be good. We are patiently waiting for your return, but you must do what is right for Mike. We will be here, ready to help any way we can. Lots of love.
>
> *Nellie S*
> Praying that you end up at the place that's best for Mike and that he gets there safely. Big hugs. Really miss you guys. Praying that I see you both across the way soon.
>
> *Megan H*
> All good news (except the anxiety, pain and throwing up part. Oy!)! Seriously, though, it's amazing. We are still wearing a bit of green every day and you are constantly in our thoughts. Thank you for the update.

*Shelley De*

*Karen, you are an amazing woman. The pillar of strength is incredible. So glad Mike is progressing. A big operation of his nature takes baby steps. Wow, being able to swallow is great. Hopefully in a week or two he will be able to be moved to a hospital closer to home. Prayers and hugs are sent daily for Mike's recovery and your enduring strength as you pull him through. Stay strong, rest and keep letting Mike know there is an army of supporters behind him. Thanks so much for the updates.*

*Becky C*

*Karen you are soooo amazing and so strong. I'll keep praying for you guys. Xoxo*

*Monique E*

*You're so strong, Karen. I admire you and have always looked up to you, but now in so many more ways. You two are inspiring. Love you and keep the strength.*

*Jenna L*

*Fear not! So much progress! This is all so amazing and a testimony that God is present! We continue to pray and believe in complete healing! You are both so strong. I was just thinking when I read your post about the scripture reading at your wedding ... Faith, Hope and Love and the greatest of these is Love. Your love is inspirational and your faith and hope are strong! May God give you his peace!*

*Elizabeth H*

*Praying that doctors will receive wisdom in making decisions for Mike's well-being. I know that you know where your amazing strength and courage come from. Continued prayers offered up on your behalf. Your West Virginia Connection.*

*Les K*

*Great news! Good thing is Mike's on his way to healing! Praying for his healing and your peace of mind. You've been through so much!!! God bless and hang in there:-)*

# Laughter

*By Karen Turnbull — Jan 29, 2015*

It has been so long since Mike and I truly laughed together. Today we celebrated by laughing! I think we are turning the corner. Today was actually a really good day. I think we have figured out his medicines to make him feel the least amount of pain with the least amount of side effects. He had occupational therapy, where he stood up out of the bed and sat in a chair for a few hours. He did hand exercises as well as vocal chord exercises. He also had a visit with the lead doctor of Head & Neck Robotic Surgery. He used a scope-guided camera to inject Mike's vocal cord with a filler. It basically plumped up the damaged vocal cord. Immediately afterwards he was able to swallow normally, which means he can drink normal liquids without having to thicken them. It should also help strengthen his voice. Still no solid foods as the left side of his face is too weak to properly chew. Mike also had physical therapy. He actually took a few steps forward and backwards and marched in place! These are huge advancements! Plastic Surgery also visited today. They are talking about putting a gold weight inside Mike's left upper eyelid. This will assist in the closing of the eye. From what we understand it is a very easy procedure and takes only about fifteen minutes. The hope is this could be done before being discharged to prevent any damage to the cornea.

The thought now is that we may be discharged as early as Monday. We still do not know where he will be transported for rehab but I do feel that everyone is working to make the best decision for Mike's case. Tonight our beautiful friend Stacy came to visit when she was done with her nursing shift. It was fun to sit around, be silly and just laugh. I am grateful to be on this side of surgery!

Thank you all for your support and as always keep those prayers coming!

> ***Kathy A***
> *So much love to you both!! Lots of prayers and love coming your way for a speedy recovery! Keep LAUGHING :)*
>
> ***Abby A***
> *So glad to hear this joyous news. Much love to you both!*
>
> ***Cindy E***
> *Karen & Mike, we are so glad it was a good day. The first of many more to come! Thank you for updating this so often. We*

*anxiously wait every day to know how you are doing. Miss you. Lots of love.*

### Nellie S
*That is wonderful news! Praying that every day gets better and better. I know there will be many, many days of laughter up ahead!*

### Kelsey P
*Laughter is the best medicine!!! Love you both!*

### Frank S
*That makes me so happy to hear that you guys had a little laughter and lightness ... yay for that!*

### Kenneth S
*Hey Mike, Rita and I are praying for you. Laughter is so good for the soul. Look forward to playing with you again ... miss your smiling face.*

### Karine Z
*Such wonderful news, Karen!! Thank you dear friends, you are such a gift to us all!*

### Jennifer Z
*Karen, this is wonderful news! You and Mike are still in my prayers.*

### Antonette L
*As they say, laughter is medicine for the soul ... so laugh on, friend!!*

### Linda Q
*How truly wonderful! What a great blessing to be seeing and feeling so much progress so quickly! Laughter truly is a gift to be savored always, and especially during such a time as this. Much love and prayers continue.*

### Rocco B
*We are all so happy to hear that Mike is progressing. We are praying that he gets the best of care and that he is able to rebound from this. Mike, you are a superhero!!!! Keep up the fight, my brother. Not one day goes by where you aren't thought of and prayed for. Please know that we all care about you and want to see you in good health. By the way, when the doctors were in your brain, were they able to tighten that one screw we talked about? lol :) Thanks again, Karen. You are amazing!!!!! Praying for all of you.*

*Melin F*
*Your one-word headers make opening and trying to absorb the information so much easier. We all have been worried and filled with prayer for you and Mike, and to see "laughter" lightens the information. This whole journey feels like it's coming to fruition. The next steps will be hard work but progress will show every day. We will be with you and we send the Swedish Prayers.*

# Outside!!!!

*By Karen Turnbull — Feb 1, 2015*

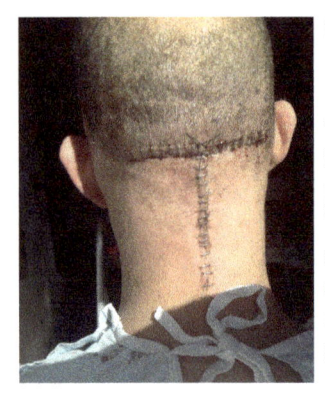

Today was huge! Mike had the wrap from his head removed ... thirty-nine staples forming a perfect T. Mike's words were "T for Team Turnbull!" The site is healing beautifully. Also, he received patio privileges so we got to go outside! This was the first adventure outdoors since December 29th! It was extremely emotional and amazing. To sit in the sun, feel the breeze and hear the birds was miraculous and awesome.

Mike is starting to get off some of the medications, which is helping him feel more alert and less out of it. We will find out in the morning where he goes from here. The hope is that a bed opens up across the street at UCLA's Neuro Rehab unit. He will stay for about two weeks and receive between four to six hours of therapy a day. This will include physical, occupational, recreational, speech and eye-training therapies. It will be hard but also really good. This will keep him close by his doctors as he recovers and builds his strength. Oncology came by today and said pathology is still working on Mike's case. Radiation oncology will be by tomorrow to discuss what they feel is best. It sounds like it could be just a few radiation treatments to act as an insurance policy to make sure there are no remaining cells, so today we are grateful for skilled doctors who have made healing patients their life work.

Last Sunday was incredibly long and scary. Thank you my amazing friend Frank (who flew in from NYC to be with me) and Shari (Mike's aunt) for keeping me company all day. I couldn't have done it without you. And, thank you everyone for holding Mike, me and our family in your hearts and prayers. This is definitely a team effort! I continue to wear green and keep my hope alive! Hope, prayers, love and light! Keep it all going strong! Love to you all!

### *JoLayne G*
*I have thought of you all day because the sermon at church was all about finding joy despite the hard things in life and how joy comes from gratitude to God. Then he used a story about a little girl whose father had cancer and about how she wanted to run through the rain while all the adults around her were worried about getting wet. Maybe I will try to find it and send it to you because it made me think of you going outside when it was raining and your motto of dancing in the rain. I can't imagine how tough things have been, and I am not suggesting you haven't had dark times, but your determination to keep looking for the joy is wonderful. Today I thanked God for the ability to just close my eyelids and I prayed that those simple things we take for granted will be restored to Mike.*

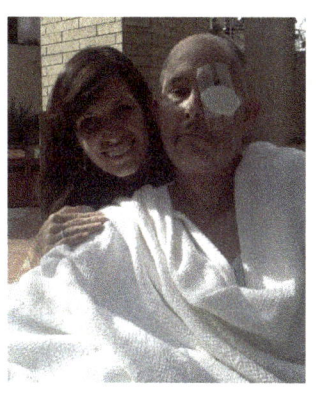

### *Sara I*
*Yours and Mike's unwavering Faith, Strength and Courage is Amazing and is serving Team Turnbull well! Know that we all Love you so much and you're Always in our thoughts, prayers and hearts!!! Much Love.*

### *Cathy M*
*What a difference a week makes!! So grateful for all the improvements and the simple pleasure of being outside today. Thank you for the detailed update. We hang on every word. We're encouraged by all the progress that Mike has made. Kudos to you, Karen, for all the tender loving care you give him, which no doubt increases his healing. Always with you on this journey. Much love.*

### *Jayme R*
*Praise God! What a day for Mike to feel the sun!! The rain clouds are parting!!!*

### *Joni S*
*Love this post, Karen! So glad to hear that he got to go outside and enjoy the beautiful weather and his beautiful wife. Still praying.*

*Margaret H*
Go Team T! We love you!

*Rocco B*
May God bless you both! Mike, hang tough brother. You are doing amazing!!!!! Karen, I can see where Mike's strength in you gives him the determination to fight! You are amazing!!!! We pray every day that he is blessed with health and well-being, giving him the opportunity to be the husband, father and friend that he is so deserving of. Much Love to both of you!!!!!

*Denise M*
Sending you showers of prayers, love, healing light and Reiki today. "See" Mike healed, healthy, whole and complete with full liberty of his mind, body and spirit.

*Adrienne S*
So happy healing is progressing smoothly. Way to go, Terrific Team Turnbull! Love you bunches and sending huge hugs!

*Lisa L*
Kind of a cool scar. So happy all is going well.

*Wesley M*
Love to you, Karen and family. What wonderful news. Team Turnbull!

# Rehab!!!

*By Karen Turnbull — Feb 3, 2015*

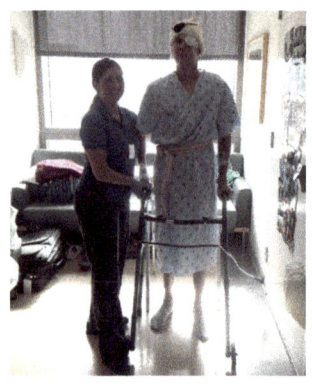

Oh my gosh! I cannot believe it. Tonight we moved Mike into the rehab facility here at UCLA. It is a small unit of a maximum eleven patients. Therapy will begin tomorrow morning at 7:00 AM! Right now he is in a semi-private room but he has no roommate at this time. I am able to stay in the room with him and there are even laundry facilities! Therapy will be hard and intense, but he is excited and it feels good to take this next step. He will have physical therapy, occupational therapy, speech therapy, recreational therapy and even pet therapy! Yes that's right, pet therapy! Every Thursday a black lab is on the hall to interact with patients. Mike will also receive zen therapy, which can include massage, Reiki and aromatherapy. So this next step, as hard as it will be, seems a lot better than where we've been. Thank you everyone for all you've done for us.

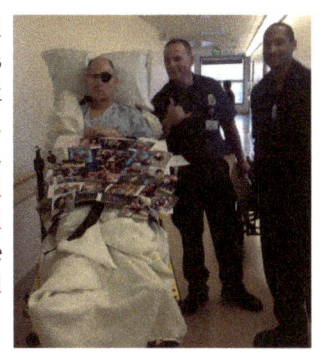

Please continue to surround Mike in your love and prayers as he begins this next chapter.

### Franz C
*Wonderful news. I'm sure Mike will thrive there! Ongoing prayers :)*

### Ellen F
*Fantastic news!! We are thrilled to hear this. The therapies are varied and seek to touch every part of Mike's being. I love it! Karen, please try to take care of yourself the best you can. You sound terrific, but we know this is hard on you. We pray for you and Mike and your whole family every day. God bless and thank you, Pastor Dave for watching over this wonderful family!*

### Antonette L
*You've got this, Mike ... Think of it as the beginning of Fiesta Island during the San Diego Marathon ... You are beyond tired, it's blazing hot, the water stops are spaced much too far apart, BUT you can hear everyone cheering you on and even though you can't see it the finish line is near. Some steps are going to be harder than others, but remember you ARE STRONG! And if there are moments where you can't find your strength, lean on your coach and your team and use their strength. I/we believe in you and are cheering you on ... GO TEAM TURNBULL!*

### Jason V
*I AM SO HAPPY FOR YOU GUYS!! This is great news!! Please send Mike my best regards. I'm sending more thoughts and prayers. This is a hard next step for him, but I know he can do it. He's strong!*

*Gary A*
*Always good to start the day with great news from Team Turnbull. All the best of thoughts and wishes for Mike in the beginning of this next phase. Team Turnbull is AMAZING!!*

*Issa F*
*Whew! Very exciting! I have to say, though, Mike ... There are less dramatic ways than major brain surgery to get an awesome "T" shaped scar on the back of your head ... just sayin'.*

*Kelene J*
*So glad he is on the road to recovery! We are all thinking of him here :) Sounds like a great rehab facility. Dogs, zen, massages! We are praying for you! Keep up the good work! Love, the D&M dancers!!!*

## Progress

By Karen Turnbull — Feb 6, 2015

It has been quite an adventure these past few days. Mike immediately started therapy on Wednesday. He was evaluated by all the different therapy modalities and met with the doctor at the rehab unit. Even though day one was mainly for evaluation it was hard-core and he was working all day. On the first day alone, here are some of the feats he achieved: he dressed himself, fed himself (incorporating his right hand, which has been pretty much non-functional), walked to the end of the hall and back with the walker, and most amazing of all went up and down six steps! Of course the therapists assisted as needed but these are huge improvements from just a few days earlier. Also, his diet was changed to mechanical soft. This means he can eat pretty much anything as long as it is not hard or crunchy.

Thursday, day two, showed even more improvements. He was able to shower for the first time in a month! (Sponge baths are fine but there is nothing like feeling hot water hit your face!). He also got to work with two of the sweetest little doggies, Maxine and Henry. The sensation in his right hand is very dull, although he is feeling elements of pain and temperature change, which is good. The senses for soft things are still not very strong but Maxine and Henry were very happy to help him work on this by receiving lots of petting. He also worked on giving cheerio treats to them with his right hand. The speech therapy was very hard. Because of the left side facial droop it is very difficult for him to enunciate and speak clearly. The tongue exercises were really challenging but I know they will help. PT had him working in the gym, building his core and doing squats, heel raises and leg lifts. These will all help strengthen his stabilization and mobility. And in the afternoon he did an extra session of therapy which incorporated riding a recumbent bicycle. He road two miles in five minutes! Muscle memory and motivation are a beautiful combination! Then he played Connect Four with one of the other patients. It is funny how a simple game that we played in our childhood is now therapy. He was required to use his right hand for picking up the pieces and dropping them in. At first this was horribly frustrating and difficult but after two games he was moving like a pro (and he won both times).

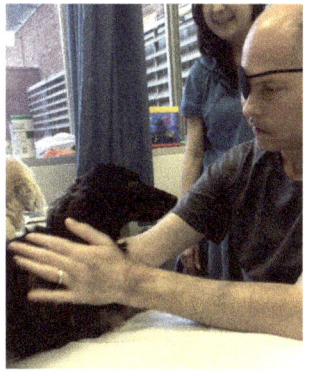

By 7:30 at night he is exhausted and snoring. His medication list is getting smaller daily. He is off of one steroid completely and the other has been lessened. This means he no longer needs insulin shots as his blood sugar level has stabilized. The only pain medicine he is receiving is Tylenol, so things are definitely improving. He is tired and at times very frustrated. The simple daily tasks that we all take for granted are now so hard. He worries about how he will function at home. He worries about how this will affect the boys. And he worries about what this is doing to me. I try to reassure him that we will get through it one moment at a time. But I'm not going to lie. It is really hard and scary to think how much life has changed.

As I write this I am sitting at LAX, about to fly home for a few days. Thank you to my friend Megan for making this possible and encouraging me to do so. For the first time in all of this, I definitely feel that I need a break. I pray Mike will be safe without me for a few days. I need to see my boys and recharge my batteries. I pray that the few days at home will refill me and give me the strength I need to face the next chapter. Mike needs our support now as much as ever.

Much love.

*Cynthia E*
Thank you Karen for all your posts. I watch daily and am so happy that Mike and your family is in the healing mode. You are the strongest woman I know and I wish I could be there to help more, but you and Mike are in my prayers daily. Love to you and yours!!!!!!! I hear it is beautiful right now in Vegas!!

*Darren K*
This is all great news that we all crave and appreciate. Go get some rest and home therapy yourself Karen, and remember, this is an exact scenario where we could fly out to be with Mike in your absence if necessary. Please don't hesitate to ask for our help.

*Dawn K*
Thanks for this update, Karen. So happy to hear it sounds like things are headed in the right direction. I hope you have a great few days with your boys, and I'll continue to keep Mike in my thoughts. I love this photo of him and his "therapists"!!

*Clare T*
Gosh, it's just simply incredible how quickly he is progressing and so wonderful. I think of you all daily and am so happy you can recharge with your sweet boys. I'm so glad Mike is getting stronger and I'll keep positive thoughts coming for continuing strength. xxxx

*Issa F*
You both are total badasses! It would be hard to leave Mike but I think God has taken a special liking to him and is right there no matter what.

*Birgit D*
I can only imagine how hard all this must be on you and the family. You are a strong woman. Prayers for Mike, you and the boys. Recharge those batteries and enjoy some time with your two wonderful boys.

*Virginia H*
Isn't God amazing? How He created us both mind and body, how we can relearn, retrain and recapture our basic functions. I am so amazed at Mike's progress. Keep up the hard work, you have two boys awaiting your homecoming. Karen, take time to regroup and rest!

*Mary F*

*What a rewarding but exhausting day for both of you! It's great to hear such positive news. I'm glad you're taking a few days to see the boys and get some well-deserved rest. You amaze me with your strength, Karen! I'll continue to pray for you and Mike.*

*Elizabeth H*

*Your great love for each other as a family will help sustain you. May God continue to help you take each new step day by day. Continued prayers lifted up among the hills of southern West Virginia.*

*Cindi R*

*Great updates. Pretty amazing in fact. So glad you get to go home and see your boys. You need to take care of yourself in order to keep taking care of everyone else. Don't feel guilty about that. Rest and play and recharge.*

*Ellen Sn*

*Stay strong, Karen. You are the central core that is holding it all together. What a wonderful girl you are, but I already knew that. It will take time but your life will go back to normal again! I am keeping you all in my thoughts. Xoxo*

*Karine Z*

*Spectacular news, Karen. What progress!!!! Enjoy your time with the boys. They will be so happy to see you!! You're the strongest family I know. You'll get through this next chapter. Love to you all!!*

*Jennifer P*

*I am sooooo happy for you guys. Sounds like you guys have an excellent rehab and attitude!!! Sending hugs and kisses!!!!!!*

*Joan F*

*Karen ... it sure sounds as though Mike is in the best place he can be right now! That in itself is a blessing ... prayers ars continuing from our family!!!*

# Homeward Bound

*By Karen Turnbull — Feb 9, 2015*

I flew back from Las Vegas today. I had an amazing weekend with my boys! We played, flew kites and snuggled! It was just what I needed. I returned to UCLA today and the decision was made that we will return home on Wednesday. It seems Mike is doing too well to stay in rehab! This, of course, is according to the insurance company. His doctors and therapists would love to see him stay one more week. After fighting for more time a compromise (if you can call it that) was met. The decision is for a Wednesday discharge. Insurance wanted to discharge him today. According to how he looks on paper, he is just doing far too well to remain in rehab. What a joke! Luckily, the doctor at the rehab facility told them that I needed trained on how to help him. He insisted that the earliest we could be released is Wednesday. Also, Mike experienced the fun of passing a kidney stone while I was gone. Apparently this is common after so much anesthesia.

So tomorrow is hard-core training for me. I will learn how to help yet not enable Mike. I have my job cut out for me. When this discharge idea was first presented to me I was furious, but I have calmed down and done a lot of serious soul-searching and praying. Now, I actually think being home will be best for everyone. Our boys need us home. It will be five weeks tomorrow that we have been away, and Mike needs to see and feel the boys' love. He will transition to an outpatient rehab facility. He still needs a lot of work. Rehab will continue to involve speech, occupational and physical therapy. I am not quite sure how the transition home will go, but I do trust that the strength we need, somehow, will miraculously show up.

Thank you to Mike's aunt Shari and uncle Joel for agreeing to drive us home on Wednesday. I don't know how I would have managed on my own and thank God I don't have to! And I am extremely grateful to Mike's mom Kathy for holding down the fort in our absence. Mike's cousin David came in when my sister had to go home. He was a great distraction and a lot of fun for the boys. Mike's sister Wendy flies in tomorrow to help as well. I don't know what I would do without these angels constantly surrounding us.

Please continue to keep us in your thoughts and prayers!

*Eric L*
*Mike's coming home!!!*

*Megan H*
"But I do trust that the strength we need, somehow, will miraculously show up." Of course it will ... your well is deeper than you think. You keep proving that. See you in Vegas!

*Monique E*
If anyone is wise enough to care for Mike at home, it's you!

*Antonette L*
Team Turnbull, you've got this! I know it's frustrating that leaving rehab isn't your choice, but think of it as running the race in your own backyard ... not the most fun because it's too familiar but it's sure to pay the most rewards because you'll end up "running" there soon enough. Mike rehabbing at home is going to get back to some kind of normalcy, and my lovely Karen you will be surrounded by people who love you. Give us chores. We are ready to help!

*Hayley M*
Wow, my goodness what a roller coaster of emotions for you both. I hope you have a safe journey home. As you said, the boys will love it and it will help with Mike's recovery. Laughter goes a long way. Thinking of you.

*Kimberly S*
Hope! Faith! Love! Trust!

*Karen K*
So glad you are heading home - what wonderful news! Your strength keeps "showing up" and because of who you are and how much you love your family, it will continue to. Please accept the help of those close by and for those of us that aren't, please know we are praying overtime! Much love to you all as you journey home. xo

# Adjusting

*By Karen Turnbull — Feb 16, 2015*

It is great to be home and to all be together again. Very special thanks to Mike's aunt Shari and uncle Joel for driving us home. They made a daunting task so much easier. Our time away was hard on everyone but especially on Evan. William, being three, tends to roll with the changes a little easier than Evan. Evan, being seven (almost eight) gets it. The fears and "what ifs", as I call them, can seem way too real and powerful. I have tried my best to be honest without overcomplicating things or being fearful, which is not an easy task. So, it is good that we have finished the "being apart" chapter. Now, it is about adjusting to this new phase. The boys have been amazing at this! They are so glad to have us home and they are so proud of every accomplishment Mike makes. We have made family game time a regular activity. This acts as 1) much needed family time and 2) therapy for Mike. He forces himself to use his weakened right hand to roll the dice or move his playing piece. It is not easy but he does it and I am very proud of him for not giving up.

Getting around the house is challenging but he is getting better at navigating with his wheelchair and his walking improves daily. He uses a half walker on his left side (the stronger side) and a special gait belt that lets me hold on to him in case he starts to tip. So far we are doing well as a team. Only when he tries to move too fast or turn too quickly does he topple a little, but I am able to gently guide him back and center his weight. We haven't moved upstairs yet but I am hopeful that we will be able to do so this week. Some friends have offered to install a banister up the left side of our staircase. Once this is in, the stairs should feel more manageable as he will be able to use his left hand to support himself. The problem with the right hand is that full sensation has not yet returned, so he has a hard time gripping and it tends to fall off the rail, which can cause his legs to buckle. Not something we want happening when trying to go upstairs! So for now the downstairs guest room will do.

Home PT and OT came to evaluate him. Thankfully they both agreed that he needs much more intense therapy at an outpatient rehab facility. Hoping for this to start this week. After the intense workouts UCLA put him through, the home visits were pretty weak. We are anxious for him to get in the rehab gym and get stronger. Our friend Franz is a physical therapist as well and he came to visit Mike on Friday. He worked him hard and it was awesome! The great thing about being challenged is the boost in confidence. Suddenly what seemed hard before doesn't seem as hard. He did things he didn't think he could do. I'm hoping that once he gets in the gym that will become the norm.

Mike's mom returned home after a long time taking care of our boys. I know I have said it before, but I honestly do not know how we would have done this without her. Kathy, I will never be able to thank you enough! Mike's sister Wendy is here but returns home Tuesday. It has been so helpful to have her here for these critical adjustment days. It is hard jumping back into life full-steam ahead. I have said before that life doesn't stop because you are dealing with cancer. Bills still need to be paid, lunches need to be packed, laundry needs to be done. I am trying to juggle my many hats. Most moments I am doing ok until the moment when I am simply not ok. But, I breathe through it, pick myself up and carry on, because what other option is there?

I have told Mike he is no longer allowed to apologize for how things are. Yes, I too am sorry that this is so hard. But the truth is that if twelve years ago on our wedding day I had been told this would happen, I still would have married him. Because even though this part is really hard, we have been blessed with more great times than I ever dreamed were possible. And we will get through this and have more. It just may take some time. I am a little worried about how I will (at some point) return to work. My FML will expire soon and I am not sure what happens then. Hoping I can apply for an extension. Until Mike is able to get around more independently my job is being with him. I try not to stress about this too much but like I said life doesn't stop just because this is going on.

I am unbelievably grateful for the gofundme.com/teamturnbull site. The money that has been donated to us during this battle is saving us more than I can express in words. If it weren't for that fund I don't know what we would do. Thank you to my amazing niece Michelle for setting it up and showing us how supported we are. Everyone who has sent us cards and checks, thank you! We are brought to tears every time we receive these amazing well-wishes. I purposely do not watch the news and haven't for years. It just tends to upset me and make me sad. I have to believe that the world is more good than bad. I have to believe that people actually want to help others. Through all of this we have seen so much kindness and generosity. I do believe in the good and I choose to focus on that, so thank you everyone for helping lift us up during these dark times. The light is showing, it is just baby steps to get there. Keep holding Mike in your prayers. This is harder on him than he thought it would be. Pray his eyes correct soon and the dizziness subsides. These are the two hardest obstacles. Pray he is able to recognize his improvements and not get too frustrated.

Thank you for loving him (and me) so much.

> *Brenda M*
> *Go Team Turnbull! Your updates are honest, heartbreaking and thought-provoking! Continued prayers and positive thoughts to you all!*

*Nathan T*
It's good to have you back, Mike! Karen, you are unbelievable. I will keep visualizing a good, strong recovery for Mike. Keep it up, you guys!

*Heide F*
Thank you for being an inspiration to all of us. This is what marriages are for ... sickness and in health ... rich or for poor ... 'til all of that do us part. Thank you my dear friend. All the best. We are so happy that you are home. With love.

*Shelley De*
Karen, you are a pillar of strength. It is hard but God gave you the power to be there for Mike and the kids. Glad you have family to give you a little break. In time Mike will get stronger. Keep encouraging him and the hugs from the boys to you and he will help. What a journey. Thanks for the updates when you have so little time. Keeping you, Mike and kids in my prayers.

*Bert V*
You continue to be in our thoughts and prayers "until forever and a day"! Much Love!

*Birgit D*
Praying for Mike and for you to keep your strength. You truly are an inspiration, Karen.

*Kristine K*
Wonderful reflective post, Karen. I am so grateful to know you. You indeed inspire me and because of you I too find strength in my life as I am approaching a new chapter. Yes, life goes on and we must be in it facing it head-on in its true reality. Love love to Mike. Love to your boys and strength, honor, respect and love to you, dear Karen.

*Melin F*
What a trooper you are, Karen. I know it's difficult at times and hard on Mike and the boys but you are the glue. Keep up the good work, keep the little boys happy and keep the big boy busy ... that's all??? Sounds simple, doesn't it? We send our love and I pray the strength you need to carry on will always be with you.

*Karen P*

*I just found this quote on my daily calendar and thought of the two of you: "Being deeply loved by someone gives you strength, while loving someone deeply gives you courage." Lao Tzu.*

*Joni S*

*I am so glad you are home and with your adorable boys. You and Mike continue to inspire me every day with your strength and love. You know we are always here for you. Praying for continued recovery. He is doing great!*

*Lisa L*

*So proud of both of you. You both are truly so special and strong!!!! You're always included in my prayers, for I do believe.*

*Lou G*

*Evan is a very, very brave kid. I hope this time is the last, scariest, harshest time he will ever have to get through all the rest of his days. I'm proud to know him, although he probably barely remembers when we met, if at all. You all have great courage and big hearts. Thank you for sharing the triumphs. Always sending a prayer and hope your way. Love from down the road.*

*Jenna L*

*Awesome news that you guys are home with your boys! The boys are the best medicine! You are both amazing! We are in awe of the progress Mike is making and the fact that he is home is a testimony of his strength and will and God's presence and healing! We continue to pray for complete healing and for the dizziness to end. Stay strong! You guys are doing great!*

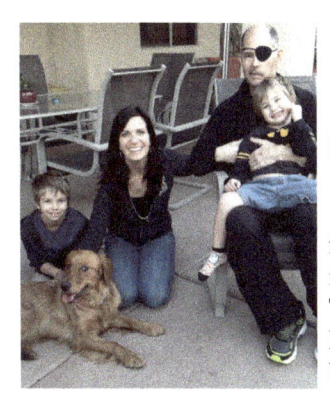

# Next Chapter

*By Karen Turnbull — Feb 24, 2015*

Today Mike and I met with and toured the NCEP (Nevada Community Enrichment Program) facility. This is an outpatient neurological rehabilitation facility here in Vegas. He starts tomorrow! This will be a 9:00-3:00 Monday through Friday rehab experience. It is much like UCLA's program but also focuses on getting him back to his pre-trauma self by incorporating outings and activities such as grocery shopping, cooking, bowling, fishing, woodworking, shows, etc. We laughed a little because he will go on different field trips each Friday! There is also counseling (available to me as well) and massage. We were warned that most clients hate the first two weeks (guessing because it is a lot to take in) but that then it gets better. The average stay is three months but depends on progress and of course ... insurance. We have fifty-seven days before we get booted by our insurance. Hoping that will be all he needs. I think it will.

Mike has made incredible progress at home just on his own. Since our friend Jimmy installed a stair rail, he has been using the steps about twice a day. Thank you Jimmy! He is also speaking clearer and napping less. Big improvements! His eyes are still frustrating him with the double vision, although with the eye patch it does seem to be clearer. He was able to participate in family movie night with us this weekend for the first time in months!!!

Also, we have added a new member to our team. A beautiful angel doggie named Baylee literally was delivered to our door. She needed a home and we needed some furry joy. Thanks Loree for choosing us to be her forever family! Since she has come into our home there are lots more smiles and giggles from everyone. I truly believe she was sent to us to bring some much needed healing. With Mike heading to "school" every day I am hoping this eases my transition back to work, which is fast approaching. I am hoping I can figure out how to juggle all the schedules, lunches, homework, etc. I may have to start cashing in on all the offers from friends and neighbors to help out. I don't know what I would do without the support team we have.

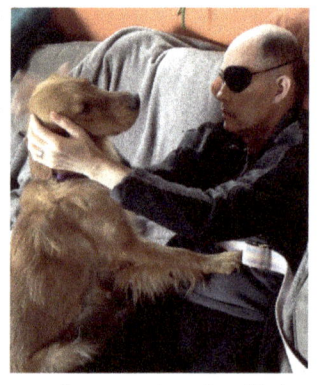

We head back to UCLA the beginning of April for follow-up appointments. I told Mike my vision is of him walking in to Dr. Martin's office with only a cane and no eye patch. Anyone care to join me on that? The representative at the rehab facility was shocked at Mike's story. The idea of a trombone player who came back after thyroid cancer invaded his trachea and now who, one month after brain stem surgery, is going up and down stairs made her shake her head and call him "Iron Man." I could only smile and nod ... yes, he is on his way back!!!

Keep all the amazing prayers, thoughts, meditations, energy and love coming! Much love to you all!

### Matt J
*Great news!! A beautiful family graced by a new addition. More prayers are in order. IRON MIKE: Onward and Upward!!*

### Alan R
*Dear Karen and Mike, I am so inspired by your progress and tenacity. I see you have the strength of your Grandmother Louise who is very happy about your progress and can't wait to see your whole family once more! I am sending prayers, good thoughts and healing all your way as well as friends who have shared your story. Your love is your key to healing and it is quite powerful. Just know that I am hoping and praying for your recovered health and happy future. All my love as always.*

### Susan S
*You are an amazing family. God is with you all the way! Lots of prayers going your way!*

### Christina P
*I literally woke up thinking about you and look what was in my inbox! All I want to do is holler "#$*# Yeahhhhhhhh!" None of us will ever truly know the strength, courage and fear that both of you face every day as you move through this journey, but know in your hearts that there is a sea of us out here loving you, cheering for you and crying with you, too! On the really hard, awful days know that you are loved and that you are warriors! Many loves and hugs to all of you!*

### Karen P
*We are SO glad about the new rehab facility. Iron Man will show them his stuff. And you, Karen, are simply amazing. I hope I never have to go through what you two have, but if so, I'll have the perfect role models. Good wishes to all five of you on rebuilding your life.*

### Mary Alice J
*Welcome, Baylee. You are such a lucky dog. You have a home with lots of love. Nice to hear good things are happening. Luvya.*

*Amy L*
You truly are an inspiration! So happy for you guys and how this journey is progressing ... XO

*Kristine K*
Iron Man! You are truly the best. Heart of gold and spirit of a warrior. Team Turnbull, looks like you're all on your way to recovery and healing. I applaud all of you. Blessings.

*John M*
Go Team Turnbull! It's exciting and encouraging to read this update and know what the team is up to now. I'm super glad to hear about Mike's progress and the rehab opportunity. Karen, you're doing EPIC work to handle everything and write these great posts so regularly. You both have so much to deal with now and I'm impressed by your determination. WAY TO GO!

*Jenna L*
Awesome! Amazing! This is great news! The progress being made is miraculous and spectacular! We are joining in the prayer that Mike walks in Dr. Martin's office with only a cane and no eye patch! I truly believe that Mike will see a complete healing! Your family together with an added new family member is the best part of the healing process. Lifting you all up in prayer as you continue on the journey! You are inspirational!

*Pete B*
Iron Mike Turnbull! You are an inspiration to us all!! Keep fighting! We are with you all the way!

# Rehabilitation

*By Karen Turnbull — Mar 18, 2015*

Well, it has been seven weeks since surgery, five weeks since returning home from UCLA and three and a half weeks of rehab. Before surgery it took me and two nurses to assist Mike out of bed even to just sit in a chair. After surgery and the initial week of recovery, he had to learn how to move his wheelchair, eat again, speak clearly and begin to find the use of his right hand. Now, I actually find myself asking him to slow down because he is walking faster than I can sometimes keep up, and I need to hold his gait belt in case he wobbles. He is wobbling less and less but it does still happen.

I don't like to be too far away when he is on the move.

Therapy is no joke! He works out daily with focus on core stability, leg and arm strength and gait training. And that is just the physical therapy. He also does writing, puzzles and drumming for occupational therapy. And then there is speech. His speech therapist, Julie, has done extra research to help him get back his embouchure for trombone. He even takes his mouthpiece with him to start building the strength back. Monday on the way home he was telling me about his day. It began with fifty sets of sitting-to-standing exercises without assistance, using his hands on his thighs to push off (last week he was pushing off the chair.) When he told his therapist, Christine, she responded, "Good, now do twenty more with your hands clasped in front of you." This came after working on the Pilates reformer, walking in a gait trainer and everything else they have him do! He is exhausted at the end of the day but has never once complained. Yes, there are moments of frustration but he is the calm, determined Mike we all know and love.

When UCLA told me that he would be out of the wheelchair in a few months I thought they were crazy. How was he going to get strong enough to walk in just a few months? Shows you what I know! The wheelchair is barely used anymore. It helps if we are out somewhere that would involve more walking than he is comfortable with, but he no longer uses it at home or at therapy. The walker has been replaced with a four-point cane, which is more stable than a regular cane but much less bulky than the walker. His facial droop has improved tremendously and his speech is getting clearer every day. His vision is clearer with one eye patched but he still fights with the double vision. He does visual exercises every day to try to get the two eyes working together. I notice a big difference in how his eyes are tracking. They used to cross pretty severely. Now they are almost tracking together. The dizziness and nausea are still there but not as often as even just a week ago. He is walking better every day and although I am there in case he wobbles, he is doing all the work himself.

We had a meeting with all the therapists last week to discuss his progress and goals. They are all thrilled with his improvements and saw every goal as something attainable. Some of his goals are driving again, taking care of the kids, cooking and playing his trombone. (I say he adds in that triathlon he started training for!). Overall he feels ok but not great. He is definitely improving and he seems to have more good moments than not-so-good moments. We are grateful for every little sign that he is headed in the right direction.

I have returned to work and it feels good to be surrounded by young artists who are glad to have me back. The school staff and my dance department faculty have been incredibly supportive and have helped make my transition back as easy as possible. The mornings are crazy as I facilitate getting everyone off to school but we are figuring it out. My parents have been here for three weeks and have been such a blessing. I think life is starting to calm down slightly and I am working on my delegating skills (which I have never been very good at!). We are developing a morning groove, and although life is far from perfect we are surviving ... one moment at a time.

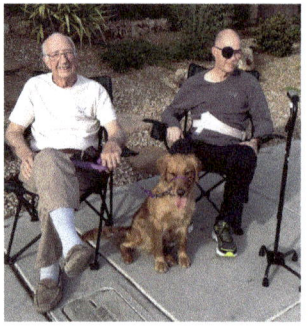

*Jim Sommer*

We meet with Dr. Obara tomorrow. It has been 100% confirmed that Mike's brain tumor was indeed Hürthle Cell Carcinoma. Sneaky cancer ... it had everyone fooled. At this time the doctors feel no more treatment is needed. Because Mike had Gamma Knife radiation to the area already, they do not want to radiate the same area again. At least not right now. His blood levels will be closely monitored and he will get current scans soon. The thyroglobulin marker was slightly higher at the last blood draw so we will see where it is tomorrow. The goal is for the number to be as close to zero as possible. The lowest was 2.0 at UCLA but it was 6.0 a few weeks ago. It doesn't mean the cancer is back, it just means there are thyroid cells somewhere. It can take months for it to drop after a procedure so we are hoping tomorrow gives us a lower number. There has been talk of oral chemotherapy drugs down the road but right now the focus is on healing. So that brings us back to the prayers, love, light, energy, meditations, etc!

I am sure you know my closing line well by now but I am going to say it anyways ... Please, keep the prayers coming! Thank you and much love!

> **Sara I**
> *Praise The Lord. His light is shining brighter than ever and your faith, strength and courage in Him have led you to his grace! Amazing news, Karen. We're so happy to hear such positive uplifting news for your beautiful family. Tell Mike that Rodney got*

back into biking and would love to go for a ride when he's able! God Bless you All! Much Love Always!!

**Curt M**
Thank you so much for this update. I had been thinking about him a lot and wondering how things were going. I am amazed at both of you and your will power to get through this. Incredibly inspiring. Thank you!

**JoLayne G**
So happy to hear of all the progress - old skills relearned, new skills developed (even yours), return to work, help from home. Praise God for all the healing, help and blessings. Still praying for continued strength, patience, healing, peace and help. Keep on dancing this dance as beautifully as you are, as hard as it is.

**Debbie M**
You guys are amazing. So glad to hear of some good news. Love you!

**Mike S**
Awesome man, awesome wife! Yay for progress. Prayers will continue.

**Fran D**
Once again, happy tears in reading your update!!! God truly has Blessed the two of you and I am sure He will continue to do so. Hopefully there is a light at the end of the tunnel and you all can finally get your lives back. Much love to you and your family.

**Jen F**
Happy tears falling! So proud of you guys and his amazing recovery. Prayers of healing will continue from our family. We love you guys!

**Tiffany P**
You guys are truly an inspiration! So glad to hear and see Mike doing so much better. Sending you all lots of LOVE.

**Virginia H**
I was so thrilled to see him walking on Sunday! It is truly amazing how far he has come in such a short time! I know your world is crazy and I hope you have time occasionally to take a deep breath and quiet your inner self. It is in God's hands now and we will continue to pray for full recovery!

*Marie K*

Simply AMAZING! What determination can do for ones soul. Prayers continue for your family!

*Suzanne P*

Mike, you are looking much better. I know this is difficult and I can't begin to imagine how you feel, but I do know that it is one step at a time and slowly, slowly you arrive at your goal. I know sometimes it can be frustrating to not be able to do what you want to do, but you are doing an amazing job of rehabilitating. You are a walking miracle! And an inspiration to us all. Remember to thank your body every day for all it has done for you. Sometimes I would curse my body when it couldn't do what I wanted it to, but it really did respond better when I was grateful. I still have to remind myself of that today. Stay strong and be as compassionate with yourself as you would with anyone you love. This is something we all know and love about you, so turn that love inward. Love you all.

*Dan S*

Thank you, Karen, for this update. We've all been waiting for some positive news and are so happy to hear it! WAY TO GO MIKE!!!! Keep it going!!! Looking forward to seeing you soon! Love you guys!!!!

*Kristine K*

Mike should be praised. He is such a warrior. He is so determined to beat this with a strong will to be himself, a vibrant, loving human being. You are a warrior as well, Karen. He could never have been through the most difficult part of this ordeal without your passionate strength, perserverance and loving kindness. I wish him steady and speedy recovery. You are both blessed.

## 2.5!

*By Karen Turnbull — Mar 20, 2015*

Our oncology appointment yesterday went as well as we could have hoped for. Thyroglobulin level was 2.5!!! Dr. Obara commented on the improvement in Mike from just two weeks ago. We go to UCLA for follow-ups in two weeks and then we will see Obara again after that. Also, yesterday at therapy Mike cooked! He did everything unassisted and made an omelet!!! In our world this is like climbing Everest!

Happy Friday! Keep the prayers coming!

**Kathy T**
*That's my son - always doing the impossible. Love you, Mom*

**Susan S**
*Yummy omelet, fantastic news, continual prayers!!!*

**Christina P**
*Displaying some of that ass-kickin' warrior strength again! All this news is fanfreakingtastic. Keep fighting the fight, Team Turnbull, and we will keep sending the vibes. Many hugs and loves to you all!*

**Avi H**
*So happy!!!!!!!*

# UCLA

By Karen Turnbull — Apr 11, 2015

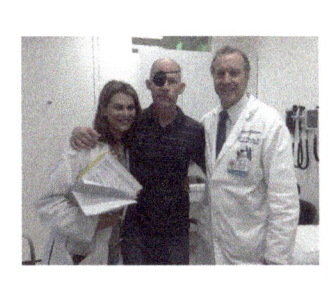

*Dr. Melissa Reider-Demer, Dr. Neil Martin*

We met with Dr. Martin and the eye specialist at UCLA last week. The MRI of Mike's brain looks amazing! Dr. Martin was very pleased with how well his brain is healing and there is no sign of any residual tumor or disease! The neuro-ophthalmologist was as amazing as all the doctors at UCLA have been. She spent three hours with Mike. After putting him through just about every test possible the conclusion is that his eyes are perfect. Each eye sees 20/20 independently. Although they are not tracking together just yet, they are improving. She was very impressed with the amount of movement his eyes now have in moving from side to side. From the pre-surgery notes she was expecting them not to move very much at all.

We were also referred to an optometrist who specializes in prism glasses. The thought is that because his eyes are changing so rapidly we should begin with a temporary prism glass. It is basically a sticker attached to the lens and can be changed as his brain heals and his eyes continue to correct. The glasses were shipped to us and Mike has been wearing them this weekend. They are not perfect. At certain distances the image is still double, and because it is a sticker the lens is not perfectly clear, making the image slightly blurry. But as he is adjusting to them, at some distances there is only one image and it is slightly better. We are actually wondering if his eyes have corrected some since we saw the doctors. We return to UCLA in June for another MRI and follow-ups with the eye doctors.

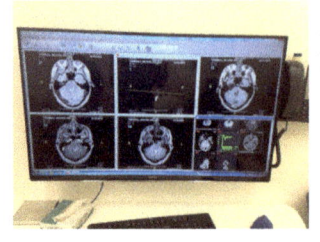

Therapy is going great. We had a family meeting with all the therapists and to quote them, "Mike is kicking butt!" He is now walking with a regular cane that just has a slightly larger base. He no longer needs someone holding him but just nearby in case he loses his balance. His facial muscles have started to move which is a great indicator that he may be able to play trombone again! And, on Friday he went on his first outing with the therapy group. It was an event called "Strokes for Strokes" and he got to golf! So, just as we all expected, Mike is working hard and proving to be the champion we all knew he was. Thank you everyone for continuing to send your love and prayers our way. We are so grateful for all that we have been blessed with.

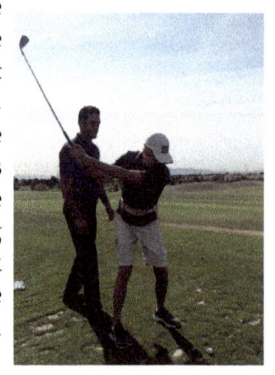

Keep the beautiful love, energy and prayers coming because every day Mike is improving. Much love to you all.

> *Stacy G*
> Fabulous news, you guys! Hopefully I will catch you in June!
>
> *Angela W*
> This is great news! I am blown away at his strength! You are amazing, Mike! Wow!
>
> *Mike S*
> So wonderful to hear! So awesome! Swimming, walking, golfing ... continuing prayers for more wonderful updates!

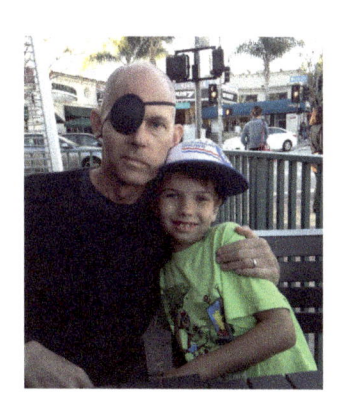

### Laura H
*This totally made our night. WOW! I'm so so so happy for you and the kids. And I'm not surprised Mike is exceeding all expectations. Please send love from Griff and Laura, and the entire 1989 Disney World All-American College Band.*

### Megan H
*Great update. Mike's tenacity and determination is inspiring, not to mention YOURS! You continue to lift all around you, Karen. No small feat. I think of you and your precious family every single day. xoxo*

### Pat C
*We are in your corner. Lead the charge, Mike! You are blessed beyond words with wife, family and extended family that will be with you through it all. Still the prayers continue.*

### Dene R
*Such an amazing story!!! God Bless you both ... and again sending you love, hugs and mega prayers from Texas!*

### Nandita S
*This is amazing news, and the picture makes me smile. Keep up all the hard work, all of you. It is paying off!*

### Virginia H
*So great to see the improvement each week at church. He and you are sure troopers and true examples of the human spirit and the will to live!*

*Fran D*
*Every time Mike pops into my head with a thought of an update, lo and behold you post one. Thank you in advance and God bless you and Mike and your family and team of doctors and everyone involved in making Mike well. This is GREAT news. God does work WONDERS, Karen. DON'T GIVE UP!!!!!!!!!! Please tell him hello for me and he is in my prayers nightly.*

*Tim L*
*What a miracle!!! Our love and prayers to all of you!!*

*Karen P*
*Truly a magnificent update! Congratulations to all of you. It's such hard work and you are doing it with such grace and style. Thank you. Our love and prayers continue to surround you.*

*Tiffany P*
*Beautiful, amazing and wonderful!!!! So happy to read this news. Keep up the good work. Love you all!*

*Ellen O*
*Wow! This is so fabulous to see! Keep it up, Mike! You got this!*

# 1.9!

### By Karen Turnbull — Apr 13, 2015

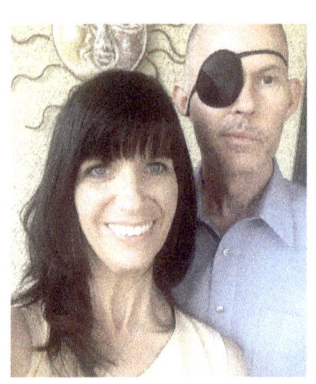

Our oncology appointment today gave us the lowest thyroglobulin level since this all began! Yesterday I was hit with a very strong feeling that this is it. It was a blind faith moment of simply believing. Something more than I can explain, just a feeling within every cell of my being. I believe we are done with cancer. Today we received the great news that Mike's thyroglobulin level is 1.9! Dr. Obara was more than impressed with Mike's improvements and said his "potential is limitless!" So, tonight we celebrate that there is no such thing as a small victory. Every victory is huge!!!

Continue the love, energy and prayers! Much love!

*Kenny A*
*This is such wonderful news!! I pray for Mike and you and the kids every day!! You have an amazing team and family!! Love to you all!!*

*Randy C*
*YAYYYYYYYYYYYYYY! Thyroglobwhatever!!! Go Mike!*

*Mark S*
*Limitless potential? That is the most astounding thing one person could say to another. Amazing. Bask in that accolade, Mike.*

*Joan F*
*Karen and Mike ... you have brought the spirit of faith and courage to all the anxious moments of your days!!!*

*Darelle H*
*Amazing! You two are the bravest people I know. Onward and upward. Love to you both.*

*Melissa P*
*So happy for you all and your wonderful news!*

## Moving Forward!
*By Karen Turnbull — May 14, 2015*

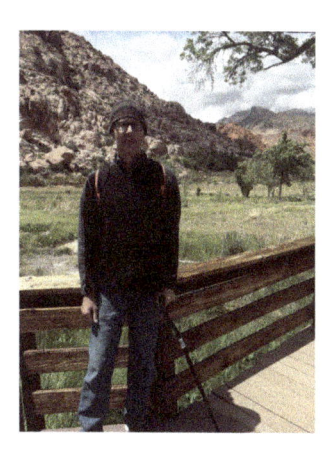

It has been awhile since my last update and a lot has happened. Most importantly, Mike is continuing to plow forward and is getting stronger every day. In fact, I began this letter yesterday explaining that he is using a single point cane. Well, when I picked him up from therapy he informed me that he is now walking with nothing! He is still a little wobbly and gets dizzy at times (although much less than before) so the decision, for now, is inside he walks on his own and outside he uses the cane! Amazing!

Mike is adjusting to the prism glasses. They are not a perfect fix and things are slightly blurry, but they do take away the double vision. We are beginning to see a vision therapist outside of his regular (six hours a day) therapy. We had an initial evaluation with her and she specializes in helping those with neurological vision problems. We liked her a lot and she seemed very encouraged by the progress Mike has made already. Her first thought was for Mike to finish his therapy program and then see her after his graduation. However, once she met him and saw his drive and determination, she left it up to us to decide whether we wanted to wait or begin now. We voted for now! After all, what are we waiting for? If we have learned anything through this journey it is that life can change in an instant. We are living in the present and making the most of each day. So, hopefully, with this additional vision therapy his eyes will continue to correct maybe even sooner than later.

We saw Dr. Obara Monday and Mike's blood work is holding strong! His thyroglobulin level remains at 1.9, which is fantastic! (The closer to zero, the better.) We have every reason to believe he is disease-free and we are surrounding ourselves with only that belief. We appreciate and thank you for believing with us!

Mike did have a slight setback one month ago. He had just passed his balance test at therapy and was feeling pretty good. He had gone to dinner with his mom while I was working with the kids group at our church. When I returned home I discovered that he had a severe fall. He had gone into the garage to look at our garage door opener, which had come off the track. His mom was on the ladder and he looked up to tell her what to do. As he looked up the dizziness hit and he fell (like a tree) onto his right side. Thankfully, the tire from Evan's bike stopped him from hitting his head. He was in extreme pain and could not put weight on his right leg. This is the side that has very little sensation. So, if he was feeling this much pain, my fear was "what isn't he feeling?" After I screamed all sorts of colorful words at him and finally calmed down I decided an x-ray was a must. The x-ray of the hip ruled out any fractures. We were then advised to get an MRI of the brain to rule out any trauma there. We did the MRI and sent the results to our doctors here as well as UCLA to get the official clear. No damage showed on the scan! It has now been four weeks since the fall and he has finally returned to about where he was in his progress before the fall happened. He still has soreness in his hip and shoulder but with massage work, acupuncture and time, that will continue to heal.

As for the boys and me, we are great! I even managed to escape home to Pittsburgh for about thirty-six hours a few weeks ago. I had the beautiful opportunity to surprise my niece Michelle for her bridal shower! It was a crazy whirlwind of a weekend and I loved it! There is nothing like family and seeing everyone recharged my batteries.

We celebrate the amazing milestones every day. The boys light up when they see Mike accomplish a new goal. The fact that they can have Daddy Grilled Cheese again is as big a gift as Christmas morning. They are his number one fans and I know they keep him going when it gets really tough. Our life is not perfect but then no one's is. So we wake up each day and celebrate that we are in our home with our beautiful boys and sweet dog. Most times our house is full of joy and lots of laughter (except when I am trying to get our eight-year-old to do his homework, or our three-year-old to stop having a tantrum, or when my husband pushes things too far and I am afraid of another setback!), but these moments pass and I am reminded that although life is anything but normal, this is our new normal and I will gladly take it. It sure beats where we were four months ago! The other great news is Mike's face is continuing to improve. His cheek is moving more and his smile is slowly coming back. Oh, how I love his smile! One day, one moment, one breath at a time. Thanks for being with us through this journey. It means more than you will ever know.

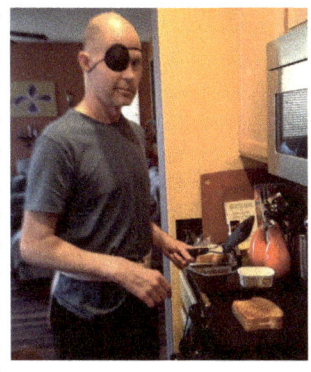

Keep all the prayers, love and energy coming! It is working miracles!

> *Vince V*
> It warms my heart and tears me up every time I read these posts. You guys are amazing, and I'm so glad Mike is progressing. Keep it up. Lots of positive vibes from us to all of you.
>
> *Brian M*
> Thanks for the update, Karen. I am awed by the courage, fierce determination and love you all have displayed through this ordeal.
>
> *Suzanne P*
> Really good news! You are right Karen, you have to take each day as it comes and live it to the fullest. It teaches us not to take things for granted, but to embrace life. Thank you for reminding me of that as well. Sometimes it is easy to get caught up in the small stuff that really doesn't matter. You and Mike keep reminding me to be appreciative. Every time I see a picture of Mike, I am amazed at how far he has come. I know to him it feels like an eternity, but he really has made great progress in a short time. I continue to send you all love and healing. xoxox

*Curt M*

*Every time I read these updates it makes me think how fast life can change and what is really important. Give our boy a hug from the trombone community!*

*Jean T*

*Thank you for the update, Karen. Your biggest blessing is each other. Hold on!*

*Tiffany P*

*Fantastic news ... so happy to read of the progress and hear how well everyone is doing. Love you guys!!*

*Jeanine C*

*Your perspective of gratitude and grace is beautiful. Think of you guys all the time and look forward to some play time with all the boys.*

*Devonee M*

*Tears of joy and gratitude reading this. You amaze me every single day, Karen. I love you all!*

*Dave W*

*Keep up the strong work, Mike! Karen, we only met once, but your strength is an inspiration to me. Your kids sound amazing!!! I think about you guys a lot and send good vibes your way on a daily basis!!!*

*Rosita P*

*We are so happy for you guys ... sending you lots of hugs and kisses. God bless you!!!*

# Big Improvements!

*By Karen Turnbull — Jun 18, 2015*

Well, it has been quite a week! Last Thursday Mike graduated from the Nevada Community Enrichment Program. This is where he has spent the last three and a half months rehabilitating. They had a lovely ceremony for him. My nieces Megan and Jill were visiting and they were able to attend with the boys and me. Mike gave an excellent speech and there was not a dry eye in the room. His heartfelt words of gratitude touched everyone. As we would all expect, everyone there came to love Mike dearly. All the therapists and many of the clients had beautiful words to share. It was quite emotional to sit in this room of humble heroes. Every person there is fighting every day to regain control of their lives. Simple things we take for granted like being able to eat with a fork or being able to stand are part of their daily fight. To hear their stories of how Mike has inspired them and how they inspired Mike was very touching. Mike's speech pathologist, Julie, shared a beautiful quote that she said reminds her of us: "Sometimes God's greatest servants have to climb the tallest mountains." We were very touched by this.

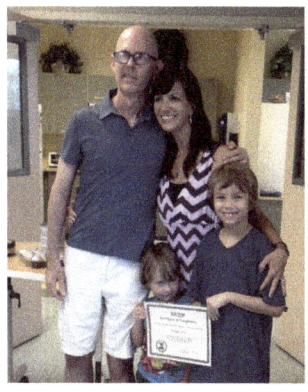

The graduation came earlier than any of us had hoped. Basically Mike is now doing so well that insurance cannot justify him being in a comprehensive program. He is now walking without any assistive device! His eyes are showing improvement, his face is beginning to move even more and his speech is greatly improved! It is a long road and he definitely still needs work, just not in such a comprehensive program so he has been doing self-rehab at home. Sometimes it gets challenging when daily distractions get in the way, but it is just a transition and we will figure it out. Come mid-July he will begin outpatient PT and OT, hopefully three times a week.

After graduation Mike and I left for the airport. He was scheduled for an 8:00 PM MRI at UCLA that night. After dealing with flight delays, airport changes and car rental mix-ups we made the appointment. Thank you to our beautiful friends, Stacy and Ferris, for letting us stay in their home. It was wonderful to catch up and share many laughs with two amazing people and their beautiful daughters! And, thank you Megan and Jill for staying with the boys while we were gone.

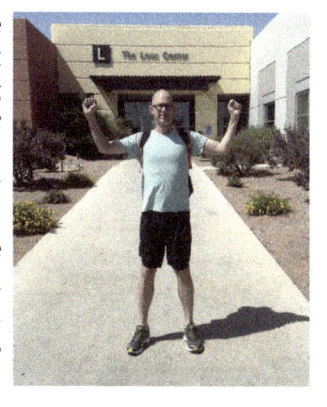

Friday morning we headed in to see the neuro-ophthalmologist. She was very pleased with Mike's progress. His eyes are tracking much better and moving more together. Although the eyes have improved, she did not feel it was time to change his prescription yet. We continue to see the vision therapist here in Las Vegas. She is excellent. She has given Mike lots of homework to help get those eyes working together. She will monitor when to change the prescription, so for now he's working with the glasses he has.

After receiving the good news from the neuro-opthalmologist we then went to see Dr. Martin, the neurosurgeon. We received wonderful news that Mike's MRI looked great! There is no sign of disease, tumor or trauma! Dr. Martin said it looked exactly as he would hope it to look! He then had Mike go through all his tests. It was wonderful to see Mike able to show off his improvements! Dr. Martin was very pleased! He then invited Mike to attend a fundraising ball they hold every October and possibly share his story and speak. Mike was both thrilled and honored! We do not know yet if he will be chosen to speak but either way it will be an honor to attend. We then shared our words of gratitude with Dr. Martin. We just don't know how to say thank you. He was very humble and said he was only part of the picture. He recognized all the hard work Mike has put in. He then said to us, "What I like to say is that we (surgeons) open the door for God to heal." Beautiful!

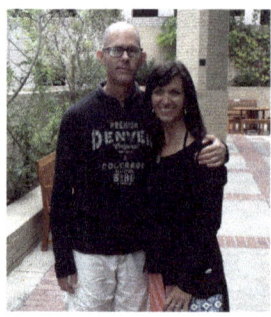

So now it is more therapy. Mike will continue to heal and retrain his body. UCLA does not want to see us back for six months! Thank you God for the amazing healing that has happened! Thank you to Mike for fighting so hard every single day and never giving up! Extra big thanks to Mike's mom, Kathy! This amazing woman came and lived with us for two months to take care of our boys while we juggled school, therapy, doctors appointments and work. Not an easy job! And thank you to all of you who have been on this journey with us. Your love, support and words of encouragement keep us going. We are forever grateful to all of you!

All of the love, prayers, and wonderful energy has worked ... keep it coming!

> *Suzanne P*
> Such awesome news ... I was thinking about you today, so it was great to get this update. I think Mike would be a great inspiration

*for others that are also engaged in the challenge to regain some sort of normalcy. I am so, so happy for all of you. I know the boys are thrilled and very proud to see their father accomplish so much. This is true success. I love you!*

### Laurence A
*Mike! Keep up the good work as I know you will. Who knew all the discipline needed to become a great musician would come in so handy! Rock on friend!*

### Rocco B
*Mike and Karen, I'm thankful for health and well-being for both of you. May you both have continued blessings of strength and wellness. You are both amazing for all that you have gone through and are still working through! You will always remain in our prayers. Love you both and I look forward to seeing you again soon!*

### Virginia H
*Such wonderful news and a big shout out to you, Karen, for having the strength to endure these past years. God has given you the grace to endure and Mike the strength to recover! Blessings on all your family!*

### Sara I
*Your family's story continues to touch the lives of so many and be truly inspirational and life-changing! I can say this because that's exactly how I feel after meeting your beautiful family only recently through the benefit at church. Now you're not just our neighbors but our friends, whom we cherish deeply. Whether or not Mike shares his story at the ball, just know that God chose your family for this incredibly difficult journey because he knew your family's strength, faith, love and trust in Him, as well as one another, would see that you triumphantly made it to the other side, all while your followers and supporters watch in awe of you. Your story isn't finished, but it continues to be nothing short of inspirational to all who love and support you, even those you've only just met!! We love you All so much Team Turnbull.*

### Shani F
*Wow! Mike, you are a walking inspiration. Literally! It warms our heart every time we see you at church. God is so good and has blessed you so much! Keep up the hard work.*

*Stacia F*
*Karen, this brings tears of joy to me. I have been praying and rooting for you all!! Continuing this practice while you and Mike do all of this AMAZING work. !! Xxx*

*Lou G*
*Still prayin' at ya. Thank you for the inspiration. Your courage and great big spirit help me every day.*

*Heidi H*
*Such wonderful news. So happy for all of you, although I too am not surprised by Mike's ability to speed up his healing and rehab schedule! Enjoy your summer :)*

## Six Months!

*By Karen Turnbull — Jul 25, 2015*

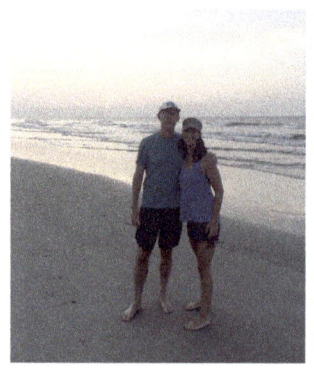

Well, today marks the six-month anniversary of Mike's surgery! To say it has been easy would be a lie, but we are most definitely in a better place today than we were then! I specifically remember Dr. Martin saying to us that he felt in six months Mike would be in a much better position. I thank God that he was correct! Sometimes the frustration hits and Mike just wants to wake up and be back to his normal self, but then we take a moment and look back at where we were. Six months ago Mike could barely see, speak, move or eat. At that time we were faced with either taking the chance on surgery or making him as comfortable as possible for whatever time he would have left. Really it was no choice at all. We simply did what we had to do. We had to trust and take a huge leap of faith. I am so glad we did! So today we celebrate! We celebrate life! We even celebrate the hard times because we believe anything is possible.

This summer we got to take a break and be with family. We traveled to Hilton Head, South Carolina for an amazing week with family. Mike walked the beach, sat in the ocean, swam in the pool and even rode a three-wheeled bike! He made everyone laugh in typical Mike fashion by just being his amazing, funny self. We then spent another ten days in

Pittsburgh with my family. We snuck in a trip to Hershey Park to see our dear friend Frank and his beautiful new fiancé, Julie! The boys got to laugh and play and be happy little kids. We went back to the mountains, to Seven Springs, where we got married almost thirteen years ago. It's been a very full thirteen years with some very hard and scary moments, but I would say "I do" all over again.

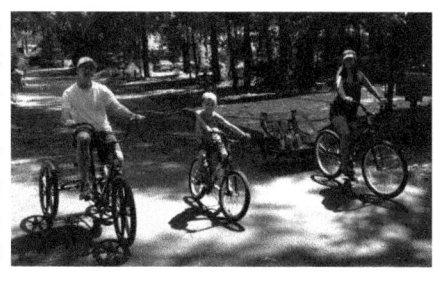

The other day Evan told me that his little friend down the street asked him where his dad was. He said this because he sees me outside with the kids but had never seen Mike. Evan simply told him the truth: "My dad doesn't come outside much because he had a brain tumor." His little friend said, "Oh wow, I feel so sorry for you." Evan replied, "Don't. He's doing great and we're ok." I am so proud of him! This is our truth. Maybe we didn't choose this path but we do get to choose how we face it. Some times are harder than others and some days are longer than others, but overall I have to agree with Evan ... we are doing ok!

Thank you all for following our story and sending your love and prayers. We are grateful for all of you. Thank you God for guiding us through this journey. I know You are with us every step of the way.

Happy six-month anniversary to the bravest man I know ... I love you, Mike! Thank you for keeping your promise to fight and not give up.

Much love to you all and as always ... keep the prayers, light, love and good energy coming. It is working!

> *Dale B*
> *So glad to hear. You both are such an inspiration. You all are in my thoughts often!*
>
> *Lou G*
> *Love to you all. Thank you for all the inspiration, light, hope and most for the incredible torrents of love you manage to get onto these short posts. Evan, you are the Man. I am so proud to know you.*
>
> *Darelle H*
> *"We're okay," and "this is our truth." And so it is ... I love you guys.*

*Jason V*

I'm so so so so happy that he is still improving!!!! This is amazing news!! The strength and courage that your family has is incredible and it's beautiful. Always sending my prayers your way!

*Christina P*

I am so proud to have strong cancer ass-kicking friends! Fight on brother and sister ... your strength and courage radiates and infects others around you. Infect on my friends. Infect on!

*Marianne M*

Happy Anniversary, Mike! You better get those dancing shoes polished. Michelle's wedding is only six weeks away!! Karen, as always, your posts make me cry - but at least this time they are tears of joy! Can't wait to see all of you again! Love, love, love you guys!

*Joni S*

You and your family continue to inspire me every day! Mike looks terrific and I'm so glad you got to have a little relaxation family time together this summer! Love you sweet friend! Continuing to send prayers and good thoughts!!!

*Gil K*

Congrats!! You are such a strong family! An inspiration to us all. Mike, I miss you more than you will ever know! Call when you're up to some Laksa! Hugs!

*Cathy M*

Happy Anniversary, Mike! This is great news! You, Karen and the boys continue to be an extraordinary inspiration to us all. You are indeed the bravest man I know and I applaud all the strength and endurance you displayed to get to this place on your journey. Sending more love, light, support and prayers.

*Shani F*

You are an amazing family! Your hope and positive outlook is contagious. Thank you for sharing with all of us. God bless you all!

*Deb S*

So glad to hear about your progress, Mike. Happy Anniversary to you both.

*Rocco B*
*Congratulations Mike, Karen, Evan, William and family for your amazing work! You have inspired so many of us to look at life in a different way. We are so proud to say that Mike Turnbull is our friend. Our prayers will always be coming your way. Love you all!!!!!*

*Margaret H*
*I love you so much! You are an incredible woman! Mike is a remarkable man! Sending you lots of LOVE.*

*Curt M*
*You are both an inspiration as a couple. It is rare to see this level of love in a family under these kinds of extraordinary circumstances.*

*Pete B*
*Your posts are probably the most encouraging thing I read besides the Bible. The strength and love you guys show reveal the true heart of God and the way you tackle every obstacle builds faith in us all. Praise God for the Turnbulls!*

*Lynne E*
*We are so happy to see Mike's progress. He is one great guy and it's easy to see why you all love him so. He is the luckiest man in the world to have you as his partner. Continued good wishes and prayers go your way.*

*Nandita S*
*I can't believe the progress in six months. Mike amazed me at the hospital with his spirit and he amazes me now. As do you, Karen! Wishing you even more progress in the next six months! Xoxo*

*Elizabeth H*
*What an amazing story. What an amazing couple you are. What an amazing God we serve. I'm so happy that you were able to be with your family back home. I will continue to keep you in my prayers.*

*Jenna L*
*What a celebration indeed! WOW. God is amazing and so are your and Mike's inspirational positive attitudes! We continue to pray every day for complete healing for Mike! So glad you were able to go to the beach and Pittsburgh and have time with family. Life is*

a celebration! Thank you for sharing your journey. You guys are awesome!!!

**Ellen Sn**
Oh Karen, it makes my heart feel full and happy to hear you speak about Mike. I am so happy you guys are exceeding limits. I keep you and Mike in my thoughts always. Xoxo

**Sharon H**
Your truth is remarkable and beautiful. Happy six-month anniversary, Mike. You are the bravest man I know, also. My love and continued prayers to you always. Aunt Muffy

# A Week of Firsts!

*By Karen Turnbull — Sep 3, 2015*

Last week was the first week of school for all of us. Evan started third grade and William began his second year of preschool (he feels very grown up and a pro!). I returned to Las Vegas Academy for the start of my eleventh year as a member of the dance department faculty. How did eleven years go by?!?! And, Mike began yet another new therapy program. For the first time since November we have no "live-in" help for the school year. I have delegated jobs out to the boys to help with the morning routine and Mike is there to help manage the chaos.

While William is at school, Mike goes to physical therapy and occupational therapy. Thanks to our amazing neighbors and friends, I have managed to figure out transportation for everyone (a task that was keeping me up at night in anxiety). Mike also attempted to drive for the first time last week. Don't worry, he will not be hitting the open roads yet but he may be trying his skills in some empty parking lots. His prescription on his eyeglasses was lowered so things are a little clearer. The new lenses did take a few days to adjust to and it felt a little like a setback while his brain adjusted. He still has double vision without the glasses but he says the images are beginning to get closer together. Instead of four eyes, he now says I have three! His face and mouth are moving more and more every day and his smile is starting to appear again. Balance continues to be a daily struggle but he is working on it. If we are out somewhere and he stumbles I sometimes smile and tell the onlookers, "He is not drunk." Other times I think, "Hey, it's Vegas. People are used to seeing people stumbling about. Let them think what they want."

Evan has been doing swim team, which has motivated Mike to get in and swim too. He is amazing! The first time he tried swimming (just a few months ago) he would get horribly dizzy when he tried to turn his head to breathe. Now he swims laps beautifully and breathes every three strokes just like our friend and coach Devonee taught him! His new therapists seem to be good, although we now realize how spoiled we were at the NCEP program. The team of therapists, assistants and specialists there were so vested in Mike's recovery. We are definitely grateful that he was there at the most critical time in his recovery. He had a few sessions at one therapy office over the summer, but we switched last week due to insurance. Funny thing is, the physical therapist at the last office was recently diagnosed with Hürthle Cell thyroid cancer. She was not going to do anything about it until she met Mike and heard his story. So, in a weird way, we think he was only meant to be at that office a short time to help her decide to get treatment. She made an appointment the week after meeting Mike. Although I have not yet met his new therapists, Mike tells me they are very positive and inspired by his story. They are pushing him hard and hopefully more improvements are coming.

The biggest news of all is that this Saturday we will be attending my niece Michelle's wedding! If you have been following our story, then you know that Michelle started the gofundme account for us and has been a huge cheerleader for Mike. Her one wish has been that Mike be able to dance with her at her wedding. Well, the song has been chosen, his suit is packed, and God willing, Mike will dance with Michelle! (I have tissues packed, as I know my eyes will NOT be dry!). Pictures to come next post!

Thank you, as always, for keeping us in your thoughts and prayers. As Mike gets stronger he has been able to see more people. It helps so much to know that everyone is keeping us in their thoughts and prayers. The posts, texts, emails and words of encouragement help motivate and keep us focused on the future. Love to you all!

May you have a great holiday weekend and keep all the love, prayers, light and energy coming!

> *Tammy C*
> *So happy to hear all the wonderful news and progress with Mike! You are all such an amazingly strong, inspirational family! We love you all so much! Keep up the good work, Mike! Can't wait to see the picture of Mike dancing! I'm crying just thinking about it! Much love to you all! Missing you soooo much!*

*Shannon B*
*We pray every day for all of you. I know that this journey has been difficult and I know you always look at the positive side:). Love and light and we're rooting Mike on from DC!! And yes, it's Vegas so yeah, let people think what they want. XOXOXO*

*Andrea L*
*Mike and your entire family are the exact meaning of "love conquers all." I have choreographed a dance for this season with your family as the motivation. I can't wait until the dancers perfect and rehearse it so I can share it with you. Team Turnbull for President!!! Xo*

*Laurence A*
*Thanks for sharing all the wonderfulness! All of you are amazing and inspiring. Happy dancing!*

*Christina P*
*You bring my life sunshine with all this great news! We love you guys and continue to send butt-kicking positive thoughts your way! Loves and hugs.*

*Judy E*
*God has guided you through amazing trials, carrying all of you at times. There is so much praise to be given to God for answered prayers, and much admiration for the entire family for their trust and perseverance.*

*Michelle R*
*Amazing, amazing, amazing. I hope Mike continues to improve and you continue to have the strength of a warrior!*

*Devonee M*
*I LOVE YOU TURNBULLS! You are all amazing and beautiful to me in so many ways! ENJOY this time with your precious family and send us some pictures of that dancing! XOXOXO*

*James M*
*What a joy it was to read this update. Mike and your whole family continue to be in our prayers. Mike is an amazing inspiration to me. God Bless the Turnbull family!*

*Ellen F*
*Kim and I are in awe of you, Karen, and your beautiful family, Mike and the boys, as well as other members of your family we have met*

*at New Song. We continue to pray for you and champion Team Turnbull! You are all so inspiring, and we are glad to know you and call you our friends. May the Good Lord Above continue to bless you and keep you in his loving Grace. Amen!*

### Katey J

*Yeah!!!! Great news ... keeping the love and prayers coming. You all are an inspiration to many others. Know that we think of you often and no daily prayer time goes by without sending one out for you all. Love and hugs.*

### Nathan T

*That's all great news! You both are wonderful people and an inspiration to all. Keep the good news coming!*

### Laura T

*Have a terrific time at the wedding!!! You inspire us so much with all you have done and continue to do. You're absolutely amazing! We love you tons. xoxo*

### Sharon H

*Just makes my heart beam with joy! I am always praying for you, beautiful family ... always ... have fun at the wedding!!!*

## Michelle

*By Michael Turnbull — Sep 10, 2015*

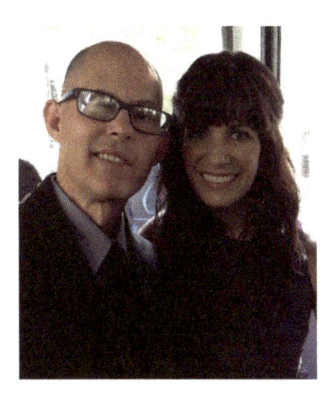

Hi! I know it has been a long time since I posted anything myself, and there are a couple of good reasons I haven't. One, I was pretty beat up a few months ago and unable to see or write, and two, Karen has been doing such a great job maintaining this site that I just stayed out of it so I didn't screw it up! Last weekend we were able to attend our niece Michelle's wedding in St. Louis. I wrote the following on Michelle's fundraising site and thought I would share it here:

To everyone who was able to attend Jordan and Michelle's wedding, thank you! When Michelle announced that almost everyone in attendance had donated to this fund to support our family, Karen and I were overwhelmed with gratitude. We considered getting on the microphone to thank you all in person, but decided the evening was not about us. Also, the dance with my niece was a symbolic gesture of thanks to all of you. There was a time just a few short months ago when we weren't sure any of that would happen. I was unable to walk, talk, see or eat, much less dance, so the fact that it all came to fruition was incredible. To be able to dance with Michelle at her wedding and therefore grant her birthday wish was truly a special moment in our lives, and something we will never forget.

To everyone else who donated through this site, thank you as well! From college friends we haven't heard from in years, to friends and family around the country, to anonymous donors and, perhaps most incredibly, to people none of us have ever met, we are again overwhelmed with gratitude. Your selfless acts of kindness have made a huge difference in our lives and in the lives of our children. As a musician and a dancer we have never made a ton of money, but we somehow managed to see the world doing what we loved. We also managed to support our boys and keep them busy, and even take an occasional trip like the one this weekend to St. Louis. Since I have been disabled, and as a result unemployed, for the better part of a year now, this fund has allowed us the ability to maintain a sense of "normalcy" for our kids. Evan and William are still involved in swimming and gymnastics, and William is attending the preschool at the church in our neighborhood. I have been able to see a vision therapist, myofascial stretch therapist and an acupuncturist, none of whom take insurance but all of whom have helped me heal and improve.

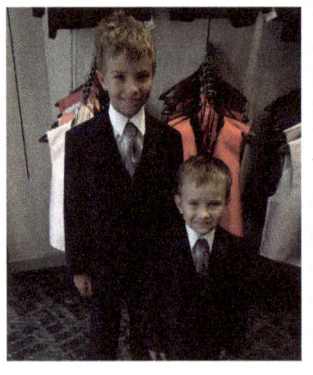

If I have learned anything during this adventure, it is that the only real important things in life are family, friends, faith and health. To be able to walk, talk and spend time with my wife and children are the only things that really matter any more. As difficult as this journey has been at times, we feel blessed in so many ways. I can't imagine going through this without Karen by my side. I have had a great life in large part due to her. She is truly an Angel on Earth and I owe everything to her. It has struck me many times over the years how similar Karen and Michelle are, so I know from experience that Jordan is in for a great life as well. Jordan, may you always remember how fortunate you are to have Michelle in your life.

There are really no words to describe how thankful we are to all of you. Hopefully, my presence at Michelle's wedding and my continuing improvement is in some small way an indication that your hard-earned dollars are being used in a positive way. We will never feel that our thanks are adequate, but please know that we love and appreciate you all, whether we've met you or not! Thank you again. With infinite gratitude.

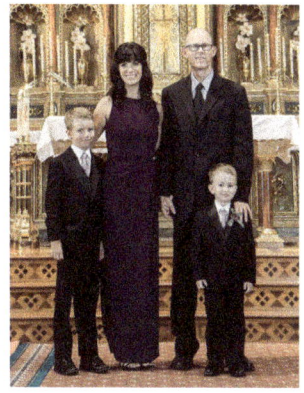

> *Pat C*
> *Life is beautiful, brother!*
>
> *Nan R*
> *Special post and pictures. It is so wonderful to see the four of you-such a beautiful, happy, connected family. Hearing the kids talk, as well as you and Karen, about this time in your lives shows that. It is also a testament to your faith and love. Thank you for blessing all of us, as you feel blessed. Blessings of support are needed, and blessings of faith and witness are essential. You four have provided the latter. May healing and all needed things keep coming to your family. Sending prayers and hugs. :):)*
>
> *Heather W*
> *This post made my day! There are no words for how truly amazing and inspiring you and your family are!!!*
>
> *Shelley De*
> *Michael's message was beyond eloquent and touching. It was such a great gift to hear that he danced with Michelle. The family picture says it all. The Turnbull family is a pillar of strength. Keep getting stronger, Mike, and Karen you are an amazing wife, mother and friend. Always in my thoughts.*
>
> *Elizabeth H*
> *Your journey through all of this has been so inspirational to so many! What a beautiful family you are! May God continue revealing His*

amazing Love and Grace to all of you. SO happy that you were able to dance with Michelle. She looked beautiful and you looked amazing!! Next event ... meeting your great nephew!! So exciting!!

**Darelle H**
That is truly amazing and wonderful. My heart swells every time I hear of your progress and see your pictures. All my love to your beautiful family and to you.

**Robin C**
What beautiful pictures and what an amazing journey you have all been through. Each week when we see you at church we are awed and inspired by you. And to see how you have kept the kids - kids - through all this is so wonderful. With and love and prayers.

# Wedding Dance

*By Karen Turnbull — Oct 11, 2015*

We had an incredible weekend in St. Louis last month. Our niece Michelle got married to her best friend Jordan, and the four of us were all part of the wedding.

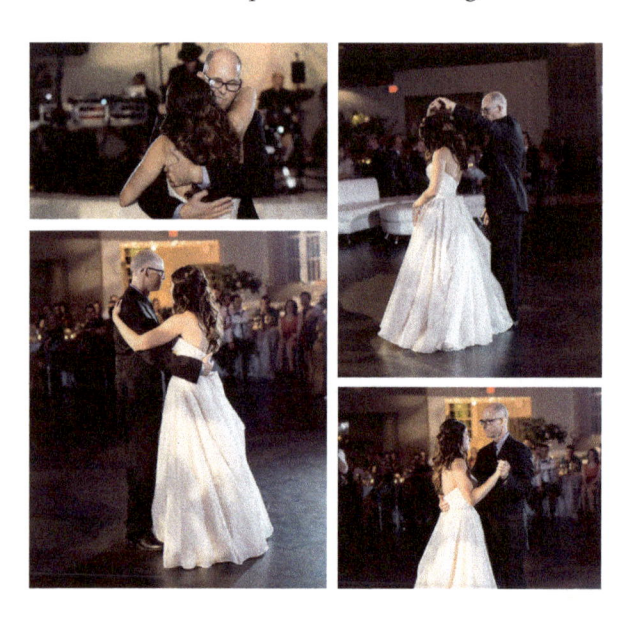

**Mark S**
*Wow! Just wow!*

**Doreen L**
*Such a reminder of what an amazing, healing God we have that you have come so far, Mike. God has blessed me by getting to know you four as you've come through this challenge with faith and love. Wow!*

**Darelle H**
*WOW, WOW, WOW! That's all I've got! You guys rock!*

# Thankful!

*By Karen Turnbull — Nov 28, 2015*

This post is extremely overdue, so for that I apologize! The months of October and November have been wonderfully busy! For the first time in a long time, life has been somewhat normal. Our days have been full of activities with the kids and we are making the best of every day.

At the end of October, Mike and I attended the UCLA Neurosurgery Visionary Ball. It was an amazing night! We didn't think we would be able to go and then at the last minute we were gifted two tickets to attend the event. So, we hopped in the car and made the drive for an amazing twenty-four-hour date! Mike and I talked the entire five-hour drive without even listening to music. It was wonderful to have uninterrupted time together. Thanks to my wonderful sister and brother-in-law's credit card points we were treated like royalty at a fancy Beverly Hills hotel (complete with a complementary BMW to take us to and from the event!). As soon as we walked in, I immediately recognized the residents that worked in the Neuro ICU. These young doctors had been by our side nonstop during the most critical time. Talking to them was a highlight of our night. It was amazing to see how rewarding it was for them to see Mike vertical! For him to be able to stand with them, hug them and thank them was so powerful.

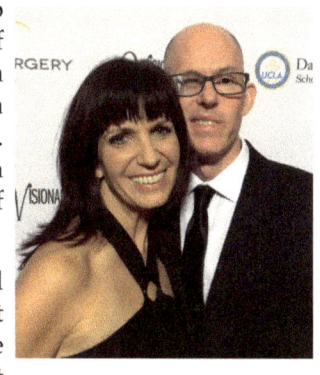

It was a wonderful evening filled with stories of hope and inspiration, and I have to say I was very proud to be in that room on Mike's arm. A few moments really stood out. One was when Dr. Martin was speaking. He said, "If you ever find yourself in the Neuro ICU at UCLA, things have gotten pretty bad. But, if you are ever in that position, you can be guaranteed we will do everything we can." This statement rang full of truth for us and many in that room. Each year they choose a few speakers. This year's primary speaker was a young man, nineteen years old, who had a rare endocrine brain tumor. As we sat there listening to his story, we thought about how awful it was for this young boy to go through so much. His parents spoke as well, and because of their donation there is now a full-time neurological endocrine research position at UCLA. Mike and I sat there feeling so grateful to be in that room surrounded by so many miraculous people.

When the event was over we went to speak to Dr. Martin. We wanted to say hello and thank him for all he has done. When he saw us he turned to Mike and said, "Next year we will have you speak." Mike, being the humble man he is, said, "I'm just honored to even be here." Dr. Martin shook his head and said, "No, your story is even more remarkable than this year's speaker." What?! It's one thing to be in it and think your situation sounds really rare. It's another thing to hear a world-renowned neurosurgeon say how remarkable and rare your case is!

On November 7th, we celebrated Mike's birthday, as well as the one-year anniversary of when all of this started. As it turns out, the Leukemia and Lymphoma Society's annual Light The Night walk was being held that night, so we walked! Mike, his mom, our two boys and me walked through the streets of downtown Las Vegas with thousands of others carrying lanterns representing hope for a day without cancer! It may not have been the triathlon Mike dreams of doing, but it sure was a start!

So, this year for Thanksgiving we were beyond grateful! This is the time of year when things started turning really bad for us. Look what can happen in a year! Mike continues to work hard at therapy. Some days are harder than others but he never gives up. Little things have started happening that prove we are still on the right road. I came home one day from work and Mike was so excited to show me that he could give William a piggyback ride! Wow, what a moment that was! In our life, the little things are not so little. Our house is fully decked out for Christmas this year. We are definitely celebrating every day!

Happy belated Thanksgiving to everyone! Merry Christmas, Happy Hanukkah, joyous Kwanzaa and any other holiday you may choose to celebrate! We love them all! May everyone be blessed with joy, health and lots of love!

I can't end a post without saying it, so here it is ... keep the prayers, love, light, energy and well-wishes coming! Mike is proof that they are all working!

*Estelle T*
*So amazing to look through the old posts and see what a miraculous outcome your journey has had. Much love to you all.*

*Matt J*
*Yes indeed ... I can see Mike sharing his experiences. Karen, you have the makings of a book. I sense that you two are going to have one whale of an adventure!! This latest update was truly the high point of my day. And yes, prayers are still being said daily. P.S. Mike ... Once a Bonehead Always a Bonehead.*

*Marianne M*
*Beautifully written, Karen! I think back on this time last year, and marvel at the progress Mike has made. God willing that triathlon is still in Mike's future!! Looking forward to a big Christmas celebration this year! Love you guys!!*

*Edward E*
*We hope and pray for you all every day!!! What a Happy post! We are as Thankful as all of you are. You are truly an Amazing Family!!! It shall be a very Merry Christmas!!! Xo.*

*Susie C*
*You and Mike are amazing! Truly an inspiration to us! Hugs, prayers and adoration to you both!*

*Nellie S*
*What a touching story. Thanks for sharing. Your family is such an inspiration and we always keep you in our prayers.*

*Gabriel F*
*Amen!! I Thank The Lord for your daily Miracles!! May God continue to Bless You All Richly!!*

*Dene R*
*It's so inspiring to read this update and to know how well you all are doing. Mike and Karen you are just awesome!! I wish I could be*

*there in person to give each of you a big hug, but alas I am sending you one via the air ... all the way from Texas! May God continue to bless and keep you both in the palm of His hand.*

### Dave W
*Words cannot express just how happy I am for you and your family, Mike!!! I think about you and your amazing story often and wish you and yours all the best this holiday season and far beyond!!*

### Gailyn A
*Your story continues to be an inspiration! We are so happy for you and hope you have continued blessings through the Holidays and New Year!!*

### Marcia M
*Wonderful news! Reminds me of how precious every moment is. Many blessings and prayers to you.*

### Joan F
*Karen and Mike ... your story is evidence that miracles happen every day! God bless you and your family in the new year of 2016!!!*

## CHAPTER FOUR

# A Break in the Clouds
## 2016

### Hello 2016, We Are So Happy You Are Here!

*By Michelle (Moulden) Bonham — January 3, 2016*

Happy New Year, everyone! It's been a long time since I've written an update, and I apologize for that, but no news is usually good news! As many of you know, Mike has been doing GREAT!!! In fact, we were fortunate enough to spend the last ten days with him, Karen, and the boys as they traveled to Pittsburgh for Christmas with the whole family. It was a true feat considering this time last year we were waiting to get word on when Mike would be airlifted to UCLA to begin surgery and treatment. It's amazing how much can change in one year, isn't it? We are so thankful for all that 2015 brought. Even the worst circumstances managed to bring so much good in so many ways. It's funny how life works that way. However, we are also SO happy to have this year behind us and move forward into a brighter 2016!

As I mentioned, Mike is doing wonderfully. He's enjoying life with Karen and the boys, and continues to make improvements every day. There are still many things that are not quite "back to normal," and may never be, but that does not deter Mike for even a second. He continues to work on his vision through vision therapy, both with a therapist and on his own, and it's definitely improved from this time last year. He got "kicked out" of physical therapy because the therapist said that he was doing so well that they were just watching him work out at this point, so he should just go and get a gym membership instead! Talk about incredible. Santa also brought him a pair of training wheels for his bike so that he can get back to training for that triathlon, and he's already put them to use!

Although things are not perfect, all that matters is Mike is here with us and thriving, despite every curve ball that has been thrown his way.

Thanks to all of you, their life has been able to remain somewhat normal throughout this journey. The boys are happy and healthy, and truly grateful for everything in their lives. Evan is a Rubik's Cube master and William is enjoying gymnastics. Karen has been able to return to work and even choregraphed an incredible piece based on this journey. The raw emotion brought us all to tears; it was simply amazing. The funds continue to be put to good use. Mike has been able to go to vision therapy and receive acupuncture treatments, both of which are not covered by insurance but are vital to his recovery.

In 2016, Mike will be joining a gym to continue building his muscles and motor function. He is also hoping to attend the Balance Center to continue working on stabilizing his balance. We're also trying to convince him he should become a motivational speaker and Karen should write a book about their journey ... so stay tuned to see if we succeed in our efforts. ;) They have already encouraged so many people with their own journey. We can't wait to see who else they're able to help along the way!

Thank you for continuing to follow along on our journey and supporting us. Your thoughts, prayers, love and light have kept us going and we are eternally grateful for all of you! We wish you a happy, healthy 2016!

xoxo,
Team Turnbull

P.S. For those of you who may not have seen it on my Facebook, my birthday wish came true! I was able to dance with Mike, a.k.a. Superman, at my wedding! Warning: have tissues in hand.

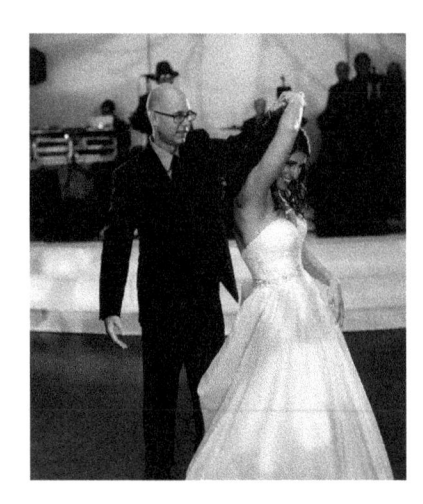

# Happy New Year
*By Karen Turnbull — Jan 21, 2016*

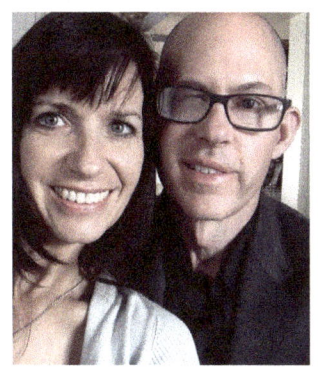

It has been about six weeks since my last post. During that time we have celebrated hard! On December 18th Mike and I headed to UCLA for his six-month checkup. The day started with an MRI of the brain and then a meeting with the neuro-ophthalmologist and, of course, with Dr. Martin. We were thrilled to hear that the MRI looked great! No sign of disease, bleeding or trauma. Mike's vision is still double, although there have been improvements. The prescription for his prism glasses has gone down twice. His eyes are looking more centered than they were but it continues to be a constant daily struggle. The glasses do improve the double vision, but they tend to make things blurry. For the most part I think he has just gotten used to it, but not being able to see well is still high on the list of complaints. Not that he complains much. It's more like a casual mention of how he can't quite see. That said, Dr. Martin was still thrilled with Mike's progress. He watched him walk, did his round of neurology tests and told Mike to continue with therapy, which is ironic because two days earlier his physical therapist dismissed him! Basically they told Mike, "We are just watching you work out at this point. Go get a gym membership."

So, we looked into that but have held off for now as Mike has started a new round of physical therapy. It is at The Balance Center, which deals specifically with balance issues and retraining the brain. He is being challenged in ways he has not yet been challenged. It is a wonderful facility where they have tracks along the ceiling that connect to harnesses that patients wear. The harnesses keep Mike safe from falling and allow the therapist to really push him to the limit. The hope is he begins to gain better balance and control. I am very optimistic that we will see great improvements soon.

We are also going to try hyperbaric chamber treatments. We met with the neurologist Wednesday and are hopefully optimistic. The ironic thing is insurance covers the initial meeting with the neurologist but they do not cover the actual treatments. Where is the sense in that? Yes, go see the specialist to see if you are a candidate for this treatment, but if you are, sorry, we're not going to help you pay for it. Oh well, I cannot let this opportunity go by. Mike is a candidate and the doctors feel it could greatly improve his quality of life, so we are going to give it a go. (Good thing I don't like designer purses or fancy shoes!). I promise I will let you know how it all turns out, but my instincts have guided me on this journey so far and I feel like great changes are ahead in this new year!

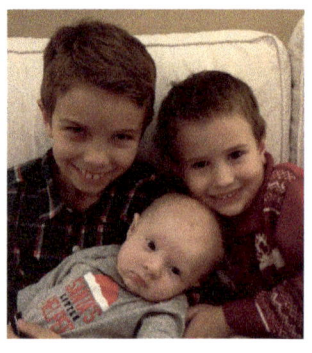

As for our holidays ... Mike, the kids and I traveled to Pittsburgh to spend the holidays with my family! It was amazing! The difference between walking through the airport in June and then again in December was unbelievable. Mike was amazing! He walked without the need to clutch on to my hand. The only difficulty was going down the gangway to the plane. The slope of the ramp was a little tricky but still much easier than back in June. The trip was wonderful. My niece Melissa and her wonderful husband Wes just had their first baby in September. We got to meet this amazing little angel "baby Ryan" as the boys call him. Evan and William could not get enough of him! They wanted to hold him, feed him and even help change his diaper. We got to be at his baptism, which was just a beautiful day full of family and love! Our visit was busy with family time, gameplaying, adventures to the science center and to see the Harlem Globetrotters! It was a fun-filled ten-day getaway!

*Evan, William, & Ryan*

When we returned home we were greeted by presents under our tree. Turns out Santa made two stops. One in Pittsburgh with small gifts that could fit in suitcases and one in Vegas with the larger items that wouldn't quite make the trip on the plane. Included in those was an adult pair of training wheels for Mike's bike! A few days later Mike put them on his bike himself (which was quite a feat) and took his bike for its first ride in over a year! Basically it was like one of those videos you see with the dad helping his young son the first time he rides a bike. There we were in front of our house, me running alongside Mike, holding on to the bike to help him get going and find his balance. By the fourth try, though, he had it! He didn't go far but he managed to make a couple loops in the cul-de-sac and it was awesome!

On January 25th we will celebrate the one-year anniversary of Mike's surgery! Amazing the difference a year can make! This month I have been reminded daily of where we were this time last year. Life is far from perfect and yes, we have our daily struggles, but it sure beats lying in a hospital bed. We continue to be so humbled and full of gratitude to everyone that has helped us on this journey. I don't know how we would have gone through the past year without all of you supporting us. Mike and I are forever grateful. May 2016 be a year of love, laughter, health and happiness! If you feel like sending Mike a happy anniversary on the 25th, please feel free! We will be celebrating our new start! Much love and as always keep the prayers, love, light and energy coming!

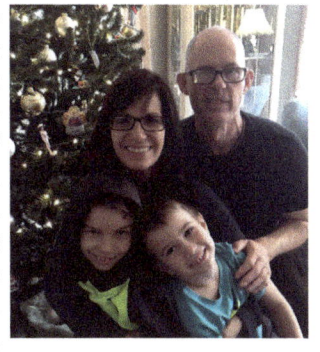

### Tammy C
*So wonderful to hear all of the positive things that are happening! What a journey you have been on! Give Mike a big hug and tell him to keep up the hard work and dedication to restoring his health. We are so happy to hear all of the wonderful things he's accomplished! Sending prayers, love, healing, light and happiness your way! Celebrating with you at how far you've come! Much love to all of you! Miss you so much!*

### Jayme R
*Awesome update!! And through this all, your faith and hope in God and each other has unwavered. Beautiful!!*

### Jason V
*Reading through all of these updates and seeing how Mike has improved makes me so happy. I can't wait to read about what he's going to accomplish next! Thank you for the updates. It means a lot. Still sending all of my love and prayers to you and your family!*

### Doreen L
*Thank you for your update! Ah, the miracle of prayer, a strong, determined personality and family and friends! Prayers continue for the vision and balance issues. You are one awesome family!!!*

### Joan F
*What a wonderful post to start the New Year! Mike's strength obviously comes from genes in his family! Your strength and fortitude comes from where?! I hope I got even a fraction ... lol! You*

both are totally amazing and have accomplished sooo much and have so much to be proud of ... I am proud to have you as my cousin!! God bless and prayers are ongoing!!

**Kristin U**
Thank you for writing with such detail that I smile and feel as though I've seen these things myself. The good news is wonderful! With much love and many prayers.

**Pete B**
Awesome update! Your continued progress and perseverance, Mike, really lifts my spirit! It's hard to get down on things when your buddy is crushing it! Keep rocking brother!

**Shani F**
You are such an inspiring family! God is using your experience to teach all of us how we should live our lives. Happy Anniversary. This next year is going to be an amazing one!

**Elizabeth H**
It was so wonderful to have seen you both in Pittsburgh, along with the boys. You have such a special family and it is so obvious how much love there is. You both are such an inspiration to so many. May God strengthen and bless you in amazing ways in 2016!!!

# Three Years!

*By Karen Turnbull — Mar 30, 2016*

March 30th marked the three-year anniversary of Mike's first thyroid cancer surgery. A lot of people would say three is a magic number. Things tend to happen in threes. When Mike's brain diagnosis happened, we thought, "the third times the charm." Well, for us things tend to happen in fours. Our first kiss was on December 4th, our address is 1204, we dated four years before getting married, we were married four years before child number one and there were another four years before child number two. So, I am now praying that the four-year anniversary is when we can celebrate being cancer-free because Mike has recently been diagnosed with recurrence number four. Stupid cancer.

About three weeks ago Mike had a PET scan. We requested it. His blood levels have been holding strong, although the thyroglobulin level has been creeping up slightly. The doctors have not been worried, in fact they have been thrilled with Mike's progress. He has been on blood thinners for about a year because of blood clots that formed in his lungs when he was bedridden. We wanted to get off of them. The best way to do that was to do a scan and take a look at how things appeared. While the blood clots are gone, two new hotspots have shown up. One is on the front right side of his neck, just under the collarbone and the other is on his sternum. I chose not to panic. I was going with the thought that the lymph node in the neck could be glowing due to a leftover cold and the sternum could be scar tissue from previous radiation treatments. A biopsy of the lymph node proved me wrong. Yes, once again we were faced with the word cancer. A thorough CT of the neck was done and it appears to be isolated to the one node. As for the sternum, it is not the same area, but right next to the previously treated area. So, Mike has already received two of the five radiation treatments to the sternum and will have surgery to remove the lymph node on Monday.

Dr. Wang will do the surgery and he expects it to take about two hours. Compared to what we've been through that sounds like a walk in the park! Depending on how everything goes, Mike will either spend the night in the hospital or he may be released Monday night. It will just depend.

We have had a hard time sharing this. We still have not told the boys. Honestly, that is the hardest part. I fear that with every one of these occurrences they're losing part of their beautiful innocence. I hate cancer for doing that! But, they are amazing and surprise us with their strength every day. I am sure that they will surprise us again. Mike and I are actually doing quite well. Our life is beautifully full with taking the boys to activities, physical therapy and enjoying every second we have.

That being said, I am not going to lie. I am angry. I am angry that we are facing this again. I am angry that I am posting this again. I am angry that I have to talk to my boys about cancer again. I am angry that instead of spending spring break at the beach or somewhere fun we were getting CT scans and bloodwork. I find myself throwing my hands up in the air and screaming "enough!," and then I calm down and I feel guilty because underneath the anger I am so grateful. I know how bad things were and I am so grateful for how things are now! Even with this new diagnosis, life is great! Sometimes hard or challenging, but great! And our family is really, really great! So, we will fight again and we will keep fighting every day. I do still believe that we are stronger than this and Mike will once again kick this.

It has been suggested that after surgery, Mike begin an oral chemotherapy drug. It has been used for years for liver cancer and has recently been approved for thyroid cancer that is stubborn. It is a target type of drug, meaning it is designed to search and destroy only the cells that are causing problems and to leave the healthy cells alone. There are side effects, of course, but we don't know which, if any, Mike will have. If we decide to try it we will closely monitor for side effects. If they get to be too bad then we will discontinue it. Going back to my idea of "fours," this would be the fourth type of treatment to try. Maybe it will be the magic little pill that keeps this from coming back.

I have forwarded everything off to UCLA to have them look at Mike's case as well. I want to be sure that Mike is being looked at as a whole and not just a piece of the puzzle here and there. We will see what they come back with. I figure it doesn't hurt to have many eyes looking at his case.

In the meantime, prayer warriors unite! Keep Mike and our boys in your thoughts, prayers, love, light and energy! We will be ok, but it sure helps to know we have so much love surrounding us!

Thank you all for your support and love. Keep those prayers coming! Much love to you all!

> *Karen P*
> *You are in our heart and prayers. Your whole family is an inspiration about just not giving up. We share your anger at "stupid cancer". We're holding you next to our hearts in love and light.*
>
> *Curt M*
> *Damn, makes me angry too. Your strength just blows my mind. It's fantastic how you can reframe all of the stuff to something so positive. It's inspirational for all of us. Mike is very strong and if anybody can get through this, it's him. Give him a kiss and a hug from both of us.*
>
> *Birgit D*
> *I agree, stupid cancer. You are in my thoughts and prayers, always. Remain strong and again you will beat this. Your family truly is an inspiration. Much love and positive energy your way.*
>
> *Rocco B*
> *There's not a day that goes by where a prayer of well-being is being said for You, Mike and the boys. Michael's road to recovery is a part*

*of our lives. We are here for you and have not forgotten. Praying for health and well-being always. May the Lord touch upon Mike and heal him from this cancer. May his doctors and caregivers be blessed with the wisdom and knowledge to treat him properly and may you be blessed with the strength that you need to do everything that you do. Peace and Love to you, Mike, your sons and family.*

*Paul Q*
*So sorry to hear this. Our family will be praying for Mike, your boys and for you. Positive thoughts and vibes from Wyoming!*

*Kerry D*
*You are a strong, amazing family. We are thinking of you and sending positive thoughts your way!*

*Jaime D*
*Karen, you are both so strong. We will be praying for you. Hold strong.*

*Nan R*
*Karen, agree stupid cancer, but your faith is strong, God's love and care is strong, it sounds like the two procedures and follow-up are strong and your family is strong- amazing, loving, united. Prayers are being sent. Hugs too. Blessings.*

*Gail R*
*It was so good to see all of you today! You all seemed so happy and healthy, and I know that is coming from inside your hearts. I love all of you and am keeping you in my prayers!!!!!*

*Kerryann D*
*Praying and sending love to you always. Number four is going to be it! I will tell you that the oral chemo my dad will take for the rest of his life to keep his leukemia away is a great comfort to me. Hopefully the side effects will be minimal or nill! I'm just so happy to know you beautiful people. You both bring me joy every time I see you. Sending hugs, prayers and anything else you need!!!*

*James M*
*Oh No!!!! Cancer sucks! Mike and your family continue to be in our prayers. We continue to fundraise money for cancer research. A cure has got to be on the horizon! In the meantime, Mike will fight this, will beat this and will continue to be blessed! Lookin' up!*

**Mike G**
*Sending lots of love and LIGHT! Xo xo xo xo*

**Kelly L**
*All the love and prayers your way! You and Mike are amazing!!*

**Candy P**
*Loving all of you and sending many hugs. Keeping you in our prayers. Go Team Turnbull.*

**Shani F**
*Darn cancer! Go away and stay away! You have both been so strong throughout this whole process. It's okay to be mad and angry. Continue to trust in our Lord for peace and strength. We pray for your family and will continue to! Your testimony and strength have been such an inspiration. We love you and we believe in your fighting power.*

**Ellen Sn**
*Karen and Mike, I am saddened to hear this news. You are the Warriors. You will win this fight. I am in your corner sending love, hugs and wonderful thoughts. Keep fighting, please. Xoxo*

**Nancy R**
*Karen, many prayers. Such admiration for your spirit and strength. You continue to be strong, and we will continue the prayers. Love and hugs.*

**Shelley De**
*Wow, Karen. This was as unexpected to read as it was for you to post. The prayers are continuous and never-ending. It has helped in the past and will continue to illuminate around your family. I hope this next round of treatments beats Mike's cancer and keeps your family's strength intact. Always in my thoughts and prayers. Thanks for letting us know how you are so we can up our prayers for you.*

**Stacia F**
*Karen, this is heartbreaking to read. But I know how strong you guys are. All my love and prayers headed your way, and don't beat yourself up for being angry. Sometimes out of anger comes great change!*

*Margaret H*
*We are sending much love from St. Louis. Everyone is lifting you up. Praying for safe and successful surgery and treatment.*

*Nellie S*
*I was not expecting this post at all. I am shocked. Mike looks great and has made so many improvements that I thought the C word was behind you all. I can't believe it. I am so sorry. We always pray for Mike and your family and will continue to do so and will focus our prayers on the surgery going well and him getting rid of this once and for all. Your strength and positivity are very admirable.*

*Elena S*
*Love you all. Your faith, strength and commitment never waiver. God bless you guys. Extra prayers for Mike Monday. xoxo*

*Christina P*
*We are so laser focused sending light and love! You are cancer ass-kicking samurai and this will be it. I feel it! Please lean on this community when you have your moments of anger and frustration. This mighty mighty prayer community can carry some of the load. Sending you all the love, hugs and positive healing light you can handle.*

*Jennifer G*
*Praying for you guys! I am sorry you are going through this again. It doesn't seem fair. My husband took an oral chemo drug and it knocked out his brain cancer so maybe this will be the miracle pill your husband needs. I am glad you are sharing your journey. Cancer is a terrible disease.*

*John V*
*Much love and prayers for you all.*

*Karen K*
*You never left our prayers, and although I am deeply saddened that you are facing such a battle again, I am in awe of your strength and faith. I pray for your unbelievable love for one another to conquer this once and for all. So much love being sent to all of you! xo*

*Anne-Corinne B*
*We are sending love to you and will continue to pray for you all. May you feel enveloped by God's love, giving you peace, strength*

and healing. We will pray for your medical team there and at UCLA to have wisdom in their care. Your family is precious. Sending much hope and love.

### Trish T
So sorry. It is definitely not news of encouragement. It is ok to be angry. It is ok to be sad. It is ok to shout out to the Lord in anger and ask why. Please know that through this storm he who travels alongside faith travels not alone.

### Tom N
Thinking and praying for all of you. Soo sorry this is happening again. Mike is definitely a fighter! God bless you all.

### Hope M
Prayer Warriors Never Sleep!! We love you and our thoughts are with you all.

### Darelle H
Damn it! Prayers unite.

### Mary Alice J
Karen and Mike, as you look at another challenge in life, the best of people in our family always said to take one day at a time. May St. Anthony keep you in his care. Luvya.

### Tom E
Mike, I hate your cancer but it's nice that you have what may be the world's greatest support system, Karen and your boys.

### Heather B
I hate it, too! We only want to hear the good reports! That said, he will kick this again! Your strong family and love and support from all of your people and God's love ... !!! Praying for you guys!

### Pete B
I know it's hard to share the tough things but thank you for sharing. We need to hear it and I'm glad you caught the hot spots early! Praise God! I will double up on the prayers for Mike and all of you. We will keep fighting this battle together!

# 4:40

*By Karen Turnbull — Apr 4, 2016*

Mike just went back for his surgery. It is 4:40 PM here in Vegas! Fire up the prayers. Thank you all! Much love!

### Jordan B
*Love you guys! Praying hard!*

### Steven L
*Full strength prayers of love and healing heading your way!*

### Alex K
*We are pulling for you, Mike, heart and soul!! May the surgery be a great success. Talk soon!! Love you my friend!*

### Stacy G
*I was going to call you today on my break. At 4:30 PM. Crazy! Love you two and firing them up. Much love and peace to you today friend.*

### Doriana S
*Sending you much love and light ... keeping you in prayer:)*

### Hayley M
*Hi Karen, as always you guys are in our prayers. Even though we are miles away from you now, we speak of you often and wish you and your beautiful family well. I agree ... cancer is stupid ... that was a very nice way of putting it. You were always more polite than me!!!! Much love. xxxx*

# Home!

*By Karen Turnbull — Apr 4, 2016*

All done! Dr. Wang got it out. It was just the one lymph node and he got clean margins all around! Mike will come home tonight!!!! Thank you GOD!!!!!!! Thank you prayer warriors! We love you!!!!!

### Shari B
*Incredibly wonderful news!! Thanks for always being so amazing about keeping us updated, Karen. You are such an amazing person*

*and Mike is the luckiest man in the world for having you as his wife! All our love.*

**Nathan T**
*That's great news!! I'm so happy to hear that! You are all on the right track. Keep living in that positive state of gratitude because it brings that healing energy!*

**Ric F**
*Great News!!!*

**Jen F**
*Praise Him for His continued blessings.*

**Christina P**
*Hot diggidy damn!!!*

**Sharon H**
*Crying with joy. Thank you, Lord.*

# Day Four
*By Karen Turnbull —Apr 8, 2016*

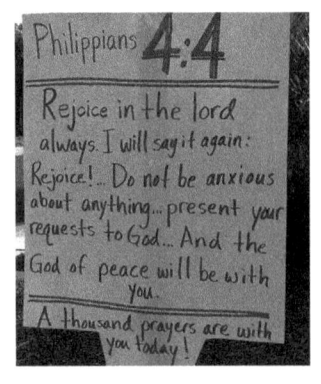

Keeping with our power of fours belief, I decided today was an appropriate day to give an update. As my friend Tammy pointed out, today is 4-8-16 (all divisible by four!). Surgery was four days ago on 4-4-16. Our friends Tom and Jen went out of their way to make sure we started Monday right and posted a huge sign of Phillipians 4:4 on the stop sign at the end of our street! It was perfect! We had a busy day with an early morning eye appointment, radiation and check-in before surgery. We were scheduled for a 3:00 PM surgery but it was pushed back slightly. That was ok, because as crazy as it sounds, Mike and I parted in the hallway, him to the OR and me to the waiting room, at 4:40 PM. We aren't positive but we are thinking it was probably right about 4:44 PM when Mike got on the operating table. We are believing in our power of fours!

So, it is four days post-surgery and Mike is doing great! To be honest, this surgery barely slowed him down at all! He was sent home Monday night and Tuesday morning he felt well enough to go to his hyperbaric chamber treatment and to radiation treatment number four. He finished radiation on Wednesday and has tolerated everything very well. Thank you Brittany and Karen, his radiation therapists, for taking such good care of him! As much as we hate the reason we were seeing you, we LOVED seeing you!

As I said in a previous post, I was dreading telling the boys about this surgery. We told them Saturday night and they were so brave and strong. They are just amazing and my wise little eight-year-old Evan put it very well when he told us, "I am a little scared but not too much because I know what we have been through and I know we will be ok." Thank you Evan for giving me strength!

Thank you everyone for your posts, comments, messages and texts! The love surrounding our family is truly amazing! And of course thank you for the continued prayers, energy, love and light! We are doing great and moving forward.

Thank you! Keep the prayers coming!

> *Angela C*
> Yay! He's such a fighter! We look forward to reading more updates about his progress to a successful recovery! Love to you all!
>
> *Shannon B*
> You will have all of the love and support to be successful in this undertaking. That is the angel meaning of number four. Angels are always around us and I know you and Michael feel the love:) Sending all of you prayers and strength!! XOXOXO
>
> *Sean H*
> Beautiful, Karen. Sending loads of love to Mike and to your family from Brooklyn.
>
> *Cindi R*
> Healing. Peace. Strength. Love. My FOUR words for you.
>
> *Belinda R*
> Holding you all in our hearts and prayers.

*Suzanne P*
I still believe!!!! What powerful words Evan gave to you! Still sending love and healing energy to you all!

*Brook D*
You guys are so strong and so good. Love love love you!

*Robin C*
Your kids are so amazing. As always I am holding you all in my heart and in my prayers. I also have Mike on my online prayer group list so lots and lots of prayers and I think the power of four is great for you guys. Love and hugs.

## Tear Duct Number Two
*By Karen Turnbull — Apr 24, 2016*

Mike is currently waiting for surgery to repair the right tear duct, which is completely blocked. The left one was done in the fall of 2014 and we have been waiting to fix this one, but obviously other issues took precedent. So, here we are back at Sunrise Hospital waiting for yet another surgery. He will probably go back in about an hour. Hopefully this will be fairly easy with a quick recovery.

As always prayers, love and light are appreciated.

*Stacy G*
May that tear duct clear up and weep tears of joy! Much love Karen and Mike!

*Karen Mi*
Bless you, Karen. I pray for you and Mike all the time and truly, please call upon me any time. I will do my best to help out in any way possible. Much love!!

## Done!
*By Karen Turnbull — Apr 24, 2016*

Once again I am saying thank you God for keeping Mike safe! The surgeon just came out to tell me everything went great! Then he sat down and asked me how Mike was doing. He shared personal stories of family and friends who are survivors and fighters, too. He was truly concerned with Mike and took time to listen. People often say how bad the doctors are here in Las Vegas. From personal experience it is just not true! We have been blessed, time and time again, with amazing medical care. I am grateful to these very smart and passionate doctors! They see Mike as a person, not just another case. I am forever grateful!

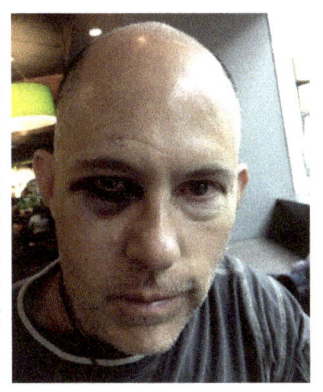

Thanks all for the love, light and prayers! Happy Sunday!

### Doriana S
*Karen, you continue to be such an amazing warrior for your husband ... you stand in faith and walk in gratitude ... beautiful, incredible:) Sending you and your family much love and light.*

### Dan S
*So glad everything went ok! Sending positive vibes as always!*

### Les K
*Thank you once again, Karen, for keeping us all updated on Mike! May blessings, peace and healing continue to surround you, Mike, Evan and William :)*

### Heather B
*That is great news! I'm so happy he has such good care ... personable and compassionate doctors taking care of him and you! Love, light and prayers!!!*

### Sara B
*Karen, it has been a while since I checked in here, only to see what Mike and you guys have been dealing with. I am sorry that he has to go through this cancer stuff again! Your son is right. After everything you have all been through Mike has got this. You are such an amazing and inspiring family. I am sending all my good vibes and mojo to you guys. Everyone at NCEP is praying for him to be 100% soon. Love and big hugs to all of you.*

# Looking Forward

*By Karen Turnbull — July 24, 2016*

Hello! It has been awhile, but here's the latest news! In the middle of June we headed to UCLA for Mike's six-month follow-ups. Mike had a beautiful MRI of his brain and everything looks wonderful! As far as Dr. Martin is concerned, he does not need to see Mike for another year! The neuro-ophthalmologist was also encouraged by the progress Mike's eyes have made, however the progress has seemed to hit a plateau. His vision has remained about the same for quite some time. So, even though he has regained more tracking and movement he still suffers from severe double vision. The prism glasses he wears help bring the two images together, but it is a blurred image. The vision problems add to daily struggles with things like depth perception and balance issues.

So, we were referred to an eye surgeon, Dr. Joseph Demer, to see what options we have. We figured we would get an appointment in a few months but as it turned out he is the husband of our neurosurgeon's nurse practitioner! Her name is Dr. Melissa Reider-Demer (Melle) and she has been one of our biggest angels during this journey. I can email this woman any time of day or night with any question or concern and she always responds quickly

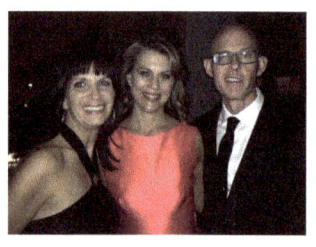

*Dr. Melissa Reider-Demer*

and makes things happen. (I am even guilty of sending her occasional pictures or videos of Mike's amazing progress). She is always happy to see how far Mike has come! When the insurance company decided that it was not necessary for us to continue going to UCLA for our follow-ups I wrote to Melle. She immediately responded with a letter to the insurance company that quickly made it VERY clear why we absolutely needed to continue our care with them. That, combined with the five-page letter I wrote to them, must have done the trick because they called us the night they received it to tell us we had been approved! Like I said, she is amazing! While we were visiting with her and Dr. Martin she said, "Let me just call my husband and see if he can see you while you are here." Next thing we know we are leaving her office, walking across the patio and entering his office! We were immediately put in an examination room and the most intense and thorough eye exam was performed. It was decided that Mike is an ideal candidate for corrective surgery! So tomorrow we are headed to UCLA for surgery on Wednesday! Please God let this work! The amazing thing is, the surgery should only take about forty-five minutes and can be done without anesthesia! The goal is to get both eyes tracking together so the brain sees one image instead of two. Like I said ... please God let this work!

During our June trip we also met with the head of Endocrinology who specializes in rare cases. He referred us to an oncologist, Dr. Deborah Wong, and Mike had a PET scan done to establish a new baseline. Thursday we will find out the results and what kind of plan they have in mind to keep this thing under control.

In May, Mike tried an oral chemotherapy meant to target and destroy. Unfortunately, he had a severe reaction that caused blisters all over the soles of his feet. It was so bad that he was bedridden for a few days. With this information we now seek out other options. Mike's brain tumor (which was kept frozen in the UCLA lab) was going to be genetically tested to see if he carries any markers that may make him a candidate for different treatments. The goal, as Dr. Wong presented to us, "Is to stay a step ahead and be smarter than it." The endocrinologist told us, "We are going to work together to ensure you are here for your children." Bring it on! We are ready!

During the first week of July our case was presented to the UCLA tumor board. This is a group of about thirty doctors all meeting to look at Mike's case and decide on a plan to battle this disease. We will meet with Dr. Wong this Thursday to see what they have in mind. We have a busy few days ahead of us. Please keep us in your thoughts and prayers.

Other than all of this ... we are fantastically great! The kids are happy and silly and make us laugh every day. We spent three weeks with my family in Pittsburgh and even managed to sneak in a family trip to Legoland between doctor appointments and PET scans. Life continues and we have vowed to keep joy in our life. We are dancing through the rain and celebrating the rainbows that continue to come out of the clouds. I will be in touch this week as we have lots happening.

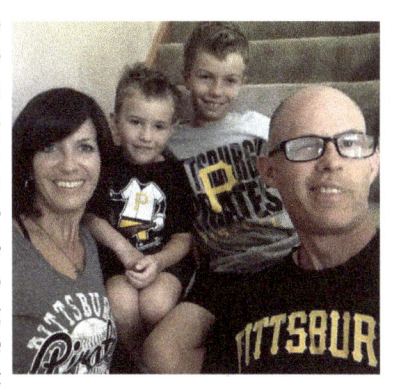

Thank you all for following our story, supporting us and surrounding us with love, light, prayers and healing energy! Much love always!

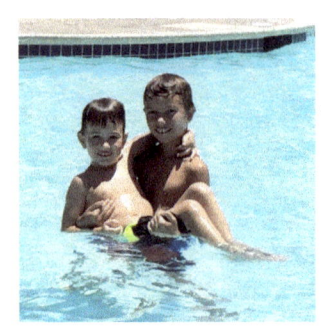

*Tom E*
*You guys are so easy to pray for because you fight SO hard. God bless all you Turnbulls!*

*Jaime D*
*Praying for a successful eye surgery on Wednesday and continued progress. Your strength and support is amazing for us all. Keep your positive spirit.*

*Christine E*
*That's amazing! Mike, you and your wonderful boys are always in our thoughts and prayers. We love you!*

*Robin C*
*Your brightness is a beacon to all of us to remember to trust God. I continue to keep you all in my prayers. Love, hugs and blessings.*

*Kerryann D*
*This is all wonderful news! Your family's light shines so bright. Sending a big hug and s prayer for safe travels! We love you!*

*Carol P*
*Oh, I'm so thrilled to hear the news and how God is working in your lives. The love, encouragement and strength you both have individually and together is pure example to me of what God has put together. Love you guys very much and thank you for sharing your journey with us. Always in my prayers...*

*Jessica H*
*Such wonderful news! We are praying for you all this week!*

*Ric F*
*"We are dancing through the rain and celebrating the rainbows that continue to come out of the clouds." Thanks for that, Karen! This is all great news. I'm happy to read all of this!*

*Melin F*
*You, Mike, the boys, the entire family of physicians and their crews are amazing. We continue to keep everyone in our prayers and are constantly amazed by the tenacity of your medical teams. Keep us informed and you will be always be in our hearts and prayers.*

*Lou G*
*Prayin' as always. In the midst of your thornbush, a beautiful rose turns up when you need one. Happy for the serendipitous meetings that bless you. Look forward to your book. You are destined to offer this journey of silver lined clouds as inspiration for all of us. Love to you all. Miss you Mike.*

*Linda Q*
*God and you got this! It seems all the right doors are opening and leading you to just whom you need. Coincidence? I think not. Hugs to all and prayers for complete healing!*

*Liese W*
*So much love and joy in this message. God is so present in each moment and we continue to pray for each step the doctors are taking to bring Mike to wholeness. Much love and joy to continue. xoxo*

*Anne L*
*Such good news ... thank you for the update! Continued love and prayers to lift you all up and guide these skilled doctors. XOXO*

*Margaret H*
*Love You All SO Much! Praying for Mike and team of doctors and medical staff tomorrow for surgery. Praying for you, my dear, sweet Karen, for strength and hope. Love to little E and W. You are amazing.*

*Karen C*
*God Bless your family! What beautiful and strong people! I miss your face and heart and think of you often! Don't hesitate to give a shout if you ever need anything! Even just a giggle or a chat. Xoxoxoxo. Sending love and light, beautiful!*

*Ellen F*
*Kim and I continue to be awestruck at you and your family's strength, resolve and positive way of looking at things. Praying that God will be with Mike's doctors and that He will give you, Karen, continued strength. Much love from us!*

*Heather B*
*Keeping you guys in my prayers! I am always amazed and inspired by your positive and gracious words! Sending our love and prayer! Give the kiddos a squeeze!!!*

# Here We Go!

*By Karen Turnbull — July 27, 2016*

Sitting in pre-op waiting to get this going! We are laughing so hard at how routine pre-op rooms have become to us. This picture says it all!

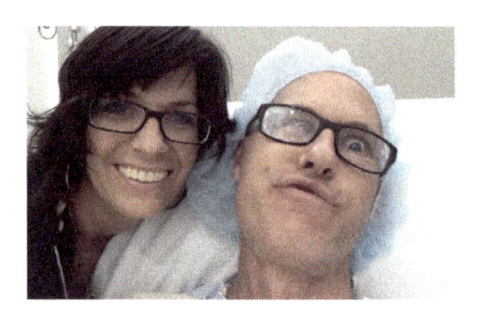

### Jeneane H
*Love, light and lots of laughter.*

### Mary Alice J
*Special people can laugh and smile through it all. Told St. Anthony this AM about Mike's endeavor this week. So it is all covered for ya. Love and God Bless.*

### Jenny F
*You two are truly astounding. Your strength and optimism is remarkable. Huge East Coast hugs coming your way.*

### Nellie S
*You guys crack me up! Your positivity is inspiring. Prayers.*

# All Done

*By Karen Turnbull — July 27, 2016*

Mike is doing great! He had the entire procedure done with no anesthesia other than numbing (lydocaine) eyedrops. This allowed him to communicate with the doctor to dial in and hopefully find the right adjustment. There is currently some blurriness due to the ointment and drops and it will take some healing to get the double vision to correct completely. For the first time in eighteen months, as we were in the car, he did not feel like cars were crossing in front of us. A huge improvement! He still has some eye pulsing so time will tell as to how much that resolves, but overall things are really good! Time for us to eat and relax!

>  **Christina P**
>  *Hot diggidy damn! Fighting through like the Champs that you are. Sending you each love and hugs!!!*
>
>  **Liese W**
>  *Amazing and wonderful!!! Sending continuous healing love and light. xoxo*
>
>  **Ellen Sn**
>  *Great news! You two are truly inspiring to others! Xoxo*

# One Week

*By Karen Turnbull — Aug 3, 2016*

We are one week post eye surgery. I wish I could say things were great and Mike's vision was perfect. I really wish I could say that. Unfortunately, we are in a rough patch. While the surgery was successful in bringing the two images together, another element has presented. It turns out that even though the images are together, it is almost as if he now has double vision with one image behind the other and the back image pulsing up and down. This pulsing is called nystagmus. We knew he had this problem when he would look out of the right eye only. What we didn't realize was that the brain had been ignoring that image or shutting it off to the point that he didn't know it was there unless he closed or covered the left eye. So now with the images being brought together the pulse is really evident. We don't know if his brain will adjust to this and maybe quiet the pulsing to the point where it is not as bothersome. Time will hopefully tell.

On top of that, a new problem has presented. There seems to be a black spot in his left peripheral vision. A call to Dr. Demer today ended with him telling Mike to see an ophthalmologist here ASAP. (He would of course see him personally but he is in Los Angeles and we are in Las Vegas). It appears this is not normal after surgery and could be a new issue, so tomorrow morning we go to see what that is all about. Praying that maybe Mike is seeing a stitch or a speck of blood pooled on the side of the eye. I have to say we're getting pretty tired of this roller coaster.

Also, we are feeling a little defeated after our appointment with the UCLA oncologist last Thursday. Genetic testing was done on Mike's brain tumor and while some mutations did show up, they were not any that would open up a world of magical healing drugs. His PET scan showed that there is a small spot on the left side of his sternum. The same spot that was already radiated. So why has a new spot developed? There are also some small spots or nodules in his lungs. Some have been there since the January 2015 pet scan at UCLA, some are new. They are very, very small but something we need to watch. So, we are feeling tired and sad. It has been three and a half years since this all began and there just doesn't seem to be an end in sight. Our future holds more doctors, more scans, trying new drugs and constantly fighting.

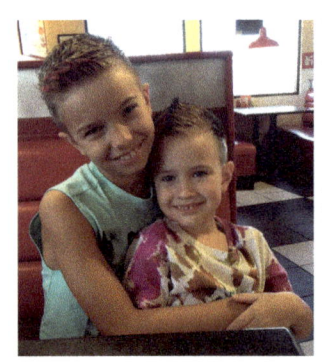

Yes, we are tired. I always try to put a positive spin on my posts, but tonight I am just tired. I am sitting at gymnastics watching my boys be the amazing kids they are. Somehow they are still full of joy and so much love. Because of them, we will get over this hurdle and we will fight and we will continue on to the next stage. Please keep us in your thoughts and prayers tomorrow morning as we visit the ophthalmologist. We are really praying this is just a small bump in the road and not a new issue to deal with. He has been through so much. I hate cancer.

Thank you for your prayers, love and light. Tonight we really need them.

*Monique E*
*My heart aches. Pit in my stomach. I am praying.*

### Marianne M
*My heart is aching, my eyes are crying and my arms are stretching across the miles to give you a hug. You, and Mike, of all people, do not deserve this card you have been dealt. Stay strong. We love you!*

### Nandita S
*You are the strongest people I know. Your grace and warmth through all has been an inspiration to me personally. I'll be thinking and sending all the vibes in the morning. Hugs and kisses to you all!*

### Shani F
*Cancer sucks! I am always praying for all four of you! And it's OK to be frustrated. Cancer is tough anyway you look at it. God loves you all.*

### Joan F
*I am and will be praying to St. Peregrine for you all! The love and devotion for each other in your family is such an inspiration ... that is a constant in this long journey! I just want to help you carry this cross ... you are loved!*

### Fran D
*Please know that we all are holding you in our hearts and sending strength along with courage to help you in this battle. Much love and prayers being sent your way.*

### Kelly C
*We are so sad, mad, frustrated and shocked to hear this news and we feel horrible for you all. You have been through enough! We know how strong you are, though, and you will conquer all of these new obstacles, too!! Our positive thoughts, prayers and hugs are coming your way from the entire Cassell family. We are all here for you!*

### Cindi R
*Ugh. We appreciate your honesty. You deserve to be sad. Continued prayers for peace and healing in the midst of this horrible storm.*

### Doriana S
*Dearest Karen, holding you and Mike and your family in a giant stream of LOVE and LIGHT! You are surrounded by angels and God's Divine Love ... Peace and Healing ... love and blessings.*

*JoLayne G*
*You certainly have my prayers- many of them. Don't ever feel bad when the sadness takes over a bit. Let the tears fall if they must. I think there is healing in tears, too. Then you will have more strength to keep carrying on. Keep putting one foot in front of the other.*

*Paula M*
*Lots of love and prayers your way! Karen, you set the bar for optimism! You and Mike will get through this bump. Everything is temporary!!!*

*Jacqueline S*
*There are no words except we love you guys and pray for you daily!*

*Randy C*
*We are praying for the answers you need, and sending our love and support your way. Here is to a quick resolution to the new issues, and love and laughter ever after.*

*Laura T*
*Dearest Mike, Karen, Evan and William, we're sending you love, prayers, hugs and strength and the hopeful wish that things will improve. We love you.*

*Stacia F*
*Oh, my friend ... Sending you support. Love. And anything else I can conjure for you.*

*Susan S*
*Please dear God be with this family. Place your hands upon Mike and give him strength and healing. We are all praying for you, Mike. You can beat this!! I know you are tired but you are strong. Keep that fight going!!! Love to all of you!!!*

*Christie P*
*Karen and Mike, we love you and pray for you. Know we are here for whatever you need.*

*Lynne E*
*Karen, I really understand your comments on the roller coaster that we ride along with you. Greg and I have gone through years of this also. Cancer, along with the numerous treatments scans and tests, never seems to end. We all deserve a time to be sad or mad or*

*hopeless, but we always seem to get up and go forward again. Our hearts and prayers to you and Mike.*

### Lance P
*Thank you for keeping us all informed, of the good and the bad. Wishing Mike and family the all best in this difficult journey.*

### Jaclyn F
*Sending so much love and many prayers! Don't lose hope. All you need is faith, hope and love. As God says, the greatest of these is love and there is plenty love between you and Mike and our whole family!*

### Rocco B
*We are and continue to pray for health and well-being for Mike, you and your children. There is never defeat in the eyes of God! Have faith and know that you are not carrying this burden alone. We are all here with you in prayer and faith. Love and big hugs to you, Mike and your boys!!!!*

### Fernanda G
*I'm so sorry. You are both so strong. God bless you and may He continue to give you strength, because I can't even imagine how exhausted you are from all of this. I pray you can be free of this once and for all :(*

### Kristin U
*I'm praying for your continued strength, and feeling appreciative of your writing. It's always great to read the positive results and progress, but we also need to remember that you both have the downers and need continual prayer.*

### Janna R
*I am screaming "ENOUGH" with and for you. I will pray for healing and comfort for you and Mike. We wish you the best.*

# Eye Appointment

*By Karen Turnbull — Aug 4, 2016*

Just finished with ophthalmologist. All is good! Hallelujah! There is a spot of condensation that for some reason Mike is seeing in his field of vision, but the retina is fine and there does not seem to be any major concern! One obstacle conquered!

Next step is follow-up scans and appointments at UCLA the end of August. Let's hope we have a few weeks of peaceful healing. Thank you all for your kind and encouraging words. Please know we read every post (many times) and are just overwhelmed with the love you all send us. It truly refuels us and gives us strength. Today is a new day!

Love, prayers and light back to each of you!

> *Michelle B*
> *Thank you God for the positive report, loving blessings and continued healing. We can all take a deep breath now while saying Hallelujah!!! Big hugs from the 'Burgh Bonhams.*
>
> *Birgit P*
> *Karen and Mike, we think and talk about you guys often. We send you strength and peace for both of you and your boys!*
>
> *Alex K*
> *Excellent news! May your vision keep improving, Mike!! Another obstacle cleared! You should be in the cancer fighters Olympics!*
>
> *Shari B*
> *Thank God!! When I saw that there was a new posting and as the site was loading I just kept saying over and over, please make sure the appointment went well today!!! XOXOXOXOXOXO*
>
> *Ellen O*
> *Great news!!! Continued prayers for continued good news and good health!*

# Point of Light

*By Karen Turnbull — Oct 19, 2016*

Hi all! It has been a while and I am happy to share some exciting news with everyone. Mike has been really busy being the awesome man I admire and love so much! In the past two months he has been able to reconnect with parts of him that, well ... make him Mike. First off, music is back in his life! No, he is not playing trombone; this time around he is playing percussion (picture of Mike on the cajon) and loving it! Anyone who really knows Mike well would agree he is a percussionist at heart. Traveling with him on our many adventures, he has always been drawn to the unique percussion instruments of the area. If you ever step into his home office/studio you quickly see lots more drums and percussion instruments than trombones!

This new adventure began by our friend Jason simply asking Mike if he might consider playing the cajon drum in church one Sunday. The crazy thing is, Jason had no previous knowledge of Mike ever playing percussion. I actually asked Jason what made him ask Mike. He said, "I just heard a voice say you should ask Mike Turnbull if he can play." Thank you Jason for listening to that voice! For me there is no doubt where that voice came from! So our home is now filled with drumming and shaking and all sorts of fun music once again! And the drumming is built-in therapy! Good for the body, mind and soul! If you are a Vegas friend and want to hear him play please feel free to join us any Sunday at New Song Church in Anthem at 10:30 AM! We have a great time and I am easy to find ... the lady in the front row smiling ear to ear!

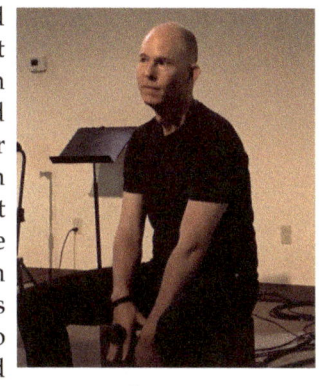

The other exciting thing that happened, just one day after Mike's first time playing, is we got him a recumbent trike. For those that don't know what that is, it is basically a three-wheeled seated bike (picture attached). It is so cool!!! After visiting our friend Terry at The Bike Shop and getting his thoughts on good ones for Mike, the search on Craigslist began. That night Mike found a post for one available in Boulder City. So the next night we drove out there and Mike got his freedom back! Now of course I asked him to go slow, ease into it, build up his strength, blah, blah, blah ... again, those that know Mike know where this is headed. The next day while driving home from work I get a call from Mike asking me if I can pick him up from the local coffee shop. I immediately said, "Of course, but why are you at the coffee shop and how did you get there?" His response: "I will explain when you get here but I am ok." So I pull in and there he is in full bike gear! Turns out he rode ten miles to the bike shop to get it tuned up and adjusted. Because he had to leave it there, he then took the city bus to as close to home as possible, leaving him at the coffee shop. His first words were, "Don't be mad at me." I laughed! He was so happy there was no way I could be mad! I asked him, "How do you feel?" He said, "Like a kid!" With tears of joy in my eyes he told me three things made him really happy as a kid: playing drums, riding his bike and skiing. Two out of three down ... now to figure out how to get him back on the slopes! He now rides his trike everywhere (provided there is a bike path or lane). He rides to and from therapy three times a week, to the store to grab lunch, to get blood work done and also just for fun. To my neighbors, keep your eyes out for him and feel free to cheer him on!

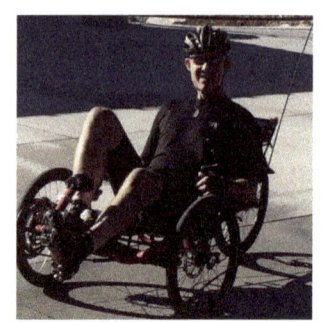

And as if all that isn't enough ... next Thursday, Mike and I head to the UCLA Visionary Ball to benefit the Department of Neurosurgery. Last year we attended as invited guests and this year Mike will be sharing his story as a "Point of Light" speaker! It will be an amazing opportunity for others to hear of the miracles that happen when beautiful minds work together. As Mike has said many times, "If I can help someone else because of this, then in some way it makes it almost worth it." Oh my love, you help more people than you realize!

As for all the other stuff ... his eyes are much improved, although he still battles with nystagmus, which is a pulsing of the eye that causes everything to look like it is bouncing. Super annoying but he is managing. The spots from the last two scans remain unchanged, so at this point they are being watched but we are leaving that to the doctors while we simply LIVE! Life is precious. Enjoy it!

The boys are awesome and gorgeous and bring more joy than words can describe! They love school, gymnastics and being silly boys! Evan completed his second triathlon last weekend and William just started hip-hop! Watch out, he's taking his moves to a new level!

Me, I am good. I am living. Right now, I feel like I can actually breathe again and enjoy life a little more fully. I am busy but happy. And I am so grateful for the amazing things happening for Mike and our family.

Thank you all for your continued prayers, love, light, energy and support. You all lift us up every day! And if I may ask that you include our dear friend Cindy in those healing thoughts and prayers. She is currently fighting the cancer fight. The Enersons are more than friends to us. We consider them family and when this horrible thing called cancer shows its ugly head we have to unite to fight hard.

Keep the prayers coming ... miracles are happening!

### Shannon B
*Wow! So wonderful to hear that things are going great. We all have so much to be thankful for:) Always sending you love and light and praying for Cindy. XOXOX*

### Angela W
*This is the best news I've heard in a while! So wonderful! I can hear the joy in your words! Love the story about the coffee shop. I bet there will be more calls like that in the future as he continues to adventure! Love it! Love you guys!*

### Nathan T
*Wow! I love to hear these amazing stories! Keep having fun and enjoying life! You guys are amazing!*

### Clare T
*You are an inspirational family and this post brought me such joy! We are so happy for you and wish you continued happiness and joy. xxx*

### Mary Alice J
*Karen, it is so special to read your post. It has to be uplifting for so many people. Continued blessings and hugs to you, Mike, the boys and Baylee. Asking St. Anthony to watch over your friend, Cindy.*

### Trish T
*You always amaze me! Mike always amazes me! Your family is a gracious gift from GOD. You all are always in our thoughts, our prayers and our hearts. Continue "living," my friend. As you already know, each day is a wonderful gift. Love you all.*

*Lynne E*
Hi Karen, what a wonderful note to read. I had tears in my eyes but this time tears of joy for you and Mike. You are both miraculous and your love for each other is so precious. To Mike I say, "keep biking and pound away on those drums at every New Song service." Isn't it great to just enjoy life without having to talk about the next "hurdle?" Prayers and love continue your way.

*Karine Z*
Love you so much!! You continue to inspire us, Mike and Karen!!

*Cindi R*
Continued love and hugs and prayers to you guys. I love that Mike is playing percussion and biking all around town! He is indeed a hero and a rock star. So are you, Karen, for being his constant support and partner. Glad you can relax and breathe and enjoy life. You deserve it.

*Sara B*
This is such great news to hear. I am smiling and have tears in my eyes for you all. You are such a beautiful family. A true inspiration to all. Stay strong and I hope to see you all soon. The big NCEP Thanksgiving is coming up soon- hope you can make it. Love to all the Turnbulls.

*Cathy M*
This news is music to our ears, pun intended. We couldn't be happier to hear of all the exciting progress Mike has made. He is truly an inspiration beyond description! Thrilled to hear that you are all doing well and living all the special moments of life. You are always in our hearts! Special thoughts, prayers and encouragement for Cindy. Much love.

*Jacqueline S*
Such wonderful news brought a massive smile to my face. Thank you for sharing.

*Heather B*
A wonderful report! Strong and beautiful family- through rough times and good- we can all learn to be more positive! Keep it all coming!!!!!

*Rocco B*
*Thank you, Karen, for this heartwarming update! I am so thankful to hear all that is positive. It is completely amazing to know that our prayers are being answered. Thanking our Lord Jesus for giving us Health, Well-Being, Guidance and protecting us on our journey in life! Much love to you, Mike and the boys!!!!*

*Kathy A*
*Such great news!! Thank you for sharing ... I love you both so much!!*

*Pam Ra*
*I LOVE this update and I love you guys. Go Mike!*

*Kristin U*
*I can totally see Mike riding ten miles to get the bike tuned up! Great writing and good news. Love, love, love and living!! So happy for you. Xoxox*

## Visionary Ball

*By Michael Turnbull — Oct 28, 2016*

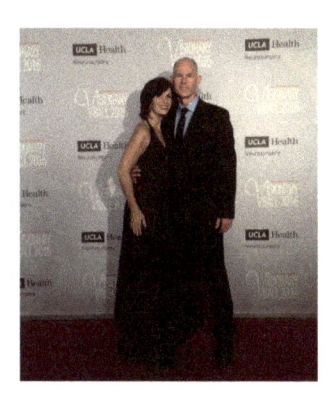

Hello, all. It's Mike. I know Karen usually writes these posts (quite eloquently, I might add) but I thought it might be nice to hear from me for a change.

The UCLA Department of Neurosurgery has a fundraising event called the Visionary Ball, which has been held annually at the Regent Beverly Wilshire for the past ten years. My neurosurgeon, Dr. Neil Martin, is the host of the event. Last night, I was honored and privileged to be asked to be one of two "Point of Light" speakers. The event had special meaning as it was Dr. Martin's last Visionary Ball. He is moving on to a new research position on the east coast after thirty years at UCLA. We were seated with Dr. Martin's nurse practitioner, Melissa Reider-Demer, and her husband, Dr. Demer, my neuro-ophthalmologist who performed strabismus surgery on me a couple of months ago, as well as my oncologist Dr. Wong and her husband. It was a magical evening, and a transcript of my speech follows below for those who are interested.

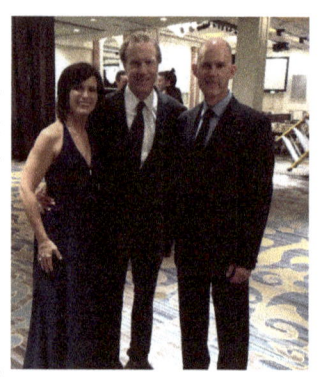

*Dr. Neil Martin*

As Karen would say, thank you all again for the love, light, support and prayers.

> Three and a half years ago I was diagnosed with stage IV Hürthle Cell Carcinoma, a somewhat rare and aggressive form of thyroid cancer. I underwent a ten-hour procedure in which I had one hundred lymph nodes removed, a thyroidectomy, a parathyroid transplant and a tracheal resection and reconstruction. I was a professional musician, so I was not familiar with these terms until the surgery, but miraculously, just six weeks later, I was back to playing trombone for Donny & Marie at the Flamingo in Las Vegas.
>
> Fast forward to November 7, 2014, which was my forty-seventh birthday of all days. I awoke with stroke-like symptoms and a series of scans showed a hemorrhage in the left pons of my brain stem, which most neurologists were calling a cavernous malformation, but they said it was in too risky a position to even biopsy. Eventually the doctors in Las Vegas said, "We are good at treating horses, but you are a zebra. We need to send you to where they treat zebras." So I was airlifted here to UCLA. Dr. Neil Martin agreed to perform a brain stem resection, although even he said he would not do so if given any other choice. Dr. Martin asked my wife how active I was prior to the hemorrhage, and she said, "Actually, he was training for a triathlon." To which he replied, "Good, he was training for surgery." From what I understand there are only a handful of elite neurosurgeons in the entire country that could do what Dr. Martin did. Surprisingly, pathology reports revealed that the mass was in fact metastatic thyroid cancer to the brain, which is highly unusual. My wife likes to say, "Can't you be

normal and boring for a change? Do you have to be rare and special all the time?" At that point I was in pretty bad shape. I couldn't walk, talk, see or eat on my own and I left here in a wheelchair, but after two years of extensive therapy here I am, so I would like to thank a few people:

Melissa Reider-Demer and her husband, Dr. Joseph Demer, have been instrumental in improving my quality of life. Obviously, Dr. Neil Martin and his staff. I don't know how one adequately expresses thanks to the person who saved their life, but he did and I am forever grateful. And of course my beautiful wife, Karen, who has been my advocate on this journey and is an angel on earth. I love you.

This is going pretty well considering I had a brain tumor! I'll close with a quick story about our boys, Evan and William. When they were able to visit us here at UCLA they were amazed and their description was "The Magic Hospital." In their eyes, it was the only place that could fix their daddy. And that's really the reason we're here tonight. So other mommies, daddies, children and loved ones can be fixed by "The Magic Hospital" and returned to their families. Thank you.

### Shelley De
*Michael's speech was eloquent. He is a walking, talking miracle. The doctors were extraordinary and restored a wonderful husband and dad. You are so lucky to have found these magicians. So happy for Michael's daily progress and for sharing his story.*

### Clare T
*What a wonderful tribute and story. THANK YOU for sharing. It really has been an incredible journey. Sending much love as always. xxx*

### Rob M
*Mike, I am and will always be amazed by your strength. You are something else, brother. And funny as all hell, too! I'm proud to call you a friend.*

### Nandita S
*You are so amazing, Mike! I wish I could have been there for your triumphant return to UCLA and heard your speech in person. You and Karen inspire me so much with your strength, attitude and love. You are my hero!*

*Mike S*
Amazing! Magical! And also quite eloquent! We love you Mike, Karen, Evan and William!

*Pete B*
Right on, Mike! You continue to amaze us all with your extraordinary attitude and perseverance in extraordinary circumstances. Wow! You're such a blessing!

*Fran D*
What a great and wonderful story of Healing and Miracles ... God Bless you, Mike, and your sweet little family!!!

*Betty S*
Great speech, Mike!!!! You are amazing!! So glad you are part of our family!! We love you!!

*Megan H*
My remarkable friends. Mike, your speech must have brought the house down. Karen, your unwavering strength and support for your beloved husband and family are examples for us all. We love you so much.

*Melin F*
I am in tears ... how brave you are and how wonderful you look. My God, what a gift you are and inspiration to everyone who even thinks they're in trouble with the diseases that confront too many today. I am so proud of you both and send prayers and love to you.

*Deb S*
You're remarkable all around. What a great speech. Thanks for sharing this!

*Rocco B*
Michael , you have done the unthinkable in this fight for your life. Out of all the people that I have met in my life thus far, you, your courage and zest for life is second to none! You are a living superhero. Not only am I so proud to have been your friend and co-musician but also and more importantly your brother in Christ. Our faith and the technical skills of your doctors, along with super strength on your part, kept you with Karen, your boys and all of us who never stopped believing! Continued Strength, Health and Well-being my brother!!!! Love to you, Karen, your sons, family and friends!

*Tim L*
*My love to you, Mike. God is so Faithful to hear our prayers for healing. Blessings to you brother!*

# Merry Christmas!
*By Karen Turnbull — Dec 25, 2016*

I hope this message finds everyone well! I just wanted to send a very Merry Christmas, Happy Hanukkah and beautiful seasons greetings and warm winter wishes to all!

Two years ago all of you helped our family through a very difficult time. I remember friends coming to my aid as I tried to get Mike from the car to the wheelchair to attend Christmas Eve service, all while keeping a three-year-old and a seven-year-old filled with the magic of Christmas. To say that was a challenge would be an understatement! Tonight not only did we attend Christmas Eve service as a family, Mike was dressed in his Christmas red and walked in proud and strong and definitely without needing assistance! Service at our beautiful New Song Church was perfect! We sang Christmas carols and filled the church with beautiful candlelight and prayers of thanks. The same friends that carried Mike from the car to the guest bedroom downstairs after service two years ago were there celebrating with us. Mike and I both found ourselves holding back tears as we celebrated how far we have come.

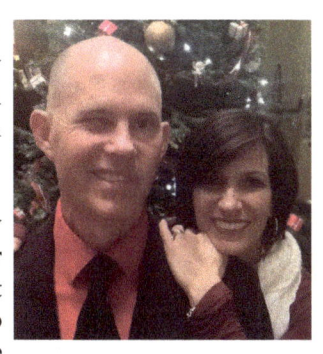

Mike's recent MRI of his brain was beautifully clean and his PET scan was remarkably unchanged! Yesterday our oncologist said we can skip our next month's appointment and he will see us in two months! While eight weeks between visits may not seem like that big of a deal, believe me, we are celebrating!

This year Mike has been able to help with all the Christmas festivities! We have baked cookies, gone to look at lights, wrapped gifts and decorated our home! We are living life and celebrating the miracles that we have been blessed with! Thank you to all of you who've held us in your prayers, thoughts and beautiful warm glowing lights of energy! We couldn't have done all this without you.

As we celebrate the beautiful magic of Christmas we wish you all the very best! Much love and as always keep those prayers coming!

Believe me, they are working!

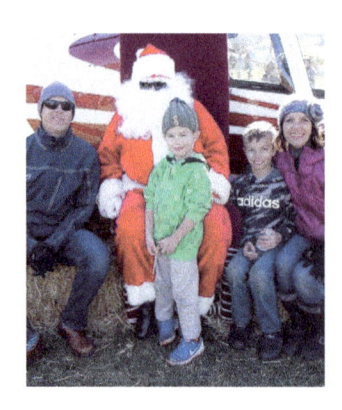

### Alan R
*What beautiful and lovely news in this update. Merry Christmas and all happy holidays. So many reasons to celebrate. Thank you for your inspiration and caring kindness. You are heroes in a world that needs you now.*

### Gabriel F
*Thank you for the updates!! Thank You, Lord, for All that has been done to bring Michael and his family this far!! Continued Blessings to you All!!*

### Suzanne P
*I am not able to hold back the tears ... I am sooooo thrilled to be reading this!!!! I love you guys so much and am so happy that you are on the road back to normalcy (whatever that is). Keep on keeping on! Such great news!!!!! Hugs and kisses.*

### Mark S
*Merry Christmas to one of the most inspirational families I know. You deserve all the goodness of the season.*

### Les K
*Merry Christmas, Mike and Karen. Sending light and love from me and my family to you and yours! I love you! All the best for 2017!*

*Nan R*

*Merry Christmas. May God's Blessings continue their gentle raining down on you. May you always have the strong Faith and Family that you have now. You are all an inspiration and a blessing to us. Thank you. Hugs. And may 2017 be your best year so far with a lifetime to follow.*

*Lou G*

*Best Christmas ever is Michael coming to the door dressed in bike gear. I was flabbergasted and so happy I couldn't speak. You inspire. I showed a few of these posts to some kids who are struggling with their health, and every one of them loves the one about goin' back to work with Donnie & Marie. Wow! is the most frequent response. They also ask about the boys. Some aren't that much older than Ev. Thank you, Mike. Love to you all from down the road.*

# CHAPTER FIVE

## Scattered Showers
### 2017

### Two Years
*By Michael Turnbull — Jan 25, 2017*

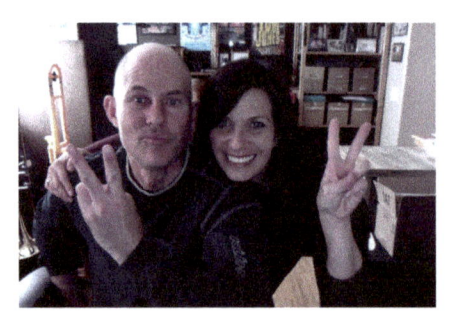

Hello everyone. Today marks the two-year anniversary of my brain surgery. To celebrate this milestone, I wanted to thank you all again for supporting my family, and to update you on my progress. There really is no way to adequately express my gratitude. All I can do is share my story and hopefully inspire others, as well as continue to improve.

The past couple of years I have seen neurosurgeons, neurologists, otolaryngologists, radiation oncologists, radiologists, interventional radiologists, oncologists, hematologists, nurse practitioners, neuro-ophthalmologists, ophthalmologists, optometrists, phlebotomists, physical therapists, occupational therapists, speech therapists, vision therapists, chiropractors, acupuncturists, myofascial stretch therapists, hyperbaric chamber technicians and others that I am probably forgetting. Many of these professionals do not accept insurance and those that do usually charge a co-pay. Your support has made it possible for me to see all of these healthcare workers. I am currently starting my seventh large three-ring binder full of medical paperwork, so the billed amount is well over one million dollars at this point. Without your help, we would be medically bankrupt.

Our children are still heavily involved in gymnastics and swimming. Evan is in a Rubik's Cube club as well as a gifted and talented program, and William is in pre-kindergarten at our local church as well as dance classes. In other words, we have been able to maintain a sense of "normalcy" for our boys thanks to you. They are happy and thriving.

As far as sharing my story goes, the last few months of 2016 were quite eventful. As I mentioned in a previous post, in October I was asked to speak at The UCLA Department of Neurosurgery's annual Visionary Ball. Only two people per year are invited as "Point of Light" speakers. This includes the entire department and every patient from the current year, and I was a patient during the previous year. To say that this was an honor would be an understatement. My neurosurgeon, Dr. Neil Martin, and his nurse practitioner, Melissa Reider-Demer, are the two people who pushed for me to be a speaker. I wanted them to be pleased more than anyone else. Melle was sitting at our table during the event, and when I returned after delivering my speech she would not stop crying and hugging me. She also told me later that in all the years she has worked with Dr. Martin, he has only been in her office a few times. He made a point to visit her the following morning to say that my speech was the highlight of the evening.

Also, Dr. Martin did a presentation about 3-D MRI imaging at the ball. He put on virtual reality goggles and demonstrated how a neurosurgeon can virtually rehearse a brain surgery before it takes place. I turned to Melle and asked her if that's what they used on me. She shrugged a bit sheepishly, and said, "Well ... the technology wasn't quite developed yet, but you've got to start somewhere!" I didn't realize I was a guinea pig until that evening.

Another amazing "coincidence" regarding the Visionary Ball was that it took place at the Regent Beverly Wilshire. While going through some old Tom Jones itineraries I discovered that we had performed for a celebrity charity event on the very same stage ten years prior. Karen said that all those years memorizing music and being comfortable on stage served me well when it came to delivering my speech.

In November, I was asked to share my story on Fyzical's website as part of their "Motivational Mondays" series. Fyzical, the Balance Center, is where I have been attending physical therapy for the past year. The director of the facility, RJ, asked if I would film a quick segment on the recumbent trike that I bought last fall. He later told me that my video has received more hits than any they have ever posted.

In December, a film crew from Tokyo came to film our family for four days. They wanted to capture our story for a TV show about dogs that has aired in Japan for twenty years. The daughter of the creator and producer has a child who is in kindergarten with William. They adore our dog and suggested that she would make a good story. She is a rescue golden retriever that we adopted one week after I returned from UCLA. The producer of the show wanted to develop the angle about how Baylee and I rescued each other, and how she has helped in my recovery.

Part of me wants to lay low and remain anonymous, but that does not seem to be my path. I end up sharing my story almost daily and it has obviously been spread far and wide. Again, thank you all for supporting us on this journey. I will continue to fight, to try to inspire others and to be here for my family.

With love and gratitude.

> *Marianne M*
> *What a beautiful post, Mike! We are all so inspired by you, Karen and the boys. We love you and keep praying daily for a full recovery for you! You deserve it!!*
>
> *Lynne E*
> *Mike, you are a true inspiration for Greg and I as we move along our journey with Mantle Cell Lymphoma. I include your wife in this comment also ... caregiver plus! Your story does deserve to be spread world-wide, giving all of us hope. Lots of love to you and your family.*
>
> *Doreen L*
> *Thank God He made me so that I can smile broadly and cry at the same time! Beautifully written, Mike, and beautiful that you are able to write it! Yes, you obviously are supposed to keep sharing your "story."*
>
> *Kristin U*
> *Wow, between your writing and Karen's you always bring me to tears. Such a beautifully written message, Mike- so YOU. Thanks for sharing. Keep sharing. With much love and continued prayers.*
>
> *Mary Alice J*
> *Mike, our prayers continue for you. We not only think you have done a great job, but hats off to Karen, Evan and William, too. Hugs*

to Baylee. Never underestimate the value of a Golden's love. Luvya.

**Debra L**
Love it! My now one-hundred-three-year-old friend still asks about you almost weekly and says she prays for you every night. So glad things are well!

**Cathy M**
Mike, you probably will never know how much of an inspiration you have been to our family. Your journey has sustained us through some dark times. We are so grateful for your living example of courage, strength and fortitude. We are profoundly touched by all you have overcome to regain your life. We are honored to know you and wish you the blessing of abundant good health. Love to you, your extraordinary, devoted wife and family.

**Devonee M**
We are so amazed by you! You are a light to us, Team Turnbull!

**Bill B**
Thank you for sharing your story! You're an inspiration to us all. God bless you and your family, Michael.

**Randy C**
So proud of you and your family! A true inspiration and a miraculous recovery! Please absorb all of the love and gratitude coming your way, and use it for more strength and courage. Your path is very difficult, but is so meaningful and important! God bless you and your family! Lots of love from the Crawford family!

**Carl T**
So glad to hear you are doing so well. Great speeches!

# Four Years

*By Karen Turnbull — Mar 30, 2017*

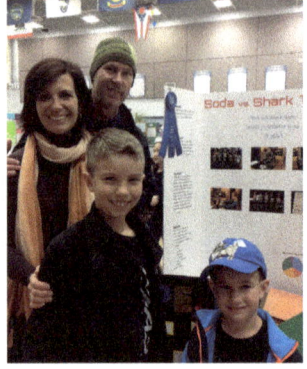

Today is another anniversary, a huge milestone. Today is our four-year celebration since Mike's initial surgery. Four years! Hallelujah! So, how do we celebrate something like this? We live life full out, loud and proud! Last weekend Mike and I got to attend our dear friend Frank's wedding. We laughed and danced and celebrated being able to share in this awesome night. This weekend Evan will present his science fair project at UNLV with all the college science projects! Wow! Today William has his fifth guitar lesson! He can already play Twinkle Twinkle Little Star by heart!

Mike and I treasure every moment, every breath, every tear and every sound of laughter that fills our life. Life is hard, messy, complicated and scary but it is also amazing, exciting, wonderful and fun! Mike works so hard every day to continue to get better. He has put nine hundred miles on his trike since September! He rides himself everywhere he can. Almost every day someone mentions to us that they see him out and about on his trike with the bright orange flag! He shares his story and inspires people every day. I am so proud of him and of our family. Today I refuse to look back and feel the fear that overcame me four years ago. Today I will only celebrate how far we have come. I look forward to many more anniversaries and celebrations. We will continue to live, laugh and love!

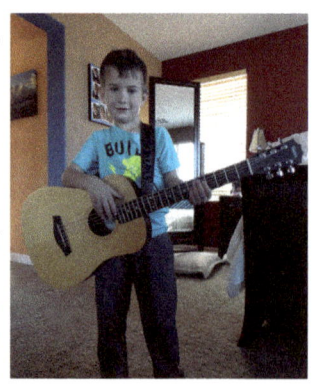

Thank you all for loving us through this journey! Today I ask you to celebrate with us! Raise a glass, make a toast, eat ice cream and know that we feel your love today and every day! Thank you God for surrounding us with amazing people who share their love with us and for giving us four years to celebrate!

And as always … Keep the prayers, energy, good thoughts, etc headed our way!

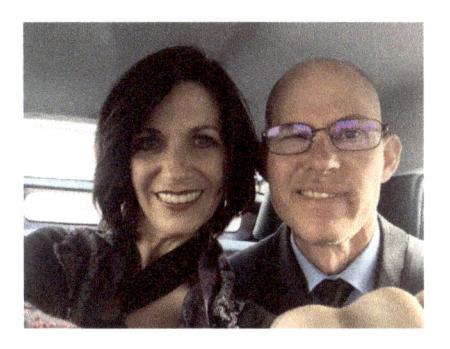

*Sean H*
*Dear Karen, you can count us to help celebrate with you, Mike and your family. You are all an incredible inspiration to us. May you continue to heal and to love. Sending a whole lotta love your way.*

*Les K*
*Thanks for taking time to reach out with this post! This is all such great news and a blessing! I love you guys and I will celebrate with you today! Always sending love and light your way! Cheers!*

*Anne-Corinne B*
*Congratulations on this anniversary as well as your celebration of life's moments every day! Your perseverance is inspirational, and we are happy for you. Thank you for sharing your joy. Sending much love and continued prayers your way.*

*Jeanine C*
*Happy to share in the joy we all feel about the tremendous progress that has occurred. The Turnbulls are a special team of love/joy/positivity warriors! Just so happy. Much love! x*

*Lynne E*
*What a great letter! Life is wonderful! We will happily share your enthusiasm and eat all the ice cream we can ... and drink many toasts to you and your lovely family. Mike is where he is because of you and your strength ... don't forget the role you play so well! God and you are a pretty powerful team.*

*Cindy E*
*Turnbulls, we love you and celebrate this day with you. You truly are our inspiration every day.*

*Jenna L*
*This is the most spectacular news!!! Congratulations and Praise God! We continue to pray for complete and continued healing each day for Mike and believe for all the good things God has planned for you and your family! You are so inspirational to us! Thank you for sharing your journey, your faith, your love and your perseverance! HAPPY FRIDAY!*

*Alicia B*
*Celebrating love, laughter and most importantly, life. May God continue to bless you and your beautiful family!*

*Matt J*
*What a miracle ... no, correction, multiple miracles!! Praise God. I distinctly remember where Katey and I were when you were in the OR. Nine hundred miles ... you are an animal!! Karen ... how's that book coming along??*

## Lavaman

By Michael Turnbull — Sep 12, 2017

On November 5th, 2014, I registered for the Lavaman Triathlon in Waikoloa Beach, Hawaii. Two days later, on my birthday, I suffered a cerebral hemorrhage which turned out to be a tumor. Obviously, I had to withdraw from the event.

I've always thought a great goal would be to attempt the event again, so I registered for it today. This may be a bit ambitious, as I can't really swim or run at this point! However, by training for a triathlon my condition will improve, my family will get to go to Hawaii and I will raise money for The Leukemia and Lymphoma Society. These are all positives! I may have to walk and it may be dark by the time I finish, but I think it's worth a try. The event is March 25th, 2018.

The Lavaman Triathlon will be symbolic for me in many ways. I will be fifty years old. It will be almost exactly five years from diagnosis. It will be a big middle finger to cancer. And I have lost many people to blood cancers, including my dad (my hero) and several friends. The last several PET/CT scans have shown several "micro nodules" but they remain unchanged. My UCLA oncologist says I will need to begin chemotherapy at some point. For now, though, I feel great and we're in "watch and wait" mode. Karen and I are living and enjoying time with our children and each other, and this triathlon is a big part of that attitude.

I know you've already given generously to my family, for which I am forever grateful, and I know there are many choices when it comes to charitable giving. However, I have agreed to raise $3200 and if you would like to donate, please do. LLS spends approximately 73% of donations on research and patient support and approximately 27% on overhead and administrative costs. Karen and I will incur all travel and lodging expenses.

Thanks for your time and for everything you've done for us!

> ### Suzanne P
> *It is great to read your post and see that you are all doing well! I really admire you and your resiliency. I know this has been an extremely difficult time in all of your lives but you have proven to be tougher. I support your decision to face that triathlon again and to do it for other people. I am with you in giving cancer the middle finger. Go Team Turnbull! Love you guys!*
>
> ### Shani F
> *You go, Mike! If anyone can do this, it is you!!*
>
> ### Kelly C
> *You are incredible and we have no doubt you'll do this! We are excited for you and you inspire us all!*

## Triathlon Training in Full Force!

*By Karen Turnbull — Oct 12, 2017*

Hi all! So I realized this morning it has been exactly one month since Mike publicly announced his goal of completing the Lavaman triathlon this March! To get an idea of what this actually means, here is the breakdown: On March 25th, 2018 Mike will suit up to SWIM one mile, then hop on his BIKE for twenty-five miles, then WALK/RUN six miles! This is no easy task for the healthiest of athletes. It requires months of dedicated training. Well, dedicated is definitely a word to describe Mike! Along with determined, inspirational and some might even say stubborn! These traits have served him well during his recovery and they continue to do so now! I have often joked that Mike doesn't really know how to do things half way. He is all-out or nothing! If you're going to set a goal you might as well make it a big one, right? This goal has been lingering in the background for three years now. Last time he registered for this event was just two days before he collapsed to the floor with a bleeding brain tumor. When Dr. Martin, Mike's neurosurgeon at UCLA, turned to me and asked what Mike's level of activity was before this happened, I told him, "He was training for a triathlon." Dr. Martin responded with, "Good, he has been training for surgery." Yes he had! That training and his fighting spirit got him through surgery, wheelchairs, walkers and canes. It got him through additional eye surgeries and years of rehab and therapy. So what's the next step for a man who clearly can't be held down? The Lavaman triathlon!

When Mike was talking to me about doing this he said to me, "This will be the hardest thing I've ever done." My response: "No it won't. You've done things much harder than this." Perspective. It changes everything.

But ... heck yeah, this is HARD! He is currently swimming three times a week. One month ago he struggled to make it one hundred yards. Yesterday he swam eleven hundred fifty yards! As I said before Mike doesn't know how to do things half way, so who is he training with? A group of elite swimmers! Each member of this group swam fifty-eight hundred yards last Friday, one hundred yards for each of the lives lost in the horrific event that has traumatized our city! UNBELIEVABLE! This group gets Mike to the pool, gives him training tips and has become an amazing support group. I am so thankful that he has them to help him on this journey.

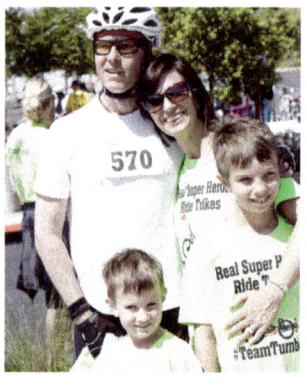

On top of this, he is out riding his trike anywhere and everywhere! We hear all the time that people love seeing him buzz by on his trike with the neon flag! He even rides himself to the hospital for his monthly blood work. The nurses all know him by name and greet him with, "Hey Mike, how's your ride going today?" They draw his blood and off he goes to grab lunch, hit the bike shop or even pick up a few groceries from Trader Joe's! Last April he completed the forty mile Tour de Summerlin bike ride. We had quite the cheering section as he crossed the finish line! Our awesome horn player friends even brought their instruments and played "When The Saints Go Marching In!" It was fantastic!

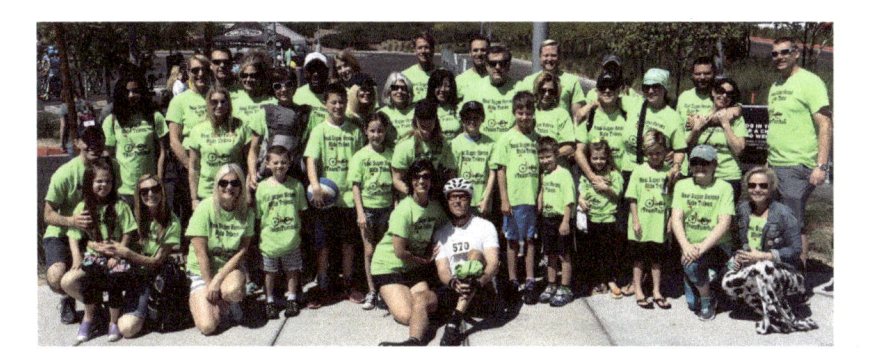

But wait, there's more ... Mike now walks the boys to and from school! He started out using hiking poles but has recently begun doing it with no poles. (Poles are legal on the triathlon, so if need be he can use them.) Talking the other day, we remembered Mike being in his rehab program and writing his number one goal on the giant white board in the conference room ... "Take care of my kids." Well babe, you are doing it! On top of the daily walks to and from school he is also out walking through the neighborhood, gaining mileage every time.

Mike is working so hard to get better and stronger every day. This triathlon is more than just an event for our family. It is symbolic of how anything is possible. Not too long ago Mike couldn't even feed himself, let alone think of swimming, riding or walking. I remember all too clearly carrying him on my back just so he could use the bathroom. Those memories fuel us now. All things are possible!

Our prayers are heavy with our city right now. Las Vegas is hurting but we are also spreading love: Life is short and precious. Set those goals Mike and know that you have an enormous support group cheering you on! More than anything, please keep loving him and surrounding him in your thoughts and prayers! Look at how far you have carried us! Keep it coming!

As always ... So Much Love!

> ### Karen Mi
> *I am in absolute awe over Mike!! This is so amazing and inspiring! I've loved seeing him in the mornings at school and I'm so happy for this continued progress of good health. You guys are truly something, Karen. I hope you have a great day!! :-)*

*Jason V*

*It is so inspiring to read everything Mike has accomplished so far and it is even more inspiring to know that it won't end here! I'm always sending your family my thoughts and prayers! Have an amazing day!*

*Nan R*

*This update is full of so much awesome, blessed, love-filled, God-filled news. Mike you are an inspiration, as is your whole family. Can't wait to hear about how you did when you come back from the Lavaman. Thanks Karen. Blessings and Joy to the Turnbull Family.*

*Kenneth S*

*Sending prayers and love to you Mike ... this is truly inspirational ... I'm looking forward to your quest and Karen, you are a beautiful writer.*

*Nellie S*

*Wow! This is the best thing I've read. I am ecstatic to hear at how far Mike has come. It is truly unbelievable. He is so amazing and inspirational! I love your family.*

*Randy C*

*Of course I'm in! I support Mike as my hero and good friend. God bless you both and Godspeed!*

*Kimberly S*

*Love, love, love this update! And Mike's tenacious spirit!! I continue to be in awe of his relentless pursuits and am grateful you both continue to bring your friends and community along for the ride (pun intended) by providing updates. Hugs and loves!*

*Yong D*

*Mike continues to amaze me. He's such an inspiration. Go get 'em, Mike!*

*Darren K*

*Such wonderful news from an amazing family. Honored to call you my close friends!*

# Happy Birthday!

*By Karen Turnbull — Nov 7, 2017*

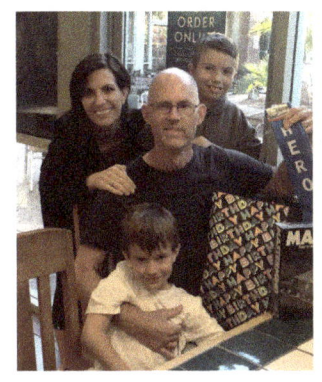

So today is Mike's fiftieth birthday! It is also the three-year anniversary of when he collapsed to the floor with what we soon discovered was a bleeding tumor in the brain stem. People have been asking us what we are going to do to celebrate his birthday. Funny thing is, we look at each other and say we celebrate every day! And that really is the truth, because we learned how quickly everything can change.

It has been a long three years! But wow, so much has happened. Mike's newest accomplishment is that this past Saturday he completed his first triathlon! This was a sprint distance, which is about half the distance of what the Lavaman triathlon in Hawaii will be. It was a great training event for him and he did amazing! He swam seven hundred yards, biked fifteen miles, and then walked over three miles! He took his time, paced himself and still managed to complete the event in under three hours! Best of all, he finished strong and was not even that fatigued the day after! His training is definitely working! Our son Evan completed the kids long-distance triathlon. It was so fun to cheer them both on and see their beaming smiles of pride at the finish line!

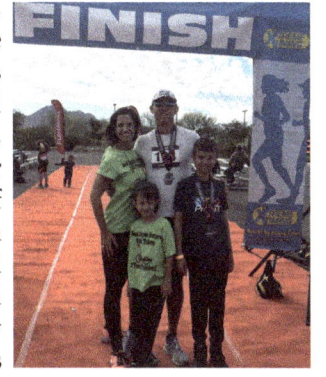

Mike and I feel so blessed every single day to be alive and have each other and our family. We count our blessings and we handle our setbacks the best that we possibly can, knowing that sometimes we just have to pick ourselves up and keep going. So yes, we are celebrating Mike's fiftieth birthday today and we celebrate the precious gift of life every day! Thank you for the love, prayers, thoughts and today especially, the happy birthday well-wishes. We love reading the comments you all leave! Please know that we read each and every one and it fills us both with the strength to keep going and to keep celebrating! Much love!

*Marianne M*
*Happy birthday to one amazing guy! I remember the day three years ago when you collapsed on the bedroom floor and I marvel at the progress you have made! Our hearts are full of happiness for you, Karen and those amazing boys of yours. Keep it going, Mike! You are an inspiration to us all! Much love to all of you.*

*Devonee M*
*Happy Birthday, Mike!! We are SO proud and impressed with you!! And we love you!!*

*Clare T*
*Happy birthday! You inspire us all to live each day as a celebration! Congratulations on the triathlon from the Tewalts. xxx*

*David N*
*Happiest of Birthdays, Mike!! You, sir, are amazing and an inspiration to us all!! Much Love to you and your family! From your Donny & Marie show family ... always thinking of you, always sending healing and loving thoughts! Cheers!*

*Heather W*
*Happy birthday, Mike! I'm always so happy to get these wonderful updates to hear you are doing well. You all inspire me immensely!!!*

*Sharon H*
*Happy Birthday, Mike! You are a warrior of the highest caliber and I love you so much! God bless you and keep you always! Love to Karen and the boys, too!!!*

*JoLayne G*
*I loved reading this post to end my day. It had been a stressful one and I was thinking I was ready to be done with the day but this is a reminder to cherish every day. Thanks for sharing so much of your journey together. Happy birthday and may God continue to bless you in all your days, whether they are the especially challenging ones or the victorious ones! I wish you many more victorious ones!*

*Sara B*
*Happy Birthday, Mike! You always amaze me. I am so proud of you and can't wait to share your news with everyone at NCEP. The mention of your name brings smiles to all of our faces. You have worked so hard and it has paid off. CONGRATULATIONS!*

Hi to Karen and the boys too. Hope to see you all for our annual Thanksgiving lunch on the 22nd.

**Steve S**
Happy birthday, Mike! So happy and thankful for your health and recovery! God is good! I think of you often with many fun memories!

**Lee H**
Happy Birthday, Mike!! You inspire me with your strength and perseverance. I wish many happy days to you and your wonderful family.

**Karen K**
You are all our heroes! I marvel at your outlook on life and your never-ending faith. You are truly walking the "walk." Much love to all of you!!!

**Katey J**
Happy, Happy Birthday, Mike!!! So proud of you and your accomplishments along with the positive can-do attitude you and your family have. We wish the best for you in the coming year ... enjoy the fifty year mark and may there be many more to come. Love always.

## Message to Karen on her 44th Birthday

*By Angelica Villarta - Nov 12, 2017*

About seven years ago, I came across this article by an unknown author and wanted to share this beautiful thought with you, Mike and the kids. Any time I would sing the song "I Hope You Dance" by Lee Ann Womack, I'd always read this letter out loud first.

When I meditated on the word Guidance, I kept seeing "dance" at the end of the word. I remember reading that doing God's will is a lot like dancing. When two people try to lead, nothing feels right. The movement doesn't flow with the music, and everything is quite uncomfortable and jerky. When one person realizes that, and lets the other lead, both bodies begin to flow with the music. One gives gentle cues, perhaps with a nudge to the back or by pressing lightly in one direction or another. It's as if two become one body, moving beautifully.

The dance takes surrender, willingness and attentiveness from one person and gentle guidance and skill from the other.

My eyes drew back to the word Guidance. When I saw "G" I thought of God, followed by "u" and "i." "God," "u" and "i" dance. God, you, and I dance. As I lowered my head, I became willing to trust that I would get guidance about my life. Once again, I became willing to let God lead.

My prayer for you today is that God's blessings and mercies be upon you on this day and every day. May you abide in God as God abides in you. Dance together with God, trusting God to lead and to guide you through each season of your life.

And I Hope You Dance!

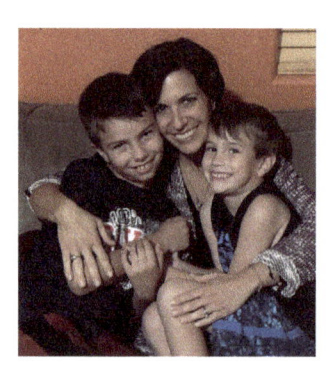

*Karen Turnbull*
*Thank you so much! You are so beautiful! Your timing with this is perfect!*

*Marianne M*
*Wow! So powerful and so true. Really makes one think. Thank you for sharing!*

CHAPTER SIX

# Dancing in the Rain
## 2018

### Happy New Year!
*By Karen Turnbull — Jan 10, 2018*

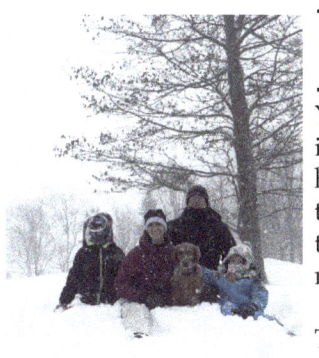

Hello! I hope this finds everyone well in the new year. We had a wonderful Christmas and New Year's celebrating in the snow with family in Pittsburgh. Mike was in his element, helping the boys build the ultimate tubing track complete with a jump! It was so fun to be together celebrating and loving every minute.

The beginning of December Mike had his regular four-month scans at UCLA. Because everything had been looking so good in his brain, it was decided that we could skip the brain MRI this time and do it next visit. Let me just say we will never do that again! Turns out we had quite a scare that sent us to that dark scary place when his PET scan showed a glowing spot in his brain. We tried to remain calm and remind ourselves that PET scans can be a little tricky to read and nothing was yet confirmed. So back he went to UCLA for the brain MRI and then we patiently waited for what felt like a very long weekend for the phone to ring. Monday afternoon came and we received the news we were praying for ... all was perfect on the MRI. Thank you God! Tears were shed and wine was drunk (by me!!)

Now, there are still those pesky little spots showing throughout Mike's body that tell us there is cell activity, but only one spot

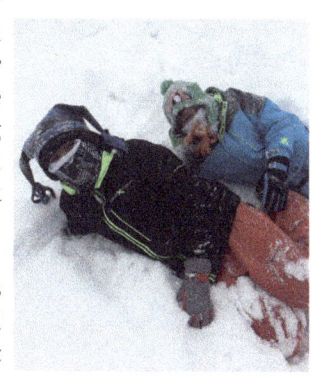

SCATTERED SHOWERS | 265

has slightly changed and the rest remain very small. All of our medical team is in agreement that Mike should live life as normal, train for his triathlon and we will repeat the scans in April after his event. Then we will decide what we need to do. There is talk of an oral chemo to knock out those spots, but we will cross that bridge IF we need to at a later date. I am hanging on to my mustard seed of faith ...

So now the really good stuff. Mike is kicking serious booty with his training! This man amazes me every day! In fact, just today as I was beginning this post he called me to tell me about today's training swim. He completed twenty-three hundred yards and sixteen hundred fifty of those were done WITHOUT stopping! Are you kidding me!?!?!? This man, who was in the ICU waiting for brain stem surgery three years ago, is breaking through all limits and boundaries to reach the highest of heights. Can you tell I am proud? In fact, he is so dedicated to his training that while visiting family in Pittsburgh he went swimming at 5:30 AM in single-digit temperatures (luckily the pool was indoors!), did a spin class to keep up his cycling legs (also at 5:30 AM) and I even joined him on a few five and a half mile walks in weather so cold that I literally had ice crystals on my eyelashes! We walked from my sister's house to my parent's for a surprise visit! Boy were they surprised when we walked in from the bitter cold! The crazy thing is it was actually fun! The trail was beautiful with snow-covered trees and I loved sharing in his determination and drive.

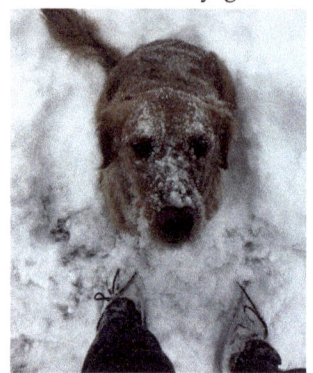

Mike is ten weeks out from completing the Lavaman triathlon with the Leukemia and Lymphoma Society's Team in Training! If you would like him to add the name of someone you love who is fighting these awful cancers to his event shirt just let us know. We will be sure to let everyone know who he is swimming, biking and running for! The boys and I will be very busy making signs and we will proudly write those names on our signs. We love cheering him on! I know you are cheering for him too, and believe me when I say your words of encouragement fuel his determination! Thank you for loving him and keep all the prayers, love and light coming! Just look at what they are doing!

*Anne L*
*So excited for the upcoming triathlon! We continue to hold you in our thoughts and prayers. We love you all. XOXO*

*Anne-Corinne B*
*Congrats on all these achievements! You are truly spectacular, Mike! We love to read the posts and give an extra cheer! We will be praying for your continued training, strength for you and your family and for continuing to find joy in each day. You all are blessings to us and so many others. Praying too for good scans in April. Sending much love and appreciation for showing such awesome determination!!!*

*Jason V*
*You all never cease to amaze me and I continue to be inspired every time I read these posts. I am always praying for you and your family! Mike, I have never forgotten about you and I hope to see you again soon! Karen, thank you for updating all of us and for your high spirits. Wishing you all the best always!*

*Clare T*
*Thank you for the updates! We love hearing your news and always feel inspired by Mike's determination and achievements. All the best for the triathlon! Much love from us all. xxx*

*Christie P*
*Amazing news! Way to go on the training! We will be cheering for you from here at home! Xo*

*Christine E*
*Amazing! I am in awe of his strength and yours. Bless your family. Big hugs and kisses and all our love sent your way!!!*

*Kristin U*
*What a great post to get to read! Keep it up, Mike! I can't wait to hear how the triathlon goes. Karen, thanks for sharing with your great writing that really paints a picture. I can almost taste that celebratory wine you drank! Thinking of you all. And sending much love.*

*Deb S*
*What an inspiration you both are! Thanks for the update. My best to Mike.*

# Honored Hero Bill Turnbull

*By Michael Turnbull — Jan 11, 2018*

WELCOME TO MY TEAM IN TRAINING (TNT) HOME PAGE! It takes more than one person to make up a team and that's why I'm asking you to donate to my TNT fundraising page for TNT!

By participating as a member of The Leukemia & Lymphoma Society's (LLS) TNT, I am raising funds to help find cures and ensure access to treatments for blood cancer patients. Your donation will help fund treatments that save lives every day, like immunotherapies that use a person's own immune system to kill cancer. You may not know it, but every single donation helps save a life with breakthrough therapies such as these. Patients need these cures and they need your support.

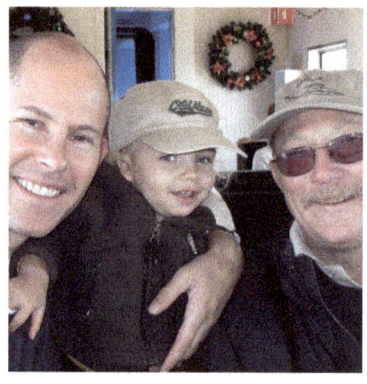

*Bill Turnbull*

Please make a donation in support of my efforts with Team In Training and help get us all closer to a world without blood cancers. On behalf of The Leukemia & Lymphoma Society, thank you very much for your support. I greatly appreciate your generosity.

Thank you!

# Five Days!

*By Karen Turnbull — Mar 20, 2018*

Hello! We are five days away from Mike's big event ... The Lavaman Triathlon in Hawaii! For the past six months Mike has been pouring his heart, soul and a whole lot of strength into preparing for this day. Just the other day he rode twenty miles across town just for a stretch session with our friend Dr. John. On Sunday morning, March 25th, the boys and I will be cheering louder than we have ever cheered, as he enters the ocean to swim one mile, then bike twenty-five miles and finish on foot for six miles! Oh my gosh he is really going to do it!! Not only has he trained like mad but he has also raised almost $7,000 for the Leukemia and Lymphoma Society!

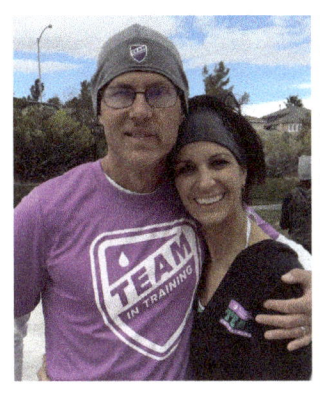

I know his dad Bill is smiling down on him and will be with him every step of the way. Bill fought hard against leukemia and it is because of him that Mike decided to do what he could to help make a difference. This will be Mike's fourth event with LLS! He has done a marathon, a half marathon, a century bike ride and now ... a triathlon! He will be awarded the "Triple Crown Award," which is given to Team in Training participants who complete a run, a bike and a swim event. All events combined have equaled over $20,000 raised by Team Turnbull for this organization!

Please keep Mike in your thoughts and prayers this Sunday. Surround him in love and light and know that you each are a part of this journey. The love and support we continue to get humbles and amazes us every day. We are full of gratitude as we celebrate life through blood, sweat and tears today, every day and especially this Sunday! Go Mike ... we all love you so much!

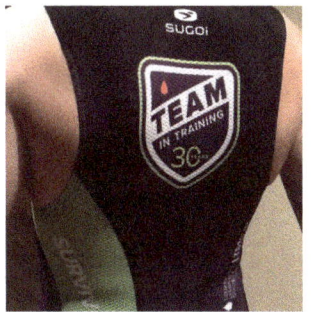

Thank you everyone for loving us! Keep all those prayers, thoughts and good vibes coming ... just look at what they have done!

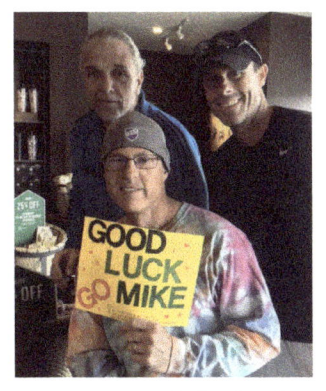

*Swim Coaches*
*Ron Fasnacht & Mike McCary*

*Betty S*
So proud of you, Mike!!! Our prayers and thoughts will be with you on Sunday.

*Anne-Corinne B*
We are cheering for you, Mike and Karen! We commend you on your goals and training! You both are inspiring and making such positive impacts on others' lives! (Like ours, giving us more hope!). We will pray, shout and cheer, and dance for you!

*Fran D*
I have not and will not stop putting Mike in my prayers every night that I lay my head down!!! Such a Miracle!!! God Bless him and his family!!! WAY TO GO MIKE!!!!

*Devonee M*
We love you SOOO much, Mike and we are SO amazed and proud of all you have accomplished leading up to this!! You are going to love this race!! ALOHA!!

*Marc H*
Mike continues to inspire us all with his triumphant warrior spirit, and his stunning lust for life! Much love and aloha!

*Marianne M*
It's so hard to believe that the time has come for you to put all your hard training into action and KILL IT on Sunday!! We are all so proud of you and wish we could be with you in Hawaii. Know that all of us here in Pittsburgh will be praying hard and cheering loud. With all our love and encouragement ... YOU GOT THIS!!!

*Laura T*
GO, MIKE!!! We're cheering you on all the way from Florida and New York! So proud and inspired by you. Sending lots of love, encouragement and hugs. Xoxo

*Sam Bl*
Thinking about you today, Mike! Love and miss you guys.

*Brad E*
We have to admire your determination. We are glad the family is there to encourage you to the finish line. Stay away from sharks in the ocean, bumps on the road and hills on the last segment.

# Happy Summer!

*By Karen Turnbull — Jun 20, 2018*

Hi! Happy summer! Since my last post Mike has continued to be all the awesome things we know that he is. First, for those that may not have heard ... on March 25th, Mike completed the Lavaman Triathlon in Hawaii, as a member of the Leukemia and Lymphoma Society's Team in Training! He crossed the finish line strong in just four and a half hours! It was an emotional day for all of us and at one point during the event, our sweet Evan broke down in tears of joy! (Sometimes we forget how much our kids have been through on this journey and then a reminder comes crashing in.)

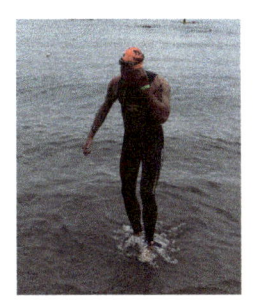

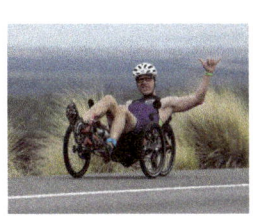

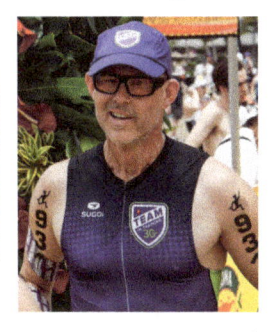

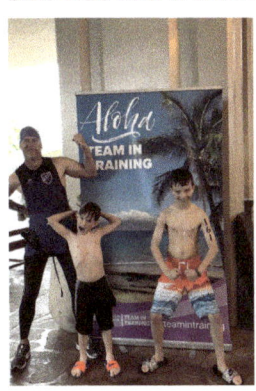

The night before the triathlon there was an amazing inspiration dinner for all the athletes involved with the Leukemia and Lymphoma Society. During this kick-off celebration, Mike was honored more than once! He was recognized for raising over $5,000 (Mike raised $7,000 for this event and together he and I have raised $21,000 for this organization!). He was then honored with the Triple Crown Award. This is a rare award given to those individuals who have completed a marathon, a century bike ride and a triathlon. Mike learned of this award eight years ago while training for the marathon (he had already completed the century bike ride) from our coach and friend Dr. John. The bug was planted and in many ways, I think the goal of the Triple Crown has been a huge driving force in Mike's rehabilitation. He has never stopped dreaming of that award! So when they announced his name and had him stand to be recognized, the pride in this accomplishment brought all of us to tears! And, finally, he was recognized for being a cancer survivor and fighter. These honored heroes were decorated with light-up leis and the room was aglow with the drive and fighting spirit they all embrace. So yes ... it is safe to assume I was an emotional wreck. The tears flowed and my heart beamed with joy, gratitude and pride in all that Mike (and us as a family) have been through.

What many don't know, because we choose not to focus on it, is that Mike's cancer has never fully disappeared. There have always been some spots that show up on his scans and in the blood work markers. A few months before the event those spots started showing signs of increased activity. We knew what this meant, but like I said we choose not to focus on those spots and instead focus on living. Fortunately, Mike's doctors were all in agreement that treatment could wait until after the triathlon. They all understood the importance of this event and felt that things were moving slowly enough that treatment could wait, so just four days after we returned from Hawaii, Mike went back to UCLA for more scans.

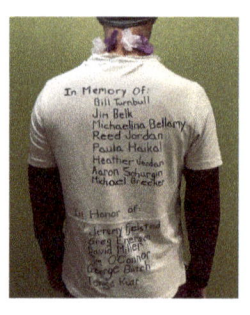

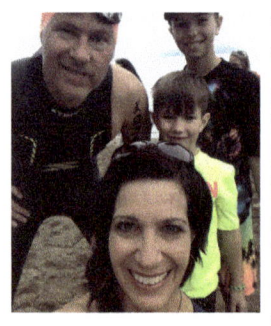

The MRI of the brain was perfect ... Hallelujah! The PET scan, however, showed increased growth and a new cluster of cells in his lungs. We weren't really surprised as we knew the blood marker of his thyroglobulin level had been steadily increasing over the past few months, so we knew there was some activity. The scan just confirmed that the time had come for the next step, so Mike began an oral chemotherapy. Now the crazy part is, we have had this medication sitting in our closet for about a year and a half. Mike never started it because the cells weren't changing and all the doctors were in agreement that there was no need to start something that could potentially cause side effects. Mike often asked me, "How will we know when to start?" I simply said, "I don't know, but I do believe we will be guided when the time comes." Well, the time came and we knew based on a few things ... the blood work, the scans, the strength he now had after completing his event and the expiration date of the medicine tucked away in our closet (April 2018!). Then we muscle tested it, which basically means we asked Mike's body if this was healing for him. He held the medicine with his outstretched arm and I pushed with all my strength to see if he was strong or weak while holding the medication. I could hang from his arm with all my body weight and his arm did not budge. To us this meant yes, this was going to be healing for him.

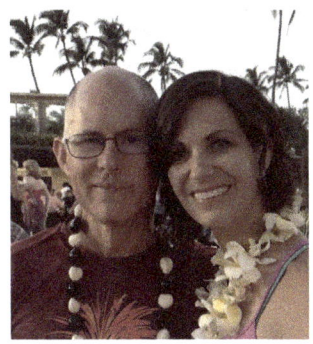

When Mike was first diagnosed in March of 2013 we prayed for a magic pill that could take it away. Well, it might have taken five years for it to be discovered but so far this is proving to be exactly that. Mike's blood work numbers are dropping in ways that are pleasing and surprising to his medical team. His thyroglobulin level was 21.3 when he began the medicine. Two weeks later blood work showed it had dropped to 9.5 and his most recent labs showed a drop to 6.2! That is the lowest it has been in two years! And Mike is tolerating it remarkably well. Side effects are really quite minimal, including occasional tiredness (although that usually comes on the same days that he swims two thousand yards!) and slight sensitivity in his hands and feet, but as we all have learned, it takes a lot more than that to hold Mike Turnbull down!

So now what? Well, we live! We celebrate life, we watch our kids grow, we take vacations, we spend time with family and friends, we savor the moments of our beautifully full life. Our motto is hung in several locations in our home and we try to live by it every day ...

*Life is not about waiting for the storm to pass, it's about learning to dance in the rain.*

~*Vivian Greene*

***So we dance, a lot, several times a day.***

We love you all! Keep all the prayers, light, love and energy coming ... just look at what it has done!

***And ... dance in the rain!***

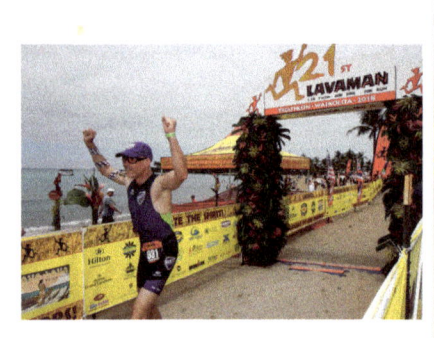

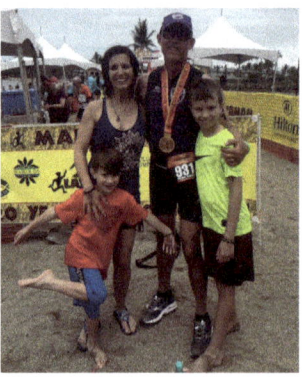

*Marianne M*

*Another beautiful, inspiring, well written post, Karen!! Your love and emotion shine through with each written word. Thank you for keeping us updated and informed! We are all so thankful that the medicine is working (but, we also all know that it is much more than the chemo pill that is helping Mike thrive!). Cannot wait to see you guys in a few weeks and celebrate at the beach. But, at least for that week can we ... dance in the sun?! Love to all of you!!*

*Trish T*

*Turnbull ... Ironically the name meaning "a man strong enough and brave enough to take on a charging bull." It couldn't be any more telling. Mike!!! Strong, yet gentle man is forever in our hearts and always in our prayers. The path that GOD has paved for you has not been one of ease for sure and I'm certain there were times you questioned the journey and the path chosen for you. None of us know our designated path nor do we know our future, but GOD always provides an open door providing you enter with the knowledge and will to allow him to lead the way. Your faith, your strength, your will and your moral compass allow you to be vulnerable when you need to and yet strong when you don't feel the strength. Great peace is available in Christ and that is more than enough to help us navigate through the journey, may it be of rough seas, deep waters, sadness and even the greatness he allows us to fill our hearts with. God is the focus. God is the reason. God is one of all greatness and because of that He will bless you all!*

*Jenny F*

*Karen, the grace and positivity you and your family exude is extraordinary. Mike is a force of nature. Inspiring beyond words. Much love from NYC.*

*Kristin U*
Thank you, Karen! You always write so beautifully and bring tears to my eyes. Keep dancing. I'll do the same as I think of your amazing family and the strength you have. Love, love, love.

*Melin F*
We are so inspired by all of you ... big and little. Our prayers won't ever stop and will follow our love and admiration every day.

*Theodora B*
Thank you so much for sharing! Rest assured of our love and prayers! Hugs.

*Cindy E*
So happy to hear that number keeps getting lower! Love you guys, and we will keep dancing with you in that silly storm.

*Shannon N*
Thank you for sharing your story, your love and your strength!

*Nan R*
The Turnbulls- such a special and amazing family: always together, always faithful, always strong (even when tears come, as our vulnerability is strength, too). Thanks for sharing your journey. So very glad you are always turning to God and full of faith that this too will pass. Rooting for you always, and praying for/thinking of/knowing that the best is yet to come. Blessings, Joy, and Hugs.

*Issa F*
I am just blown away by you guys. I am so grateful to keep receiving these updates! AMAZING!

*Lynne E*
What a wonderful note for your journal! Each and every one of you is amazing. All of us need to remember to "keep dancing!"

*Brad E*
My eyes teared up reading your journal. Congratulations on being great fundraisers for the Leukemia and Lymphoma Society. There are a lot of people praying for all four of you.

# Finding Joy

*by Karen Turnbull — Dec 17, 2018*

Merry Christmas, Happy Hanukkah, Happy Kwanzaa, Happy Holidays ... all of the above! It's been a long time since any entries have been made and here's why ...

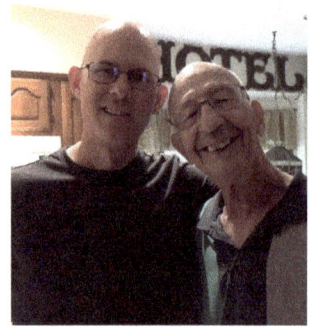

*Jim Sommer*

Many of you have commented during the course of our journey that we should consider writing a book. Well, this blog is in the process of becoming just that. My dad started the book for us and finished his portion before passing away in August. He worked on it for years, little by little, to present to us a truly beautiful project. Thank you, Dad - your love and support of us forever touches our hearts. But this project is far from done. Mike has been working on it just about every day and I help out when we have some spare time to sit together and pour through the thousands of amazing comments. It has been both beautiful and really, really hard. It was hard enough to live it once, so now reliving it has been challenging to say the least. But Mike and I both know that in book form it will serve a much stronger purpose. We both feel confident that when it is complete it will find its way into the hands of those who need it most. If our story can help others heal, then it is all worth it.

In order for it to become a book we thought it needed an ending, but the truth is it's just not that simple. Cancer doesn't just end. There will always be tests, scans, bloodwork and unfortunately, fear. We've had a lot of people asking us lately how things are and how his cancer is, so I decided it was time to let everyone know. Here is the latest update:

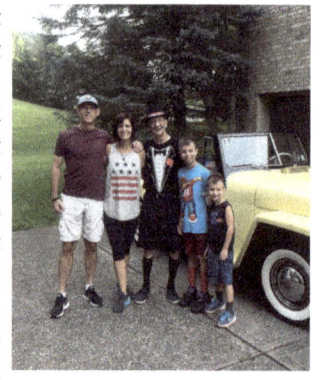

First off, we really are doing great! The kids are thriving, Mike is truly a miracle and I am finding joy in my family every day. Let's talk about Mike! He is still swimming three times a week and kicking some serious butt! He has also begun driving (only during the day and not on highways) but he has regained quite a bit of independence. He goes for monthly blood work to watch his thyroglobulin numbers. They were steadily dropping (which is what we want) until about two months ago, when they decided to increase slightly. Only by a point or two, but any increase is moving in the wrong direction. It tells us there are active cells, possibly cancerous somewhere in his body. He just had his four-month scans at UCLA. I am very happy to report that the MRI of the brain was beautiful! Couldn't ask for a better result! We definitely celebrate this news! The PET scan, however, was not quite as beautiful. It is still better than back in April before he started the oral chemotherapy, but it does show some active cells in the lungs that show characteristics of metastasis. What does this mean? I'm not really sure. It could be that the chemo just needs some time to work on these new cells, or it could be that we do nothing and watch and wait. It could also mean a new plan will surface through our medical team. We are ok with any of those options and will take it as it comes. The cells are not bothering him and they're still fairly small, so right now we wait and focus on all the great joyous things happening in our lives.

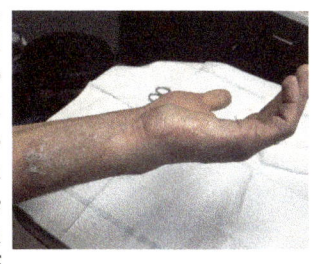

Mike and I have been talking a lot lately about how we have gotten so good at pretending that everything is fine, but then we are reminded that cancer likes to stick around (at least his does). We are really good at smiling through it all and celebrating the accomplishments, and that is because things seriously are great! Mike amazes us all every single day. He makes us laugh all the time and I couldn't ask for a better father to our boys. His favorite moment of the day is going to pick up William from school and having our sweet little boy come running and plowing into his arms. There was a time not too long ago when we didn't know if this would be something he could do again, so it's in moments like these that we find our greatest joy. Then sometimes we have a brutal reminder of how things are not so great. For example, Mike continues to suffer through balance issues. About two months ago Mike went to flip some potatoes that were on the grill, which is something he's done before and I didn't think anything of asking him to do it. But this time he lost his balance and fell onto the six hundred degree grill! This caused an intense second-degree burn on his entire left hand and forearm. That's the good hand, the hand that has full sensation and feeling in it! So yeah, that was a lot of fun! With everything he's been through I've never heard him wail like he did in that moment. Our sweet boys were right there with ice and the watering can full of cold water to keep pouring on him while I gathered gauze and supplies to wrap his hand. And that's just an average day at the Turnbull house! But in typical Mike fashion, after follow-ups with a wound care specialist, he has healed beautifully and is doing great.

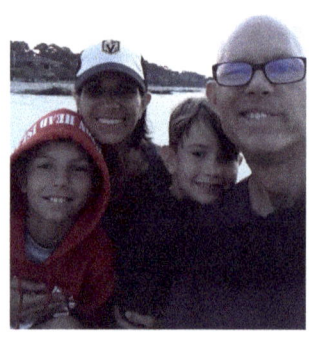

We spent a wonderful week in Colorado for Thanksgiving celebrating with family, playing games and just enjoying being together. Next week we are headed to Pittsburgh to visit with my family for the Christmas holidays. There's much to be thankful for and like I said we are celebrating and finding joy all around us. The boys are thriving in school and both are playing lacrosse. I'm not quite sure how I ended up as a lacrosse mom, but here I am spending weeknights and weekends on the field and I couldn't be prouder of them.

And for those that don't know, I decided to do something big for myself. In November I competed in my first bodybuilding bikini competition. Yes, you actually read that right, a bodybuilding competition! I trained for six months and dedicated everything to pushing and bettering myself. I am very proud of what I've done and happy to say I actually placed fourth in the Women's Masters category! (Something I never thought I could do).

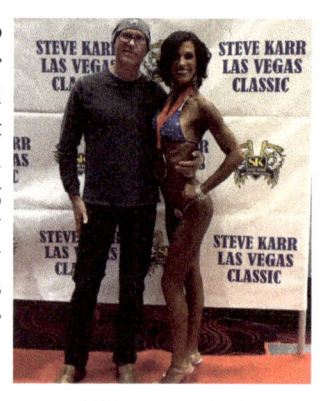

So as you can see, we are good. We're really good! If we could just get the stinkin' cells to stop showing up we would be even better, but I'm grateful that they don't cause him any problems. He really doesn't even know they're there, so if it weren't for the blood work and scans we would just go about our merry way. At least for now that's not our path, so here is what we are choosing this holiday season ... Joy! We are choosing joy every day and in all situations. My Christmas wish is that each one of you can celebrate a most joyous holiday filled with love and laughter. We will do the same, because I still believe we are stronger than those cancer cells and I am holding on to that mustard seed of faith. Together we can do anything! Much love to you all!

*Angela W*
*Karen, you are incredible in so many ways, including your writing. This is a beautiful update. I am excited to hear about this book, love that your boys are so happy and active and loving lacrosse, and totally inspired by both you and Mike and your strength of spirit and physical strength, too! What a gorgeous family you have. Thank you for the update and we are praying for good health news in the coming year! Love you all!*

*Suzanne P*
*I am always thrilled to hear from you and catch up on your latest news. I thought your arms looked awfully ripped in one of your photos on Instagram. Good for you!!! Congratulations on placing in the contest. I'm glad to know you are all doing well and appreciating so much in your lives. I have to admit it makes me tear up to learn those cells are still causing concern for all of you. It's not for the lack of fighting and staying positive. You are a model family of what it is like to fight with grace. You are the most powerful team I know. Sending you all lots and lots of love.*

*David N*
*With hope this Holiday Season finds your family rich with Love, Joy, Peace & Goodwill! Karen, you're a brilliant reporter and storyteller, and Mike an amazing protagonist of hope and endurance! Tell this story of Love. It will surely touch and heal.*

## The Journey Continues
*by Karen Turnbull — Jan 21, 2020*

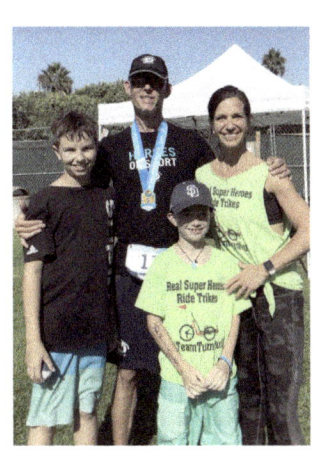

Wow! 2020! That means it has been seven years since we started this journey with cancer, and this Saturday, January 25th, will mark five years since Mike's miraculous brain stem resection surgery! To say it's been quite a journey is an understatement!

First, I would like to start by sharing all things awesome in the world of Team Turnbull, so here you go! If you've been following me on social media at all, then you have seen some pretty amazing acts of courage, bravery and remarkable athleticism from Mike. He has now completed five triathlons! Most recently he participated in the Challenged Athletes Foundation (CAF) fundraising triathlon in San Diego. CAF is a wonderful organization that sponsors paralympians, disabled veterans, amputees and challenged kids. In October the boys and I headed out to meet Mike and cheer him on. The first part of what's so incredible about this is that he actually drove himself the five hours to get to San Diego! Because his recumbent trike takes up the entire car and there was no room for us, we hopped on a plane the next day and met him there. Speaking of his recumbent trike … it's super cool! Mike applied for a grant from CAF and received money to purchase a new, faster and lighter trike. It is neon green and the boys call it the "praying mantis!" Mike used this trike to ride forty-four miles after swimming one mile in the Pacific, and then finished all that up with a ten-mile run in the hills of San Diego! I know … he is all sorts of AWESOME!

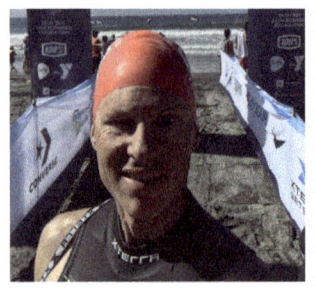

Mike also recently did a 100 x 100 swim, which means he swam one hundred yards one hundred times! That comes down to over five and a half miles!! He was in the pool from 9 AM to 2 PM (getting out only once for a bathroom break)! To refresh your memory as to how far he has come, when I first took him to the pool to try swimming in 2017, doing one lap left him clutching the wall. The boys and I were there to cheer him on as he finished that final lap and man, what an accomplishment!

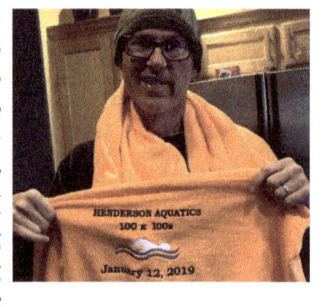

On top of all of that, daily life has improved remarkably. In fact, this past Saturday he took the boys for a fun day with Dad! What exactly does that entail? I probably still don't know all the details, but from what I've been told it included donuts and skate park hopping all across town! Evan's legs are still sore from trying out so many ramps in Las Vegas on his scooter!

Which brings me to the boys … I know I'm their mom and I'm kind of biased, but seriously they're pretty awesome! William is now eight, in second grade and reading at a fifth-grade level! If you remember he was only fourteen months old when all this began in 2013! He's silly, funny and so very sweet, and he gives the best hugs and snuggles ever (which I cash in on daily!). He is rocking out in his guitar lessons and was the only first-grader to participate in the school talent show last spring. Evan is twelve, almost as tall as me and in seventh grade. He was five when we began this journey. He is social, kind and has a special gift with young children. They are like a magnet to him and he gets such a kick out of playing with little ones. It's quite sweet to watch. He has thrown himself full-force into scooter riding and actually competed in his first competition about one month ago. After raising money by babysitting and doing odd jobs, he paid half his way to scooter camp last summer! His tricks have improved and his confidence has increased, which is the best part. The boys are our biggest supporters in life!

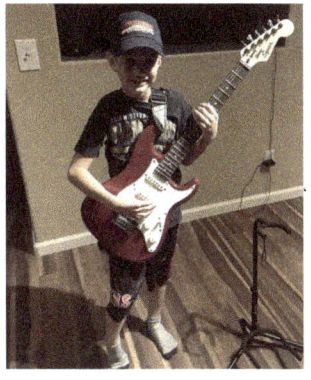

Which I guess leaves a quick update on me … well, life is funny. As I mentioned in my last post, in 2018 I had this crazy desire to do a bodybuilding competition. Never in a million years did I think that would be something I wanted to do, but that voice that won't quiet just wouldn't stop pushing me to try. So try I did! I got a coach, joined a gym and started my transformation. Since then I have actually competed in two competitions and am training for my third! I am quite proud of the work I have put in and the results that have come from it, but it's not all about sparkly bikinis and spray tans! Through the journey of training I discovered that I love nutrition! So much so that it inspired me to become a certified nutrition coach and start my own business. I have been a massage therapist since 2002 and have used my skills daily, working with a nonstop supply of injured dancers, but I decided to grow my private practice again and so in December I officially launched my LLC! "Fresh Start Nutrition and Bodywork" is in its early stages, but growing fast and strong and I'm really excited about where the future will take it.

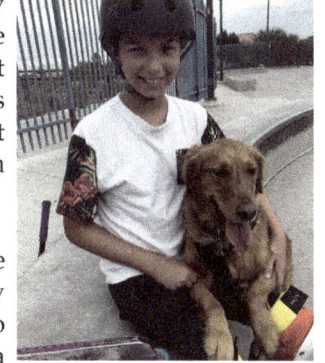

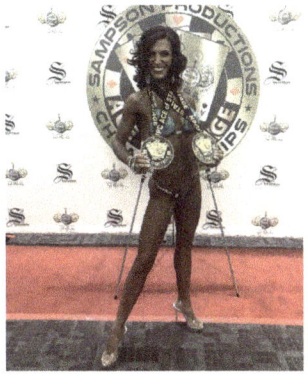

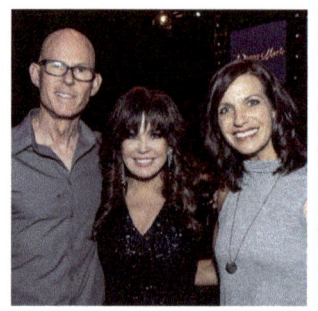

*Marie Osmond*

I should also mention that since Mike was working for Donny & Marie when he was diagnosed, they reached out to us in November to invite us to their closing night party. Their run at The Flamingo lasted eleven years! They have followed our journey since the beginning and supported us every step of the way, and they couldn't have been more gracious.

Now for the real reason for this post. The Turnbulls have been doing a lot of living! And we are really good at making it seem as if everything is great. But through all this living we have still been dealing with the world of cancer. Many people think that Mike has been in remission so I want to be very clear: we don't know that word. It has never been a part of our vocabulary. Mike has never been in remission. We have been managing and doing a very good job at it. Mike began oral chemotherapy in April 2018 and until now it has worked pretty well. It has kept the tumors in his lungs small and manageable and his brain has been clear on all scans until last August, so I'll start with that.

In August 2019 Mike flew to UCLA for his four-month MRI of the brain and PET scan of the body. The PET scan came back showing the same activity as we have always seen. Clusters in his lungs primarily, but no radical changes so no one was overly concerned. The MRI, however, showed a tumor had developed on the surface of his brain. It was superficial and in an easily treatable area, so one radiation treatment to that spot was the decided course of action. For us that sounded great! We didn't even tell anyone because in our world it seemed so small and easy, so back to Dr. Toy we went and one blast should've been all it took. He hit him with the highest dose possible as there was no risk of damage because of the tumor's easily treatable location. In December Mike returned to UCLA for scans once again (four months goes very fast.) We were hopeful that the brain spot had disappeared.

Right before the holidays we received the results of these most recent scans. Mike and I had returned home from running some errands when he got the email update on his phone. We sat in the car in the driveway as he opened it. Well, we've read enough of these now to know that when the top of the report is a paragraph in length it's not good. Quite simply, it meant there was a lot to report. The bottom line is this... Mike's cancer has spread. It is now what we call systemic, meaning it's running through his whole system. It is in his bones, lymph, lungs and yes, in the brain. Sixteen spots in the brain, to be exact. But ... before you all fall apart reading this, let me tell you we are OK. In fact, we are better than OK ... we've got this! And, while it has taken us a month of processing all this to get here, we are quite ready for whatever this next chapter brings. So here is where we are ... today Mike received his fifth of five radiation treatments to the brain. What we have learned is that the radiation treatments for Mike's particular cell type do not do what they do for pretty much everybody else. In other words, they don't shrink them and they don't kill them, but they do seem to keep them from growing. If you remember, just a week and a half ago Mike swam ten thousand yards! And that was with sixteen tumors in his brain! So in our world, if we can hold them at the size they are and stop others from developing, then that is a win! And that's our focus.

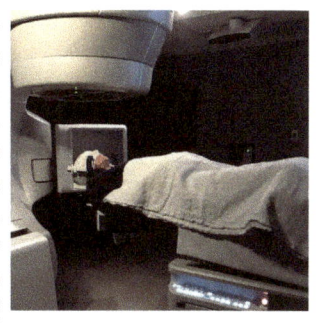

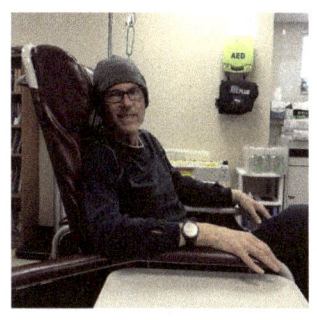

On top of the brain radiation treatments, Mike began a new course of immunotherapy today. This will involve a once a month treatment via an IV drip at the cancer center. He will go for about one hour and receive a fancy cocktail to boost his immune system to attack the cells throughout his body. He receives two different mixes: one specifically for the spots in his bones, the other to boost the impact of the oral chemotherapy that he will continue to take. We first learned about this new immunotherapy treatment last April, but at the time Mike did not qualify for it as he did not have "enough" cancer. Well, he now has plenty of cancer so here we go. We don't know yet if there will be any side effects. The hope, of course, is that there will not be. Time will tell. He is currently taking a steroid to help calm some nausea and dizziness that started to occur because of the brain tumor activity. The plan is to take it as needed and wean off when he is able. Right now it's doing the job of making him feel better and we're grateful for that.

The great thing is Mike is in the best shape of his entire life! Thanks to his fabulous nutrition coach (me!), he is eating better than ever and his physical stamina is stronger than I've ever seen. I go back to 2015, when Dr. Martin asked me how physically active Mike was before he collapsed to the floor with a bleeding brain tumor. I told him that he was training for his first triathlon and Dr. Martin said, "Good, he was training for surgery." Those words have run strong with me ever since. Yes, Mike and I train for events: him triathlons, me bodybuilding. I hit the gym every day at 4:30 AM before going in to work, and he swims, rides and has begun turning his walks into runs. But it's not about the events. Mike and I train every day for life, because that way, no matter what is thrown our way, we're ready to fight. Mike and I are stronger than we were in 2013 when this started ... physically, mentally, emotionally and spiritually. And we are a stronger team than we've ever been. Not to say we haven't had our rough patches and been faced with some serious challenges, but what could have torn us apart has just made us stronger. So we're not giving up or giving in. We're just bracing ourselves for the storm ahead and are excited to see the rainbow on the other side. And yes, we just keep dancing in the rain. Because one thing we have learned is there really is no such thing as a finish line. There is no ending, because it is life. Life keeps going and even when we leave this life here on earth there is more. Believing that helps us. Everybody has their path, their journey. This just happens to be ours. So ... the journey continues ...

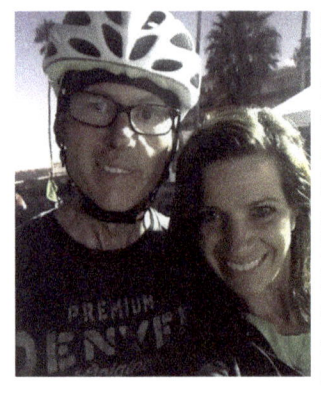

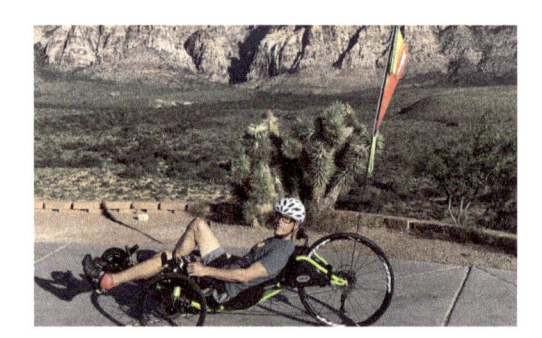

*Marianne M*
*Karen - Your words are amazing, your strength untouchable and the love you have for Mike and your family is beyond compare. Even with all that life has thrown your way, you continue to remain positive and strong. You are a true inspiration and I am blessed to have you as my sister. God has put you in Mike's life to help him on this journey and, in turn, Mike's journey has created one*

heck of a wonderwoman in you. May God's grace continue to guide both of you through this next chapter. My love to you and the three amazing guys in your life.

*Clare T*
Karen and Mike, how incredibly inspiring you both are. I've been thinking about you a lot recently and missed our "check- ins." You have truly been an inspiration to me and I am inspired by your journey and the love your family has. I truly believe you can conquer anything together. We are sending you much love and strength through this next chapter.

*Shani F*
You are both such an amazing testimony to the life God wants us to live! And Karen, your way with words is such a blessing. Some day I will sit down and read the book YOU have written because your story can't be told in just a few pages! Thank you for the update and for the inspiration you give to us and others. Love to all four of you!

*Jenny F*
Your words, your choices, your outlook - absolutely astounding. To say you are the strongest warriors and bravest souls I know is an understatement. Huge hugs from us in NYC.

*Dawn K*
I love you all so much, and respect and admire how you have handled everything leading up to now. I know this will be no different. I'm incredibly sad and horrified to hear this news but since you can still seem to add a spin of positivity to it, I certainly can too. I'm sending you and Mike and the boys all the love and good vibes I can.

*Megan H*
X*&^$%J ()*O. #$%E$#$%% and also (*&^ @#$@### *(&** !!! Okay ... now that I've gotten THAT off my chest. With the love, hope, optimism and grit you, the boys, your family and (duh) Mike possess ... I've no doubt you've "got this." We are here for whatever ... whenever. And ... we love you.

*Shannon N*
We're always so in awe of you both. You are an amazing family with an even more amazing spirit that radiates off you both! We are lucky to know you. You will continue to kick butt!

*Jaime D*
You are all, including the boys, a true inspiration to us all on how to live life to the fullest, enjoy every day and always work hard for what you want. I am praying for you all and for a successful response to the immunotherapy.

*Curt M*
I have never known two people as strong as you in my life. You are both so inspiring! All our love coming your way.

*Kelly C*
Prayers, love and big hugs are coming to you from the Cassell Family! You are both amazing, strong and the most positive people we've ever met! We are here for you anytime through this journey. You've got this!!

*Alicia B*
Wow. I am sitting in the DMV reading this and trying to stop tears from rolling down my cheeks. I'm not even sure if they are tears of sadness because your writing brings comfort to us when we should be giving you words of encouragement. Your family has always been superheroes to me. Each one of you show more courage than anyone I've met. May God heal Mike's body and continue to bring your family joy and comfort through your next chapter.

*Brian M*
Karen and Mike, you provide a definitive guide for the rest of us on how to approach life! I love your family and will be holding you all in my thoughts.

*Shannon A*
Your family is an inspiration to our world! Love you all so much! You are in all of my prayers! God bless you all!

*Jeanine C*
Continually inspired by you and your beautiful family! I love how you have each reminded me to get busy living. Cheering you all on and following your example!

*Wesley M*
Mike, you and your family continue to be a true inspiration for me. Never giving in. Never giving up. Giving it all you have and loving deeply along the way. Thank you. Much love and healing vibes to you and the entire Turnbull family.

***Heide F***
*Mike and Karen, the two of you must write a book of your journey. It will be an inspiration to all. Thank you for sharing your stories. I am inspired to live and love.*

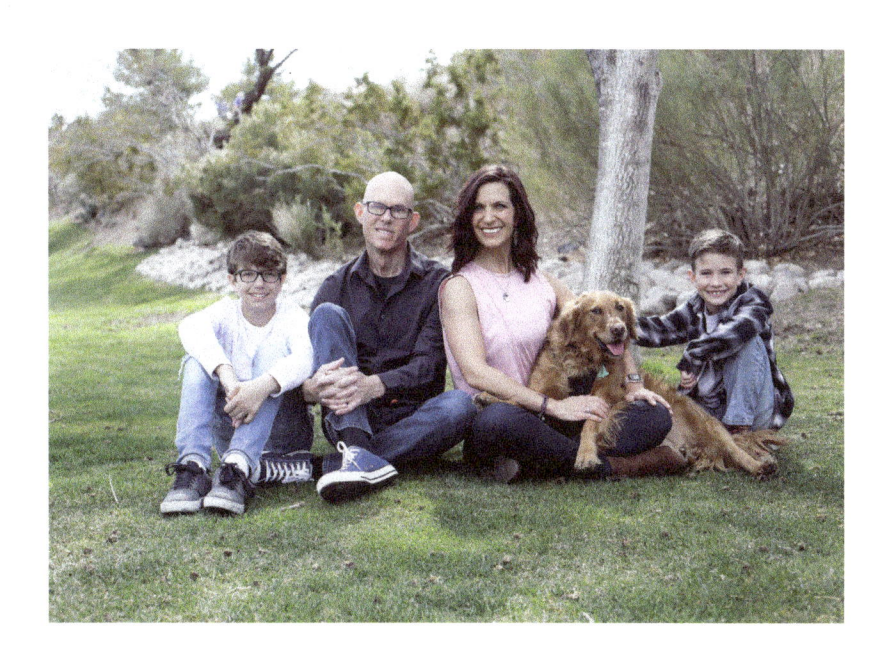

# CHAPTER SEVEN

# Signs, Symbols and Voices
## 2019-2020

The following are stories that were a big part of our journey but didn't make it into our journal for various reasons. We thought they were worth sharing here.

## Money Stories
### by Michael Turnbull

When I was in the hospital after my first surgery, my friend Gil and Marie Osmond's wardrobe assistant, Jennifer, had passed a hat around at work. The cast and crew for Donny & Marie donated whatever spare cash and change they had to us. Gil lives by the hospital, so he came to visit us and handed Karen an envelope. Just a few days prior, I had received a bill in the mail to keep my health insurance current. If I didn't accrue enough hours, I had to self-pay to make up the difference. Since I was in the hospital and couldn't work, I received said bill. It was for an odd amount, like $741. When Karen opened the envelope, it was exactly that amount to the dollar.

In October of the following year, Karen went to throw some pumpkins in the garbage bin. We had carved them for Halloween but they were beginning to rot. When she pulled the bin away from the wall she noticed that the drywall was bubbling. Our water heater had failed and was leaking into the wall. Our neighbor Rick, who happens to be a contractor, was watching football with a buddy at the time. When Karen called him they were at our place within a couple of minutes. They disconnected, drained and moved the water heater to the curb immediately. The next day they installed a new one. With the labor it was not cheap, around $1400. That same night Karen's sister, Marianne, called to see if we had checked the mail recently, which we had not. Marianne and her husband own a photography studio in Pittsburgh. One of their former employees, Shari, is a breast cancer survivor and hosts an annual fundraising event. That year she decided to give us the proceeds. When we opened the mailbox, there was a check from Shari in the same amount as the water heater.

My dad passed away from leukemia several years ago. We were told by an energy worker friend of ours that when we saw pennies it was his way of communicating with us. Right after we were told this we were at Red Rock Canyon at the overlook. The boys went over the edge to play near a tree, and the tree and the ground underneath it were covered in shiny new pennies, probably over one hundred of them. Since then, we find pennies often. Usually it is when I am facing something frightening, like right before my scans at UCLA. A couple of days before the Lavaman triathlon in Hawaii, I was out on a training ride and on the way home I stopped by the studio where William takes guitar lessons to say hi to my family. I was wearing cycling shorts that did not have pockets. When I got up from my recumbent trike, William noticed a quarter on the seat. It was a brand new Hawaii state quarter.

## Unexpected Angels
*by Michael Turnbull*

We have always valued the many friendships we have made over the years. We have friends all over the world and feel so blessed. The following are a few stories of friends who helped us when we needed it the most.

After the manubrial recurrence surgery that Dr. Robert Wang performed, our friend Marc was waiting outside the hospital to help me to the car. He is very high up in the Henderson Police Department, and he gave me a coin which represents bravery. This coin is difficult to get and is usually reserved for police officers. Marc also carried me from a wheelchair to the car on Christmas day. Those small gestures made quite an impact on me.

Our friends Rodney and Sara own a catering business and live down the street from us. They were gracious enough to come to our house and prepare dinner for us when I was not doing well. Also, Rodney is an executive chef and he invited us to his restaurant on the four-year anniversary of the brain stem resection. Their food is incredible and I still remember their acts of kindness.

Our friend Annie is an extremely gifted massage therapist who is always learning new modalities. When she was learning a treatment that involved crystals, she would come to the house every day to practice on me. I was bedridden, but she brought so much joy into our house. She would bring donuts for the boys and I really believe she helped me heal.

Our friend Stacy was a dancer in New York with Karen. It had been years since we last talked to her as she had moved to Los Angeles. The day we arrived at UCLA, we were told we had a visitor. We were a bit puzzled by this, as we hadn't really invited anyone. It turns out that Stacy had become an OB/GYN nurse, and was working one floor below the Neuro wing! She brought pastries to share with the nursing staff (being a nurse herself she knew how appreciated that would be) along with doing Karen's laundry when our stay was longer than intended. She was so sweet and helpful and she visited us regularly. It was very comforting to see a familiar face there. Stacy even let us stay in her apartment in Santa Monica when we had follow-ups at UCLA!

When I was in the Neuro wing, it would take three nurses to get me from the hospital bed to the chair next to it. There was a charge nurse named Chuck who was very strong and he could do it himself. Karen was always relieved when she saw Chuck coming. He was great at his job, very knowledgeable and compassionate. I went to see him a couple of years later to thank him and let him know how well I was doing. He literally jumped for joy!

During my radiation treatments with Dr. Toy, I had a great radiation therapist named Brittany. Her kids and ours took swimming lessons from the same people so we got to know her socially as well. Karen could text her any time with questions and she made a difficult situation less so. See her picture below with Dr. Toy.

# In the Shower

## by Karen Turnbull

It was late. The boys were sleeping at a friend's. Mike was in the ICU in Las Vegas and I escaped home to shower and grab some clean clothes. The shower was where I could scream, cry and let it out. No one could hear me or see me. I was safe to fall apart if only for those few moments. I had just been told that they could do nothing for Mike and it looked like they might discharge him. They had tossed out the suggestion of me driving him to the ER at UCLA because they couldn't turn us away. Really … that is the best you can do? Me, drive my husband with the bleeding brain tumor (who can't sit up without vomiting) four and a half hours on my own. Ok. And let's not forget that I had a 7-year-old and a 3-year-old to take care of too. I was maxed out. I had nothing left. My faith was all but gone. If you know the story of the mustard seed I honestly don't even know if my faith was that size in that moment. I remember saying out loud, through screams and tears, "God, if you are real, you need to show me because I don't know if I believe in you." Clear as could be a voice said, "If you don't believe then who are you yelling at?" I remember I actually laughed outloud.

The next morning I geared up for whatever was ahead and went to the hospital. On my way down the hall of the ICU I ran into the doctor and he said, "We are going to get you there. We are in talks with your insurance to get it scheduled. Just hold tight."

Ok God, you win. I may only have faith the size of a mustard seed but I will clutch onto that.

## When I Stopped and Listened

*by Karen Turnbull*

There have been several times during this roller coaster ride of emotions when I thought I was at my breaking point. It was in those moments after crying, screaming or finding myself with no sound at all, that I was guided to the next step. This story is one of the most powerful moments that brought me back off the edge and gave me the strength to continue. I am reminded of it often when life turns upside down and I need to power up and get things right side up again. It was December 2014, when we were still at home waiting for some sort of plan with Mike's brain tumor. It was before radiation and well before surgery even seemed like an option. We still didn't know what was going on but I knew we were headed in the wrong direction. Mike's symptoms were progressing rapidly. It had gotten to the point where he couldn't leave the bed, and even to just get him to the bathroom I had to carry him on my back.

There was one night in particular that the tinnitus in Mike's ears was so intense that he couldn't rest. Even the prescription sleeping meds did nothing to calm the intense ringing coupled with the constant sense of dizziness and motion sickness. The only way he was able to find any calm in his body was if he laid his head on my lap and I held him, much like I did our then three-year-old William. I remember sitting in the bed with his head on my lap, gently stroking his head and holding him tight as he finally drifted off to sleep. The tears started streaming down my face and in the quiet of that moment I asked God why. "Why was this happening? Why did you bring us together? Why would we feel a love this deep and strong and create these beautiful children and then experience this magnitude of heartache and pain?"

Through my own tears I finally drifted off to sleep. I remember waking up and looking at the clock. It was 3:30 AM. Clear as could be I heard the words "to get him through it." Immediately a calm came over me and in that moment I understood. You see, this was always going to be Mike's path. I don't know why, but it just was. And in that moment, I was able to step away and see the bigger picture. I was able to see the events of our lives bring us together and unfold to carry us through this. God brought me to him and him to me because, for whatever reason, he had to live this and I was the one strong enough to get him through it. That moment changed everything for me. It powered me through not just that moment, but many moments thereafter. And it still does to this day. I still don't understand all the "whys" to any of this, but I know that we are a team. None of this is easy, and there have been many days and nights where I truly didn't know how I was going to find strength. But I do know, with everything in me, that the strength always comes and I would live through it all again if I had to. Because God doesn't make mistakes, He makes miracles.

## Green Tree

*by Karen Turnbull*

When we got the go to fly to UCLA, life started moving very quickly. I ran home to grab my bag and kiss the boys goodbye. I didn't know what was ahead or how long we would be gone. I came downstairs with a green scarf around my neck. My friend Annie was there and she commented, "Perfect! Green ... the color of hope." From that point on I always had something green on. I was determined to hang on to the little hope that I had remaining. Off I went and then, off we went. It was 9:30 PM when we arrived at the Neuro ICU at UCLA. We were whisked into a room and immediately action was happening. Scans were being done, labs were being drawn, and Mike was being stabilized. The "angel nurses," as I fondly called them, helped set up the recliner chair so I could try to get a little sleep.

In the morning they gave me towels and toiletries and told me how to get to the shower facilities they had for the families of ICU patients. When I returned I was told I had a visitor. I was puzzled as I hadn't reached out to anyone and we had not even been there twelve hours. When I looked over to the waiting room chairs I saw my friend Hope. (Yes, that really is her name!) She was the wife of the drummer, Herman, that Mike had played with when working for Tom Jones. She had read my post, knew I was there, and decided to come see me. She knew I may not be able to visit but she didn't care. She told me she was prepared to wait and be there when I had the chance to see her for a few moments.

You see, the thing is Hope is a cancer survivor. She gets it. The fear, the mind games, the head spinning, the land of "what if?" that I was now living in. She told me that when she was in treatments for her own cancer, she would start to spin and go to the land of "what if?" as well. She needed a word to ground her. Something real. One day she was sitting in a courtyard before her treatment and the mind spin began. Her friend told her to pick something real to focus on. Hope chose a tree. Tree became her word. And now it was mine too. Hope handed me a necklace. A beautiful tree on a silver chain. She told me I could wear it or not and when I felt the time was right I could gift it on to someone else who found themselves in the land of "what if?" Someone who needed a little grounding, a little reminder of what is real. The crazy thing is, my niece Ali had gifted me a beautiful tree of life necklace for Christmas. In the rush of the moment I had not brought it with me but after Hope's visit I asked my sister to bring it to me when they came to visit a few weeks later.

In those next few weeks leading up to surgery I silently nicknamed myself the gypsy of UCLA. I always had a green scarf on, I always had crystals and rosary beads around my wrist (I was taking all the good spiritual energy I could get) and I always had my tree around my neck.

Finally, surgery day was upon us. My dearest friend Frank had flown out from New York to be with me and Mike's aunt Shari had driven in to spend the day with me as well. They kept me calm (well, as calm as can be expected), they made sure I ate whatever little bit I could and they loved me and held me through the treacherous hours of that day. I had been warned that surgery would be about fifteen hours. The catch was that if things turned bad they would close early, because it was more important to keep Mike alive than get it all out. At hour ten the phone to the surgery waiting room rang and the nurse informed me that Dr. Martin was getting ready to close. She couldn't tell me any more than that, so I went to the land of "what if?". That horrible place of fear. Shari went to grab some coffee and Frank and I sat in the waiting room, him holding my hand, neither of us saying anything. A small woman walked into the room where only Frank and I sat (it was a Sunday evening and we were the only ones there). She began to place books on the tables and then quickly made her way out of the waiting room. She made no eye contact and said nothing. When she left, I stood up and went to a table, picked up the book and caught my breath. I sat down next to Frank and said, "Look at this." It was a green Bible with a tree on the cover. Frank immediately grabbed my hand and said, "Here comes Dr. Martin." Dr. Martin sat down in front of me and said, "We got it all. It couldn't have gone more beautifully." I immediately began to cry tears of gratitude. Pathology showed that it appeared to be positive for cancer and that would mean close follow-ups, but we were used to that. They got it all! Mike was alive.

That green tree Bible came home with us. It is the only Bible I will ever need.

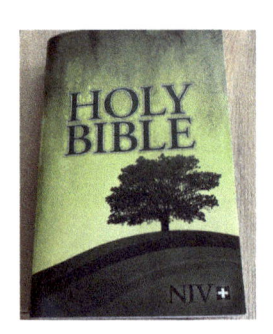

# Our Current Medical Team
*by Karen Turnbull*

Thank God for smart people!

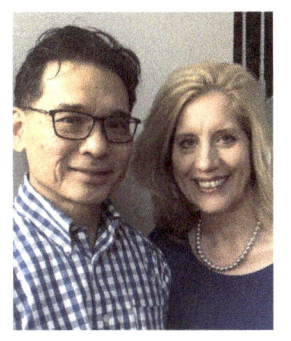

*Dr. Robert Wang and
Dr. Annabel Barber*

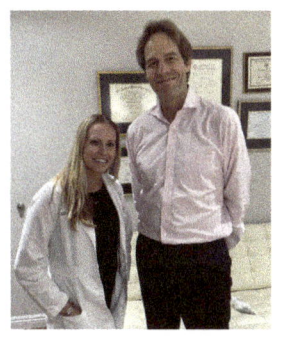

*Brittany Sims Hunter and
Dr. Beau James Toy*

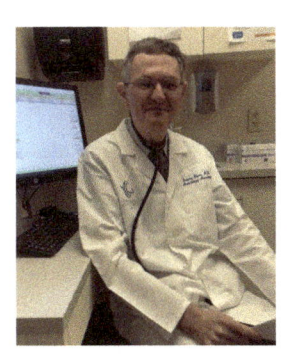

*Dr. Gregory Obara*

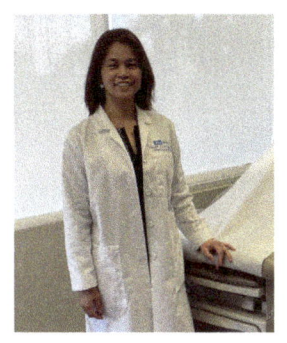

*Dr. Deborah Wong*

# CHAPTER EIGHT

# Comments

*Thank you everyone!*

Abby A 89, 93, 121, 162
Adrienne S 82, 166
Alan R 179, 248
Alex K 223, 238
Alicia B 119, 135, 157, 256, 286
Amy K 157
Amy L 140, 180
Andrea H 68
Andrea L 70, 88, 99, 104, 126, 129, 202
Angela C 20, 225
Angela W 89, 105, 186, 241, 279
Anne L 231, 267
Anne-Corinne B 18, 65, 221, 255, 267, 270
Annie W 72, 122
Antonette L 30, 138, 153, 163, 167, 173
Arthur F 67
Avi H 104, 185
Becky C 161
Belinda R 225
Bert V 158, 176
Bessie D 149
Beth B 135
Beth G 78
Beth L 100, 130
Beth S 13, 100, 127
Bethany B 47, 59, 67
Betsy A 82, 126
Betty S 71, 102, 119, 120, 125, 145, 146, 156, 246, 270
Bill B 152, 253
Bill C 8
Birgit D 84, 87, 118, 146, 170, 176, 218
Birgit P 9, 96, 125, 147, 238
Brad E 270, 275
Brandon T 129
Brenda M 17, 46, 71, 101, 108, 175
Brian M 8, 16, 20, 58, 69, 89, 191, 286
Brian P 32

Brie D 13
Brook D 140, 226
Candy P 139, 148, 150, 220
Carl T 253
Carol B 108, 110
Carol P 230
Carolyn S 31
Catherine J 96
Cathy M 10, 20, 34, 59, 76, 84, 88, 96, 100, 107, 109, 122, 139, 155, 165, 198, 242, 253
Charles D 121
Christie P 103, 236, 267
Christina P 8, 67, 72, 102, 179, 185, 198, 202, 221, 224, 233
Christine E 127, 230, 267
Cindi R 76, 84, 89, 159, 171, 225, 235, 242
Cindy E 102, 106, 130, 162, 255, 275
Clare T 94, 170, 241, 245, 262, 267, 285
Colleen S 105
Curt M 81, 94, 136, 137, 183, 192, 199, 218, 286
Cynthia E 67, 170
Dale B 197
Dan C 65
Dan F 14
Dan S 16, 29, 82, 96, 105, 126, 147, 156, 184, 227
Darci P 132
Darelle H 11, 32, 68, 81, 99, 129, 189, 197, 206, 207, 222
Darren K 122, 136, 170, 260
Dave G 31
Dave Ri 34
Dave Ro 30, 64, 68, 80, 126
Dave W 57, 124, 192, 210
David N 55, 73, 84, 262, 279
Dawn K 28, 76, 144, 170, 285
Deb S 198, 246, 267

Debbie M 89, 158, 183
Deborah P 9
Debra L 131, 253
Dene R 27, 48, 64, 156, 187, 209
Denise M 166
Devonee M 18, 95, 137, 150, 192, 202, 253, 262, 270
Doreen L 89, 99, 125, 144, 150, 207, 215, 252
Doriana S 223, 227, 235
Doug M 59, 131
Dwight S 38
Ed R 12
Edward E 77, 107, 126, 209
Elena S 121, 221
Elizabeth H 105, 157, 161, 171, 199, 205, 216
Ellen F 127, 167, 202, 231
Ellen O 188, 238
Ellen Sn 88, 120, 171, 200, 220, 233
Ellen So 20, 78, 93
Eric L 172
Eric T 11
Erica M 49, 70, 80, 143
Estelle T 88, 114, 209
Etsuko M 144
Fernanda G 88, 104, 110, 237
Fran D 183, 188, 235, 246, 270
Fran H 35, 49
Frank L 13, 15, 20
Frank S 12, 30, 50, 55, 69, 81, 163
Franz C 132, 167
Frederick W 15, 20
Gabriel F 16, 209, 248
Gail R 31, 143, 219
Gailyn A 95, 210
Gary A 22, 168
Gil K 11, 198
Greg N 31
Gregory R 139
Hayley M 59, 95, 105, 141, 152, 173, 223
Heather B 38, 222, 227, 231, 242
Heather L 70, 84, 91, 135, 156
Heather W 135, 149, 205, 262
Heide F 107, 176, 287
Heidi H 196
Hope M 9, 23, 115, 137, 145, 222
Issa F 57, 59, 119, 144, 149, 168, 170, 275

Ivy W 71, 109
Jaclyn F 147, 237
Jacqueline S 107, 236, 242
Jaime D 219, 230, 286
James M 131, 202, 219
Janna R 74, 82, 158, 237
January F 71, 77, 104
Jason H 7
Jason M 118
Jason V 167, 198, 215, 260, 267
Jayme R 87, 102, 165, 215
Jean T 55, 127, 192
Jeanine C 51, 70, 94, 126, 192, 255, 286
Jeff L 95, 138, 151
Jeff W 8
Jen F 105, 183, 224
Jen K 9
Jeneane H 78, 155, 232
Jenna L 127, 147, 152, 161, 177, 180, 199, 256
Jennifer A 134
Jennifer G 221
Jennifer M 131
Jennifer O 53
Jennifer P 153, 171
Jennifer S 45
Jennifer Z 163
Jenny F 9, 93, 232, 274, 285
Jessica H 230
Jessica S 88
Jill G 29
Joan F 82, 138, 171, 189, 210, 215, 235
Jodie M 18, 67, 115
Joey F 102, 132
John M 90, 105, 108, 143, 156, 180
John V 221
JoLayne G 88, 100, 143, 144, 155, 165, 183, 236, 262
Joni S 130, 165, 177, 198
Jordan B 103, 129, 223
Judy E 118, 129, 150, 202
Julie Y 94
Kacia B 34
Karen B 16
Karen C 231
Karen K 70, 79, 94, 102, 146, 173, 221, 263
Karen Mc 13, 97
Karen Mi 129, 226, 259

Karen O 148
Karen P 89, 114, 126, 130, 177, 179, 188, 218
Karina B 124
Karine Z 20, 21, 24, 38, 78, 138, 142, 163, 171, 242
Kate P 15
Katey J 24, 44, 55, 71, 76, 96, 114, 135, 203, 263
Kathryn L 31, 125
Kathy A 9, 77, 108, 130, 162, 243
Kathy L 126
Kathy M 125, 135
Kathy T 59, 185
Katie C 95, 119
Keith N 97, 147
Kelene J 168
Kelly C 152, 235, 257, 286
Kelly L 220
Kelsey P 17, 76, 163
Ken P 108
Kenneth S 163, 260
Kenny A 22, 110, 189
Kerry D 219
Kerryann D 219, 230
Kim B 12, 70, 78, 84
Kim F 156
Kim M 110, 119
Kimberly S 173, 260
Kristin U 108, 114, 216, 237, 243, 252, 267, 275
Kristine K 91, 94, 100, 176, 180, 184
Lance P 134, 237
Lanie F 150
Laura H 107, 187
Laura T 14, 24, 137, 203, 236, 270
Laurence A 50, 67, 130, 195, 202
Lee H 263
Les K 18, 22, 24, 43, 140, 161, 227, 248, 255
Liese W 114, 137, 144, 152, 158, 231, 233
Linda Q 163, 231
Lisa L 21, 57, 76, 80, 119, 166, 177
Liz S 148
Lou G 43, 81, 138, 177, 196, 197, 231, 249
Lynne E 131, 148, 153, 199, 236, 242, 252, 255, 275
Magally L 79, 95
Marc H 132, 139, 270
Marcia M 210
Margaret H 67, 166, 199, 221, 231
Mariana R 73
Marianne M 14, 77, 106, 120, 145, 147, 151, 198, 209, 235, 252, 262, 264, 270, 274, 284
Marie K 184
Marie O 141
Mark M 12
Mark S 15, 72, 77, 189, 207, 248
Marsha R 151
Mary Alice J 40, 159, 179, 222, 232, 241, 252
Mary F 96, 171
Mary P 9
Matt J 14, 20, 95, 119, 134, 149, 150, 179, 209, 256
Megan A 90, 135
Megan H 42, 45, 50, 53, 69, 79, 101, 120, 151, 155, 160, 173, 187, 246, 285
Megan M 29
Megan S 16
Melin F 20, 34, 51, 63, 96, 114, 141, 153, 164, 176, 230, 246, 275
Melissa M 13
Melissa P 189
Michael M 12, 57, 81
Michele R 155
Michelle B 114, 146, 238
Michelle M 30
Michelle R 108, 202
Miguel R 104
Mike G 29, 85, 220
Mike S 100, 140, 183, 186, 246
Miles P 118
Monique E 101, 149, 161, 173, 234
Nan R 205, 219, 249, 260, 275
Nancy R 118, 126, 220
Nancy W 23, 91
Nandita S 32, 48, 57, 59, 84, 107, 187, 199, 235, 245
Nate K 11, 80, 83
Nathan T 122, 143, 147, 176, 203, 224, 241
Nellie S 95, 156, 160, 163, 209, 221, 232, 260
Nicole B 156
Pam Ra 16, 71, 243
Pam Ro 131
Pam S 89, 99

Pat C 87, 129, 187, 205
Paul Q 219
Paula M 236
Pete B 180, 199, 216, 222, 246
Ralph P 153
Randy C 47, 93, 118, 155, 158, 160, 189, 236, 253, 260
Ric F 152, 224, 230
Ro K 114
Rob M 11, 245
Robin C 130, 142, 206, 226, 230
Rocco B 18, 70, 125, 145, 163, 166, 195, 199, 218, 237, 243, 246
Ron J 65
Rosita P 18, 25, 73, 104, 192
Roxane G 130
Sam Ba 127, 137, 148
Sam Bl 270
Sandy B 53, 79, 137
Sara B 227, 242, 262
Sara I 80, 87, 102, 115, 131, 134, 159, 165, 182, 195
Sara O 12, 57, 62, 87
Sean H 225, 255
Shani F 195, 198, 216, 220, 235, 257, 285
Shannon A 286
Shannon B 202, 225, 241
Shannon N 275, 285
Shari B 12, 15, 24, 55, 74, 223, 238
Sharon H 8, 64, 67, 82, 119, 126, 130, 138, 140, 144, 152, 200, 203, 224, 262
Shawn M 153
Shelley De 101, 136, 149, 161, 176, 205, 220, 245
Shelley Dr 14, 16, 105
Soeren J 17
Sonny H 84
Stacia F 11, 100, 196, 220, 236
Stacy G 186, 223, 226
Steve S 263
Steven L 223
Susan S 179, 185, 236
Susan V 104
Suzanne P 8, 32, 76, 80, 102, 121, 132, 147, 152, 184, 191, 194, 226, 248, 257, 279
Susie C 209
Tammy C 14, 25, 94, 142, 148, 158, 201, 215
Tara F 115

Teri C 20
Theodora B 275
Tiffany P 99, 183, 188, 192
Tim C 21
Tim L 115, 125, 148, 188, 247
Tina B 95
Tom E 83, 121, 222, 230
Tom N 222
Tom P 15
Trish T 94, 107, 138, 222, 241, 274
Vince V 58, 65, 90, 191
Virginia H 154, 170, 183, 187, 195
Wesley M 166, 286
Yong D 44, 260

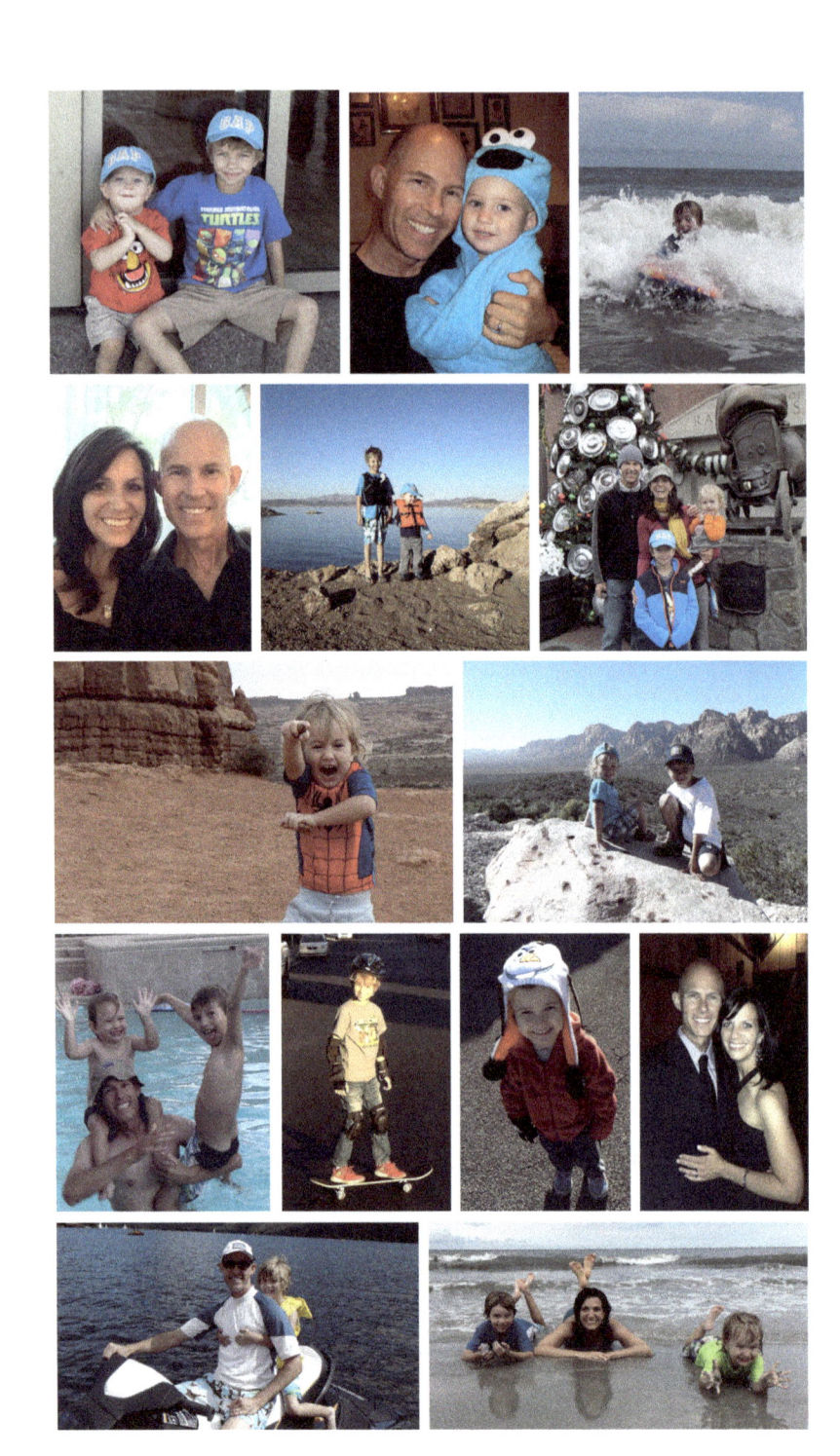

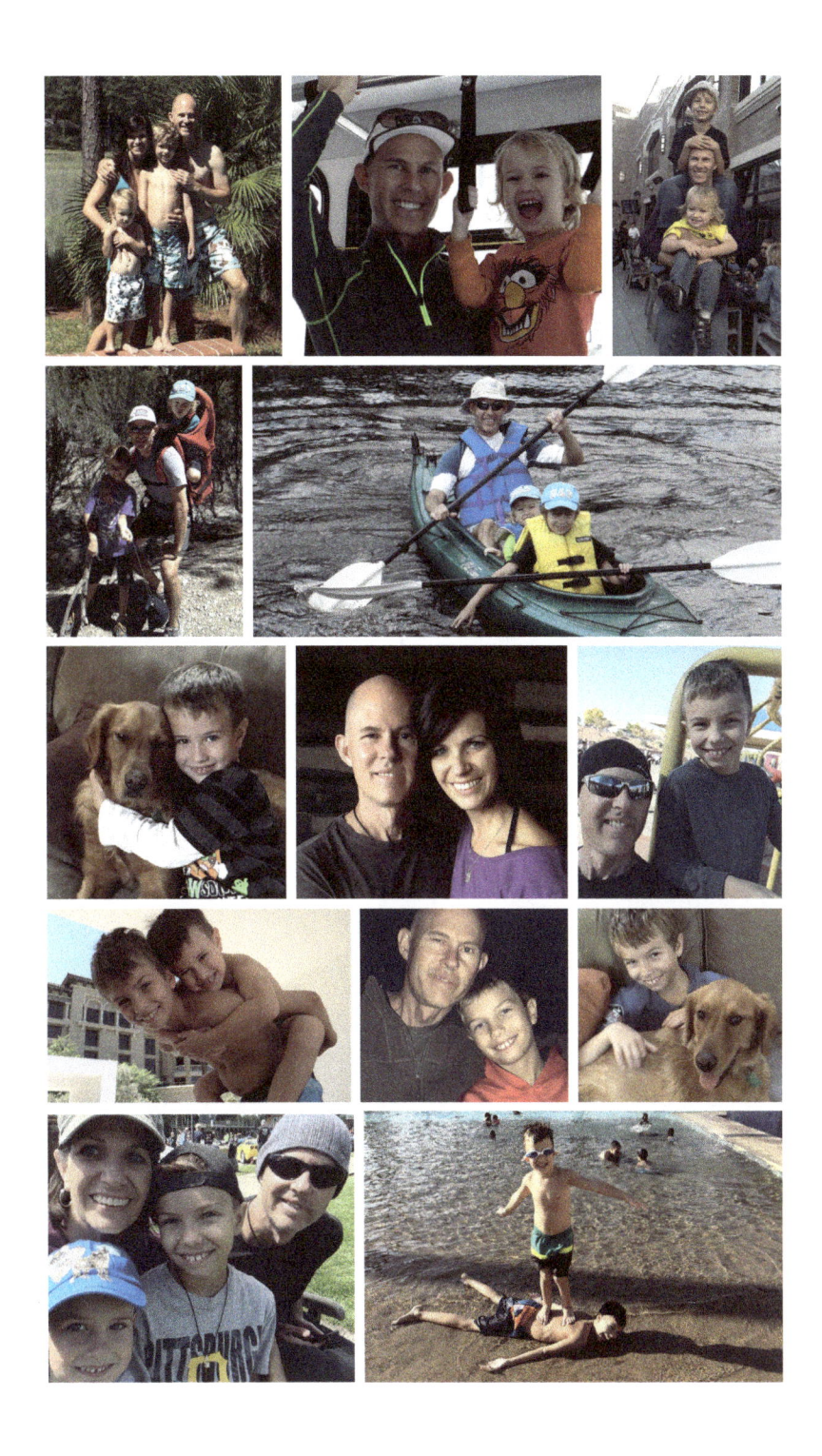

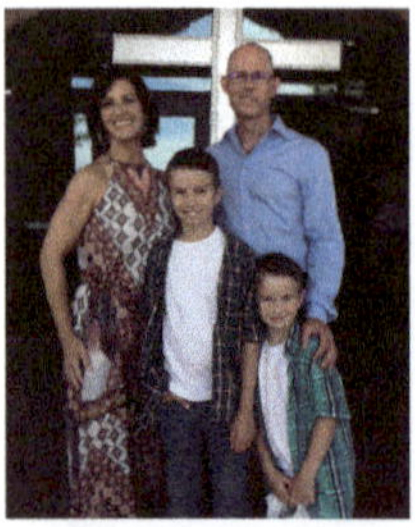
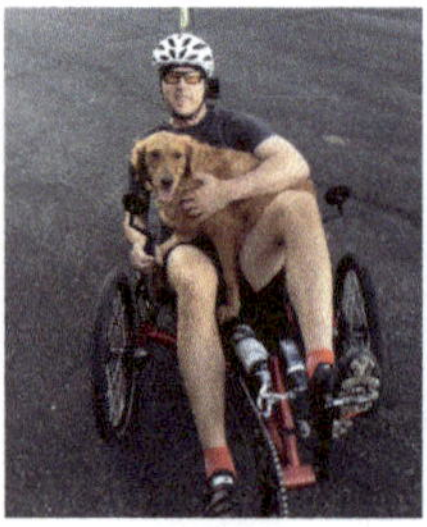
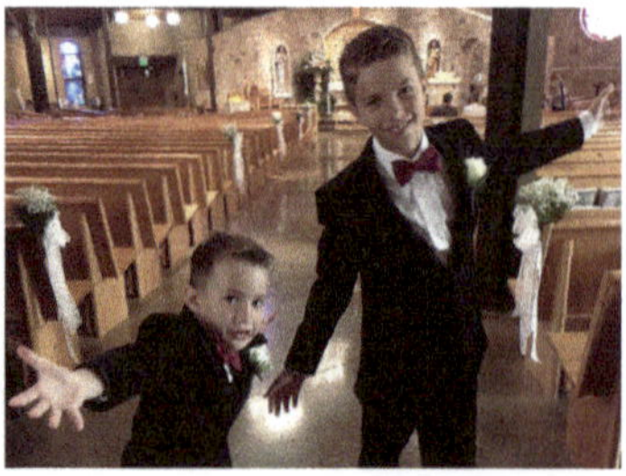
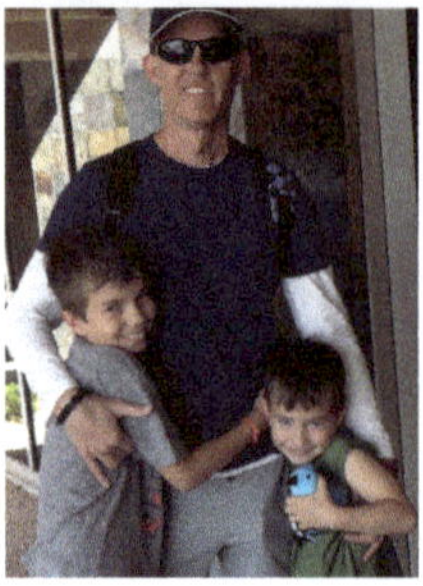
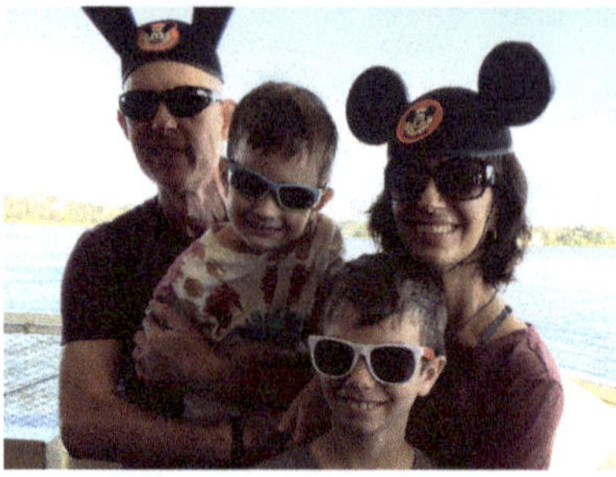
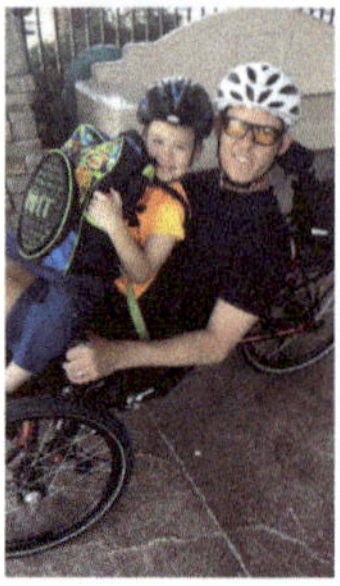
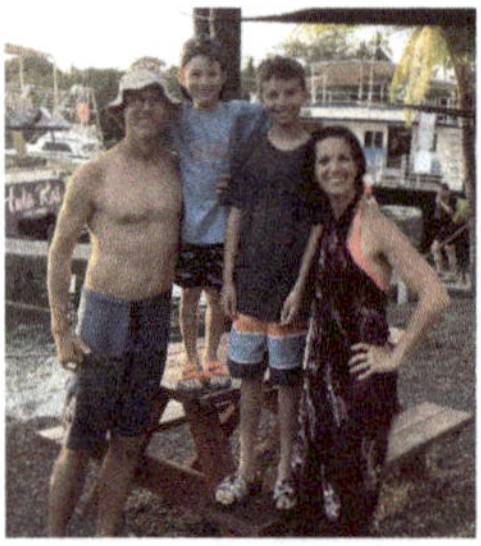
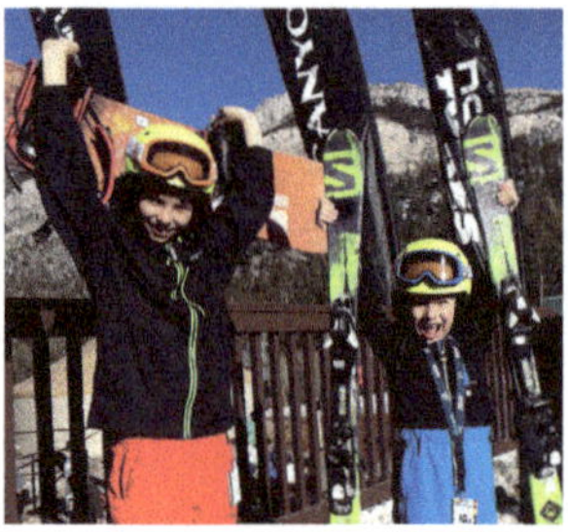
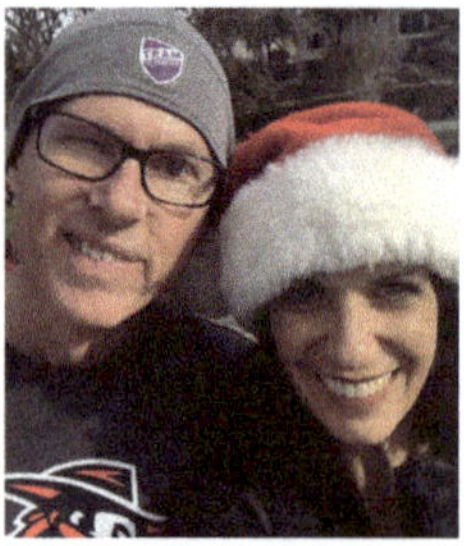
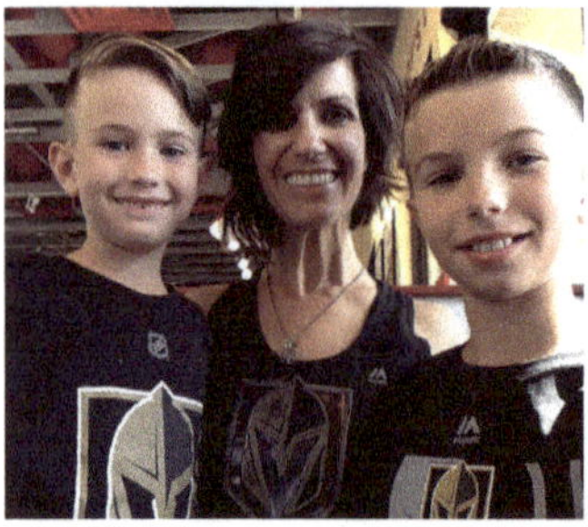
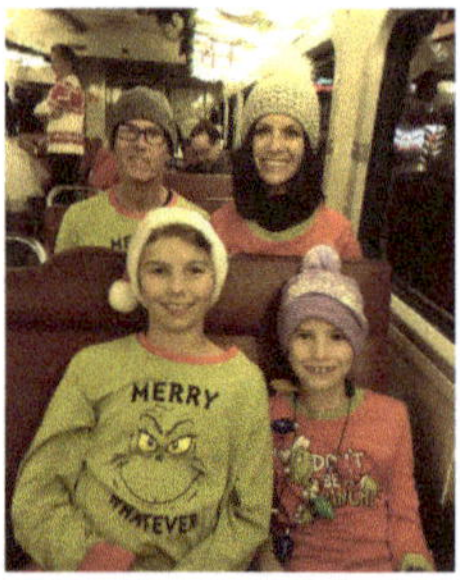
MERRY
WHATEVER
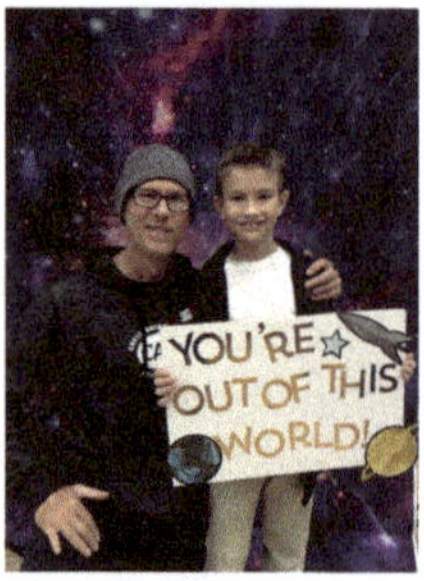
YOU'RE
OUT OF THIS
WORLD!
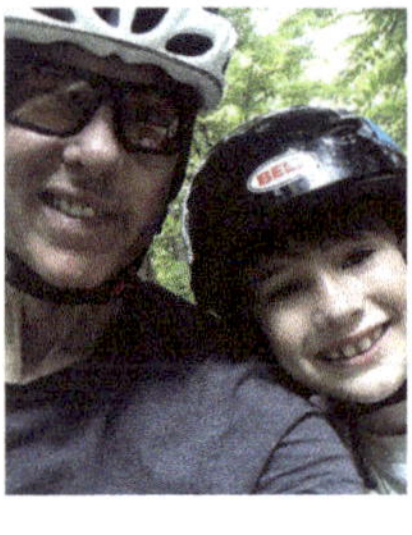
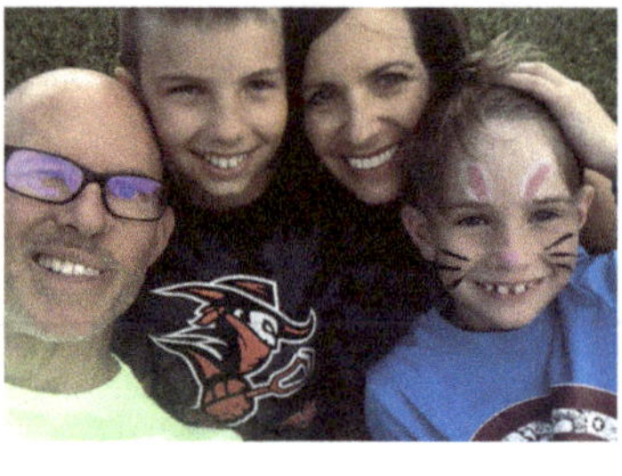
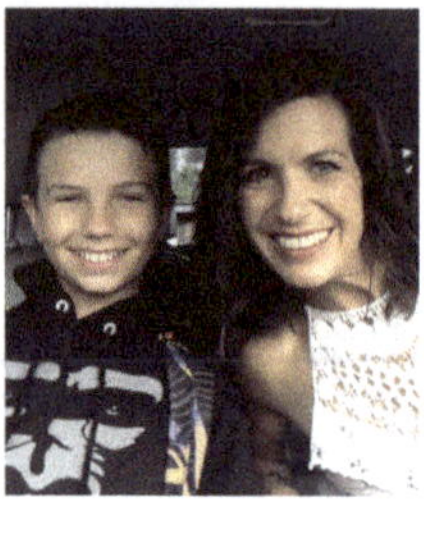

303

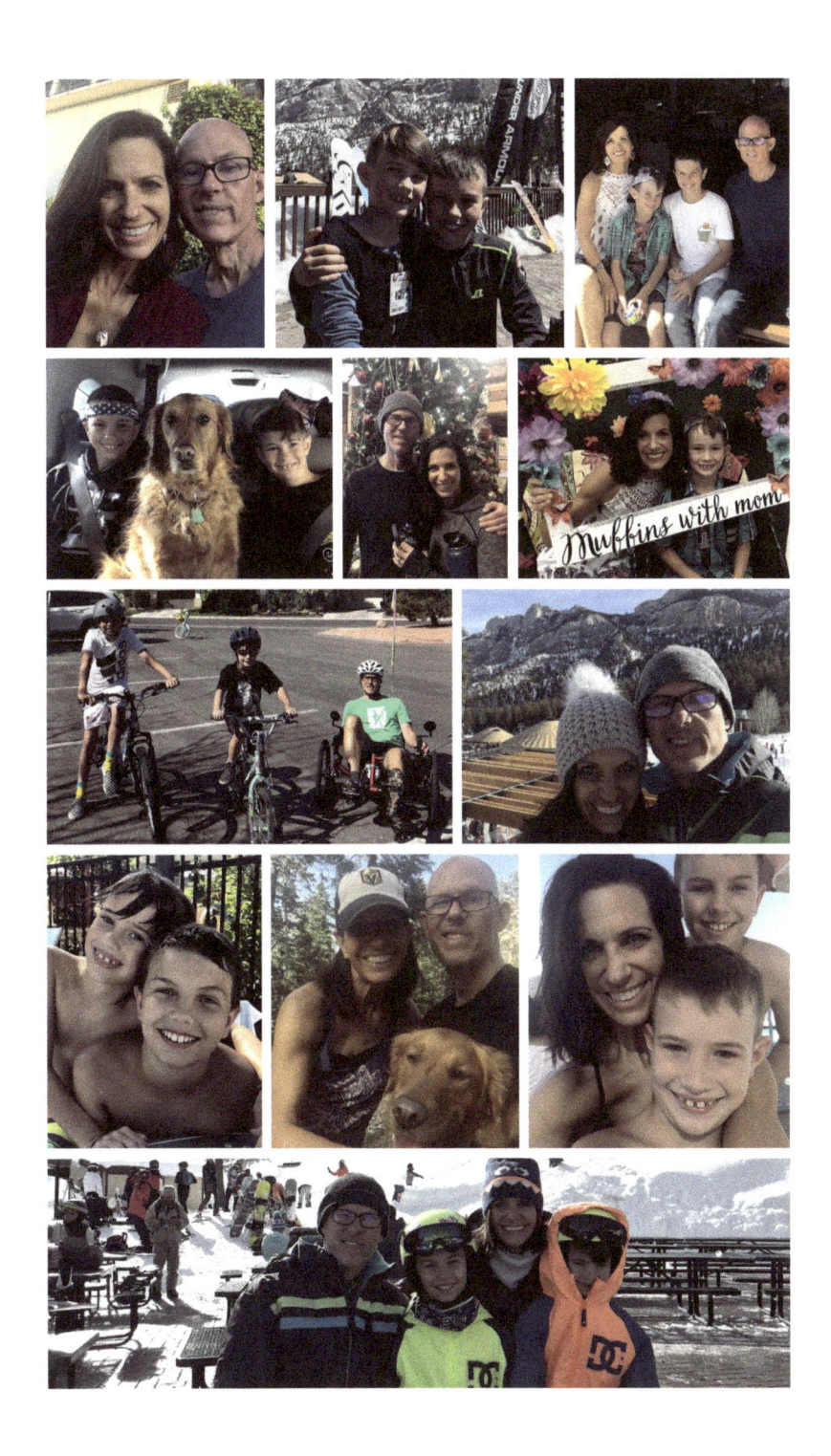

*Mike Turnbull was a professional musician for thirty years, and had the good fortune of traveling to over one hundred countries.*

*Karen Turnbull was a professional dancer and dance educator. She is currently the CEO of Fresh Start Nutrition and Bodywork, LLC, practicing massage therapy and nutrition coaching.*

*Mike and Karen met in 1998 while performing on a world cruise. They were married in 2002, and their sons were born in 2007 and 2011. In 2013 Mike was diagnosed with Stage IV cancer, which is when this story begins.*

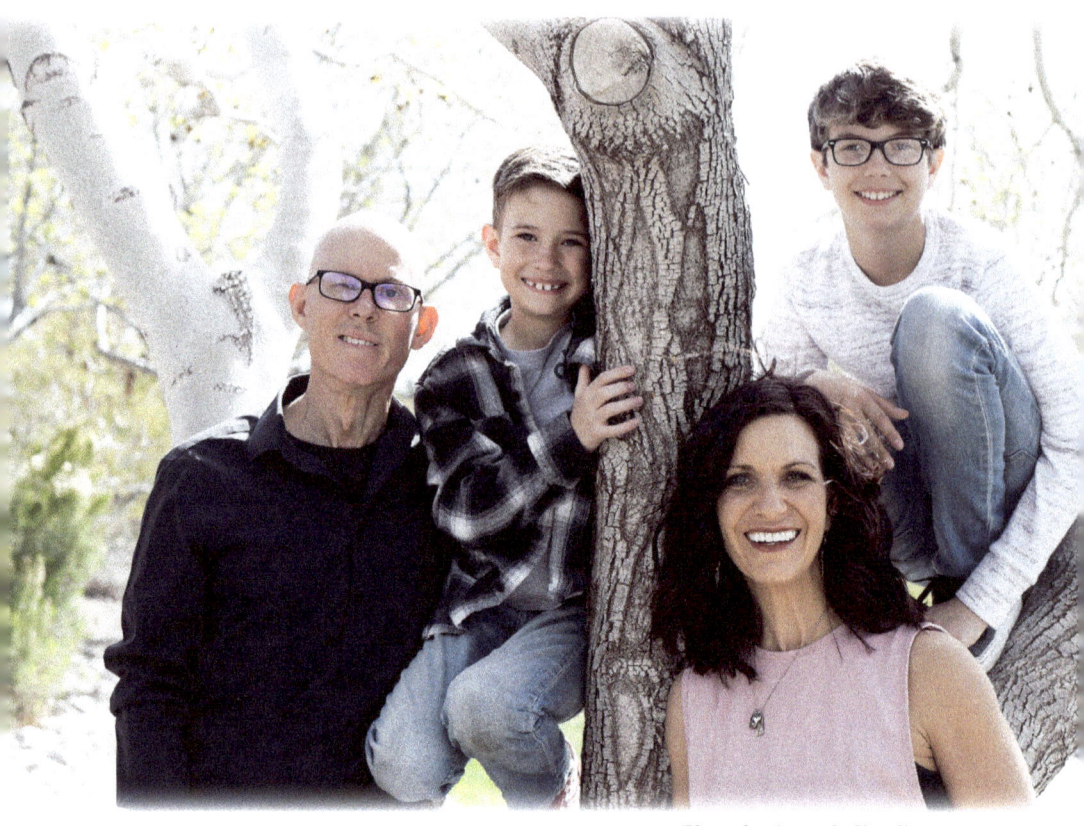

Photo by Amanda Ventling

*What you hold in your hands is a true story. A story of one family's fight against the odds. One family's story of resiliency and determination. It is a true account of Mike Turnbull's battle with a rare and aggressive form of cancer. The story is told primarily through the eyes of Mike's wife Karen, and details how her and the Turnbull's two sons fight to keep joy in their lives. From Mike's career as a professional musician to being wheelchair bound after cancer spread to his brain stem, to becoming a five-time triathlete, this story is raw, unfiltered and, although at times unbelievable, all true. It is above all else a story about how faith, family, friends and the power of prayer continue to strengthen this family.*